HOT AND BOTHERED

Women, Medicine, and Menopause
in Modern America

JUDITH A. HOUCK

HARVARD UNIVERSITY PRESS

Cambridge, Massachusetts, and London, England   2006

Library of Congress Cataloging-in-Publication Data

Houck, Judith A. (Judith Anne)
    Hot and bothered : women, medicine, and menopause in modern
America / Judith A. Houck.
    p. cm.
    Includes bibliographical references and index.
    ISBN 0-674-01896-6
    1. Menopause—Social aspects—United States—History—20th century.
    2. Menopause—Treatment—United States—History—20th century.
    3. Middle aged women—Health and hygiene—United States—History—
20th century. I. Title.

RG186.H7792 2006
618.1'75—dc22   2005051265

For my parents,
Warren J. Houck
and Rhea L. Houck

Contents

Acknowledgments

The idea for this book was hatched during my first year of graduate school at the University of Wisconsin, Madison, while I was enrolled in the class "Women and Health in American History." That course, taught by Bonnie Blustein, sparked my interest in the history of medicine and introduced me to the academic conversation about menopause. The manuscript was completed as I taught the same class, again at the University of Wisconsin. During the intervening years and my circuitous journey away from and back to Wisconsin, many people have helped move this history of menopause from an idea into a book. I eagerly take this opportunity to offer my thanks and acknowledge my gratitude.

I'd like to thank my dissertation advisor and colleague Judith Walzer Leavitt for her faith in this project and for her continued encouragement of me. Her belief that I could write this book, teach and inspire students, and be a historian was contagious. The model of her teaching and her scholarship continues to inspire my work. Further, by embracing my transition from student to colleague without missing a beat, Judy has helped my own metamorphosis. Other faculty at the University of Wisconsin have similarly eased my transition from student to colleague. In particular, Jeanne Boydston, Tom Broman, Gregg Mitman, Ronald Numbers, Lynn Nyhart, and Nancy Worcester have made coming home a pleasure. Other faculty members of the Women's Studies program, the History of Science and History of Medicine departments, and the Women's History community, most notably Warwick Anderson, Nan Enstad, Linda Hogle, Rick Keller, Mariamne Whatley, and Susan Zaeske, have provided a collegial place to work and learn.

I'd like to thank the University of Georgia Franklin Teaching Fellows program and the history department at the University of Georgia for turning a historian of medicine loose to teach American history to unsuspecting undergraduates. It was an exhilarating experience for me (and I think the students survived). In particular, I'd like to thank Sylvia Hutchinson, who ran the program; Edward Larson in the history department, who offered advice and support; and the fellows, especially John Moser, who helped make the year memorable, delightful, and invaluable.

After one year at Georgia I had the opportunity to return to Wisconsin under a National Institute of Aging Training Grant run through the Center of Excellence in Women's Health. Molly Carnes, co-director of the Center, believed that a historian could contribute to current concerns about women's aging and gave me the opportunity to prove her right. In the years I have been affiliated with the Center (now known as the Center for Women's Health Research), I have been amazed by Molly's inexhaustible efforts on behalf of women's health professionals and the health of women. Indeed, the faculty position I now occupy as a Women's Health Research cluster hire was created in part because of Molly's efforts. My association with the Center has been enhanced by the efforts of Gloria Sarto, Judee Bell, and Stephanie Lent.

This history could not have been written without the archival collections that helped me discover women's experiences at menopause. I am indebted to the collections and the archivists at the American Medical Association, the Sophia Smith Collection and Archives at Smith College, the Arthur and Elizabeth Schlesinger Library and the Henry A. Murray Research Center at Radcliffe College, the Manuscripts and University Archives of the University of Washington, the National Archives and Records Administration, and the Wisconsin State Historical Society. Further, Micaela Sullivan-Fowler, the historical librarian at the Ebling Library at the University of Wisconsin, Madison, responded to my requests for help with encouragement and good cheer. Finally, graduate students Dan Hamlin, Bridget Collins, and Libbie Freed provided last-minute research assistance that made me believe I could finish the project. Libbie also named the menopausal women, offered editing advice, and helped me negotiate the world of permissions.

Many people over the years have read bits or all of this work and helped it become what it is. When I was struggling to wrestle this project into a dissertation, my graduate student colleagues offered rigorous criticism and collegial support. For their careful readings of several chapters, I would especially like to thank Ralph Drayton, Evelyn Fine, Hae-Gyung Geong, Tomomi Kinukawa, Craig McConnell, Sarah Pfatteicher, David Reid, Louise Robbins, Karen Walloch, and Hsiu-yun Wang. Their suggestions and our conversations helped me to discover what I know about the history of menopause and to find ways to tell my story. Further, their devotion to their own work made my own fascination with menopause seem normal. My dissertation committee—Vanessa Northington Gamble, Judith Walzer Leavitt, Ronald Numbers, Lynn Nyhart, and Nancy Worcester—offered guidance on the first version of this work and suggestions for its next incarnation. Jeanne Boydston, Michelle McClellan, Leslie Reagan, Lisa Saywell, and Lisa Tetrault read the entire manuscript, offered helpful insights, and asked valuable questions. Anne Enke read most of this manuscript, sometimes on a very tight schedule, and provided trenchant criticism and unflagging enthusiasm. An anonymous reviewer for Harvard University Press also guided the transformation of this project from a dissertation into a book. I would also like to acknowledge Judith Norsigian, Cynthia Pearson, and Barbara Seaman, whose impassioned reaction to the manuscript reminded me of the political importance of history. While their views of events did not always mesh with mine and the direction in which I wanted to take this book, I nevertheless am grateful to them for sharing their fresh perspectives. They pushed me, and I pushed back, and I think the book that emerged is stronger and better for our exchanges.

As I have taken this project public in different forums, various scholars have offered inspiration, criticism, and encouragement. Rima Apple, Charlotte Borst, Ling-fang Cheng, Daiwie Fu, Janet Golden, Daniel Horowitz, Susan Smith, and Elizabeth Watkins have all contributed, in ways big and small, to this project. I also appreciate the invitations from Tomomi Kinukawa, Hsiu-yun Wang, and Kirsten Gardner that allowed me to bring my work to new and exciting audiences.

My students at the University of Wisconsin and the University of Georgia have taught me a great deal over the years, reminding me constantly why I love history and demonstrating that a study of the past can illuminate the present and influence the future. Their willingness to struggle with challenging ideas encourages my own historical investigations. More recently, as I have been increasingly absorbed by this book, my students have patiently listened as I would say, "Let's look at the example of menopause" without ever rolling their eyes (at least not that I could see). I appreciated their forbearance.

My editor at Harvard University Press, Ann Downer-Hazell, has supported this project for several years now. Her patience has been greatly appreciated, but she was perhaps most helpful when she urged me to let it go, insisting that I would feel better. Indeed I do. Susan Boulanger provided terrific copyediting and promptly responded to my many queries.

Beth Withers and Sara Davis at the press have made the publishing process less mysterious.

Many people have contributed to this project in intangible ways. Sarah Pfatteicher has reinforced for me the value of friendship, breakfast, and a trusted hand on the other end of the rope. Lisa Tetrault has reminded me that a hunt for birds, a walk with dogs, and a swig of beer could make time in front of the computer more productive. Anne Enke has been an all-around good egg, sharing hockey games, live music, and the joys and anxieties of junior-faculty status.

I dedicate this book to my parents, Rhea L. Houck and Warren J. Houck. They gave me a childhood of fossil hunting, star gazing, and bird watching, thus nurturing my love of the natural world. They also gave me a childhood full of books, which encouraged my love of words. Their varied forms of support have made this career and this book possible. My siblings, Emily Houck, Susan Houck, and Robert Houck, have encouraged and been curious about my academic work, but they have been most useful in keeping me grounded in a world where the fine points of historiography matter not at all. Lyn and John Pauley launched my academic career with a champagne party after my first day of kindergarten and supported my continued efforts. They lived to see the dissertation; I regret that I can't share the book with them. Finally, my gratitude to Lisa Saywell knows no bounds. Note cards from the first paper I wrote on the history of menopause bear her handwriting, and she stayed up late with me as we put the manuscript to rest. In the intervening years, she has supported this project and distracted me from it. She has helped me understand the history of menopause and has reminded me daily of life's nonacademic wonders.

HOT AND BOTHERED

Introduction

In July of 1970, the Democratic Committee on National Priorities considered its agenda for the coming year. Committee member and congresswoman Patsy Mink urged her party to make the fight for women's rights a priority. Dr. Edgar F. Berman, Hubert Humphrey's personal physician, vehemently dismissed Mink's suggestion, insisting that women's physiology disqualified them from high level positions of authority and influence. To reinforce his claim, he implored his party to consider the consequences of a "menopausal woman president who had to make the decision of the Bay of Pigs." Imagine a bank executive, he continued, making a loan under the influence of "raging" menopausal hormones.[1] Berman's comment sparked a national debate over the biological qualifications for political power and economic influence. The popular media turned to other members of the medical profession for further clarification and comment.

Berman apparently found little support among his colleagues. They vociferously condemned his position as "out of date," "nonsense," and a "male put-on." But even those physicians who disputed Berman's claim revealed unflattering expectations of menopausal women. A specialist in industrial medicine, for example, reassured the public that a menopausal "woman might be bitchy as hell," but her ability to "swing a $10-million loan wouldn't be affected." A San Francisco psychiatrist claimed that a woman's erratic behavior at menopause was not caused by her biology but by her changing social niche and society's disregard for older women. Ending on a positive note, he added that "our way of thinking about men's and women's roles is starting to change. It's going to be a new ball game." Endocrinologist and enthusiastic member of the National Organization for Women Shepard Aronson took a different tack. By insisting that menopause was "most upsetting in women who stay home and think about it rather than do a good day's work," he encouraged women to

1

move beyond home and hearth. These physicians did not dispute that menopause affected women's behavior, but they disagreed on the cause of that change and what it meant for women's participation in society.[2]

In the midst of the hoopla, Berman resigned his position with the Democratic Party, but he remained unapologetic about his position. At a press conference, he insisted that if physicians didn't know that there was an "abnormal psychologic condition known as menopause, then they better go back to medical school." He pleaded for the public to understand, however, that he didn't consider women inferior, just "different." Indeed, he found women quite capable of fulfilling their "greatest job": raising the next generation. And, as if the frying pan were not bad enough, he lamented that Mrs. Mink lacked a sense of humor.[3]

This episode illustrates several issues bearing on women's relationships with their bodies and with their social roles. First, according to some social commentators, biology sets the limits for women's participation in public life. A woman's relative weakness, her childbearing potential, and her physiological cycles are thus seen as disqualifying her from life outside childbearing and housekeeping. Second, because it allegedly affects a woman's body and her behavior, menopause provides a vulnerable target for those hoping to reserve political and economic power for men. As a result, menopause has both social and political implications for women. Third, physicians, widely regarded as experts on all things bodily, are asked to arbitrate conflicts that are essentially political, rather than medical, in nature. Finally, middle-aged women, freed from the familial demands that frequently hamper younger women's careers, pose a particularly potent threat to the status quo. Although Berman's comments were galling enough in 1970 to make the evening news and to force his resignation, the issues this incident raised are not unique; indeed, they characterize consistent themes in the history of women's bodies in the United States.

Over the past twenty-five years, academics and activists of various stripes have focused attention on the meanings of menopause and its evolving treatments both in the United States and abroad.[4] In general, this scholarship makes two broad, sometimes overlapping, claims. First, it suggests that the experience of menopause is forged in the interaction between biology and culture. Neither the biological "symptoms" nor the social meanings of menopause exist apart from a cultural context and a social understanding about the nature and role of women. Margaret Lock's remarkable comparison of menopause in North America and in Japan, *En-*

counters with Aging (1993), for example, demonstrates how the cultural discussion of menopause was also a conversation—a debate—about "what women are for."[5] Second, much recent menopause literature claims that medicine has come to dominate what had once been (and what many of these authors think should be) a natural, physiological transition.[6] These studies tend to focus on the medical construction of menopause as a "deficiency disease" and on the emergence of hormone replacement therapy as its cure.[7]

My investigations build on this rich literature to place the medical construction of menopause in the twentieth-century United States in its historical context. Many questions about the cultural meaning and personal experience of menopause remain unanswered. What has menopause meant to women? How have women coped with their physical symptoms and their changing social roles? How have doctors viewed their menopausal patients? How has medical theory shaped medical practice? How have cultural and technological developments influenced the answers to these questions? In exploring these issues, I address the relationship between menopausal women and their physicians, the interaction between cultural developments and physiologic change, and the connection between aging women and their bodies.

These women's changing bodies, in particular their loss of fertility, inspired society's anxious consideration of women's roles and the meaning of womanhood. Women have long been considered the more embodied sex, vulnerable to the bodies' cyclical upheavals, frustrated by its complicated physiology, constrained by its reproductive demands, controlled by its voracious appetites.[8] Changes in the nature of the female body consequently suggested changes in the nature of the female. In this book, I argue that the bodies of menopausal women have served as a cultural canvas for delineating some of the larger questions about the nature of women, the breadth of women's roles, and the nature of medical practice.

The medical and cultural constructions of menopause were not foisted upon women solely by male physicians and social commentators. Women, too, have participated in the cultural assessment and construction of menopause. As physicians, they have contributed to the medical conversation about menopause and have advised other women on how to cope if the going got rough. But menopausal women outside medicine contributed to the popular understanding of menopause, as well. Whether welcoming or dreading menopause, ignoring hot flashes or rushing to doctors for treatment, keeping their trials to themselves or swapping their stories with bridge partners and sisters in struggle, women have contributed to the meaning of menopause and to society's assessment of menopausal women.

The women whose stories are covered here are for the most part white, middle- and upper-class women. There are several reasons for this. First, while the earliest medical sources suggest that identifiable groups of women experienced menopause in predictably different ways, by the twentieth century, discussion of group variation had largely given way to consideration of individual variation. Thus, although physician Andrew Fay Currier wrote in 1897 that "savage and barbarous women, peasants, Germans, Scandinavians and Russians" complained little at menopause while the French, the Irish, and "the highly organized, nervous, city-bred women" were liable to find menopause particularly disagreeable, such claims became increasingly rare.[9] For most of the twentieth century, the popular and medical accounts of menopause depicted menopausal women as married, reliant on their husbands for economic support, and occupied with keeping house, playing bridge, and contributing to worthy causes, that is, implicitly, as white and middle or upper class. Second, the popular sources generally targeted a middle- or middle- and upper-class audience. Domestic health guides, articles in the periodical press, marriage manuals all appealed to the interests, concerns, and expectations of economically comfortable women. Third, the medicalization of menopause is largely a story about women willing and able to access medicine for nonemergency health care. Women who sought medical care at menopause and left their doctors' offices with prescriptions were generally affluent women. Finally, the women who shared their experiences for this book are overwhelmingly white, married, and middle or upper class.[10] There are exceptions, particularly with regard to class, and as we will see, the economic position of these women influenced their attitudes toward and experience with menopause. But, in general, the women appearing in this story encountered menopause from privileged positions.

Attitudes toward menopause in the United States unfolded along two trajectories. Therapeutic options affected medical attitudes and the lived experience of menopause, and the social backdrop, particularly the ebb and flow of feminism, influenced both popular and private perceptions of aging women. By using the changing social and political landscape as a frame, this study aims to illuminate how menopause was viewed by physicians, articulated by medical writers, and experienced by women.[11]

Mapping the Terrain

On a purely biological level, menopause marks the end of menstruation and the concomitant end of fertility. Most women experience menopause when they are between forty-five and fifty-five years old. The years before and after menopause have long been associated in the United States with a wide range of physiological changes and emotional challenges. These larger changes are technically referred to as the *climacteric* or *climacterium* (or, more recently, *perimenopause*). In both medical texts and the popular imagination, however, the word *menopause* has been used to encompass both the end of menstruation and the sometimes difficult adjustment by body and psyche to life beyond reproductive cycles. In western settings at the beginning of the twenty-first century, menopause is often associated with mood swings, hot flashes, and memory loss. The biological consequences of menopause, however, are not universal. The physical and psychological experiences considered menopausal depend on the cultural and historical context.

The history of menopause in the twentieth century falls into three eras defined by developments in the treatment of menopause and shifts in the public lives of women. These occurred roughly between 1897 and 1937, 1938 and 1962, and 1963 to the present. The edges of these boundaries are not decisive; they do not mark the beginning of immediate and radical change. Rather, they indicate the beginnings of new conversations and concerns.

In 1897, Andrew Currier published the first book by an American physician to focus exclusively on menopause.[12] Between 1897 and 1937, hormone treatments, known at the time as *organotherapy,* made their appearance on the medical and popular scene. These hormones' crude refinement, high cost, and dubious efficacy prevented their widespread use, but the development of hormone therapy did encourage increased medical attention to menopause. Yet despite having this new weapon in their pharmaceutical arsenal, physicians failed to embrace menopause as an event of particular medical consequence. Although doctors believed that middle-aged women should consult a physician regularly to check for early signs of serious illness, menopause itself did not in their opinion warrant its own visit. Nevertheless, some women robbed of sleep by hot flashes or frightened by copious bleeding, did turn to their physicians at menopause. Physicians generally treated these patients with education and reassurance, supplemented, perhaps, with prescriptions for bland food, sensible fashions (no corsets), and temperate living. Women physicians, in particular, discouraged too great a reliance on medicine. They maintained that a smooth passage through the storms of menopause required self-control rather than medical intervention.

Around 1938, however, hormone therapies gained both legitimacy and increased use when a British biochemist developed diethylstilbestrol (DES), a synthetic form of estrogen. This biotechnological development created cheaper and apparently more efficacious hormone treatments and thus increased their viability. In theory, these therapies did not immediately supplant earlier treatment strategies. Because they regarded menopause as both a social and a physiological transition, physicians writing in the medical literature declined to rely exclusively on a medical solution. As a result, most physicians (at least most of those publishing in medical journals) still recommended reassurance as the treatment of first choice, supplemented if necessary by sedatives to ease patients' anxiety. These doctors advised hormones only if less invasive measures failed to relieve women's difficulties.

But medical theory fails to reflect precisely medical practice. At the same time some physicians were advocating pharmaceutical restraint in print, others were freely prescribing hormones and sedatives in practice. Consequently, hormones and "nerve pills" played a significant role in the menopausal experience for many middle-class women in the middle years of the twentieth century. Women themselves encouraged the use of hormones during this period. Inspired perhaps by hormones' promised miracles, as championed by the popular literature and their bridge partners, some women specifically asked their doctors for hormonal therapies.

After 1963, physicians and women increased their reliance on hormone therapy, spurred on by the work of Robert A. Wilson, a Brooklyn gynecologist. In a series of medical and popular articles, culminating in the 1966 book *Feminine Forever*, Wilson promoted estrogen replacement therapy (ERT) from "puberty to the grave" to treat the "deficiency disease of menopause." First establishing menopause as a disease, Wilson then touted estrogen as the key to its prevention and cure. Wilson's message (and responses to it) exploded in the media as popular periodicals and menopausal women tried to pinpoint the true promise of hormone treatment. Although most physicians dismissed the most radical of Wilson's claims, his campaign revolutionized the treatment of menopause; the prescription rates for menopausal estrogen therapy quadrupled between 1962 and 1975. The popularity of estrogen therapy fell sharply after 1975, however, when medical studies suggested that ERT caused endometrial cancer.[13]

Hormonal replacement therapy was down in the late 1970s but not out. By adding progestin to estrogen, physicians and drug companies claimed to eliminate the risk of endometrial cancer, and by the 1980s, the fortunes of replacement therapies rose again by promising to prevent thinning bones and heart disease. Further research in the 1990s and into the twenty-first century, however, eroded the case for the benefits of ERT and strengthened the case for its dangers.

The eras bounded by biotechnological developments roughly coincided with significant shifts in women's participation in public life. Between 1897 and 1937, the New Woman ascended, won the vote, and lost public attention to the less political (but more fashionably coiffured) flapper. Physicians, both collectively and as individuals, were not of one mind about the New Woman and her legacy, and their uncertainty emerged in discussions of menopausal women. On the one hand, most physicians welcomed the broadened social opportunities earned by the demands of the New Woman and her determined sisters. These physicians saw menopause as the biological marker of decreased familial responsibilities, and they urged women who had once dedicated their lives to family to enter community life more fully. On the other hand, some physicians worried because, in their view, as women moved beyond their homes, their behavior became distinctly unwomanly. In particular, these physicians worried about the masculine, sexually aberrant, and selfish behaviors they felt some women displayed, and they mapped these anxieties onto the bodies of menopausal women. These physicians, focusing on what they saw as alarming mental manifestations, feared that as menopausal women shed the physical and symbolic impediments of fertility, their behavior would come to mirror the activist "spinsters" who rejected domesticity in favor of public life. By labeling such behavior as symptoms of mental disorder, these physicians intended to encourage menopausal women to hold tightly to their femininity even as they moved into roles previously reserved for men.

After 1938, as the New Woman retired and receded into public memory even while women continued to stream into the workforce, the popular media, including books, movies, and women's magazines, considered the role of the modern woman. On the one hand, women, at least white, middle- and upper-class women, were encouraged to find complete fulfillment in their roles as wives and mothers. On the other, the popular media acknowledged that a life devoted to domesticity could be isolating, frustrating, and dull. These contradictions led to a wider discussion of women's roles. Should a woman try to have a family and a career? How much time and attention did a woman owe to her family? Could childless women be fulfilled? These questions about women's status influenced physicians' interpretations of menopause in the 1940s and 1950s. Publishing in popular books and magazines, many physicians promoted the view that menopause "liberated" women from the most demanding aspects of family life, but they insisted that only women who had followed the rules of domesticity when they were younger would reap the rewards of their newfound freedom. Still, these physicians insisted, gendered expectations remained in effect, even for menopausal women. They urged women to cope with their menopausal symptoms by ignoring their own difficulties and donating their housekeeping skills to the broader community.

Many women apparently agreed with the medical advice promoted in women's magazines. Some middle-class women considered menopause a trivial transition, a normal process that merited little concern and even less conversation. They scolded women who wielded their menopausal symptoms to garner sympathy, regarding such self-indulgence as pitiable, particularly given the world's more serious problems. They advised other women to acquire worthy pastimes and ignore the petty inconveniences of menopause.

Finally, by 1963, women across the country had begun reassessing their roles in the home and in the workplace, a trend that culminated in the "women's movement," or second-wave feminism. Robert Wilson, in promoting his treatment for menopause, capitalized on both the fledgling women's movement and the sexual revolution. Aging women, he suggested, needed estrogen therapy to prevent the "horror of living decay" and to secure the gains of feminism, but, further, recognizing the increased competition that middle-aged women faced in the sexual marketplace, Wilson recommended hormones to keep women "fully feminine" and sexually attractive. Wilson thus argued that hormones benefited women both when they donned their business suits and when they took them off. Wilson's views of women, menopause, and hormones did not go unchallenged, but, aided by the popular media, he set the terms of the medical and popular debate that ensued.

Between 1963 and 1980, women evaluated menopause and its treatment against the feminist backdrop. Inspired by feminism's insistence that women should participate actively in their medical care, many women sought information about how to cope with the symptoms of menopause.

Turning to women's magazines, public libraries, friends, and even the American Medical Association, women tried to determine the best way to control their changing bodies. Some women demanded hormone treatments and shopped around until they found doctors who would provide them. Other women refused to see menopause as a pathological process and rejected medical intervention, claiming that women's liberation supplied the only therapy they needed. Most women chose from a wide variety of options that fell somewhere between these poles. Feminists themselves debated the merits of Wilson's regimen and his characterizations of middle-aged women. Although they disagreed about the value of hormones, feminists nevertheless insisted that women, not doctors, must control their bodies and their health.

After 1980, many feminists stepped up their opposition to the routine prescription of replacement hormones; menopausal and postmenopausal women, however, impressed by their alleged role in securing healthy aging, used hormones in unprecedented numbers. Nevertheless, throughout this period, most women relied on nonmedical interventions (or needed no intervention at all).

Menopause Matters

In exploring how gender's evolving expectations were mapped onto menopausal women's bodies, I build on important scholarship in medical history, women's history, and American social history. Tackling issues from criminality to insanity to motherhood, historians have shown that the normative views of womanhood matter a great deal in the construction and perception of bodily experiences.[14] Although medical views of menopause were clearly influenced by social forces, it is crucial to remember that the power of cultural norms is not absolute and that cultural views of women are not monolithic. I do not claim, therefore, that culture determined medical perceptions, but rather that physicians' views of their menopausal patients resonated with larger social themes. As historian Ann-Louise Shapiro argues in her study of women and criminality, "The medical story gained its authority from its linkages with other, widely diffused ideological assumptions and cultural concerns."[15] Shapiro reminds us that physicians were not merely foot soldiers for a hegemonic culture, wielding medical expertise and treatment to prevent women from venturing outside their prescribed role.[16] Doctors, while internalizing cultural and medical values, could and did promote meanings of menopause at odds with the dominant cultural expectations of women.

But physicians are not the only actors in medical history. In 1985, Roy Porter challenged historians of medicine to "lower the historical gaze onto the sufferers," to do medical history from the patient's perspective.[17] Too often, Porter claimed, historians and sociologists generalized about the nature of the medical encounter and the power of the medical profession without looking at the objects (patients) of the medical gaze. If patient perspectives are not consulted, many claims about the nature of medicine will remain unconfirmed.

Since Porter's call to action, many valuable patient-centered histories, using a variety of strategies, have been published. Some historians have read medical accounts "against the grain" to piece together the experiences of the patients themselves.[18] Others have let the sick and ailing speak for themselves, often demonstrating that sufferers can and do achieve understandings of their affliction quite apart from the medical view.[19] My study combines both approaches, gleaning clues about women's experiences from medical and popular literature while relying on women's own voices whenever possible.

Historical claims about the reach of medicine in the lives of ailing people can best be examined by considering the views of patients. In his important synthetic study, Paul Starr argues that, by the dawn of the twentieth century, physicians had gained cultural authority, "the authority to interpret signs and symptoms, to diagnose health or illness, to name diseases, and to offer prognoses."[20] The relationship between physicians and their menopausal patients can serve as a test case to determine the strength of this claim for medical authority. In part, the example of menopause fits Starr's model. During the twentieth century, physicians increasingly claimed menopause as a medical concern, and women at menopause increasingly turned to their physicians for advice and treatment. As a result, menopause shifted from a normal life transition, well outside medical purview, to a medical event.

In some very important aspects, many women never abdicated control of their bodies, but rather forced physicians to share their authority.[21] These women decided for themselves whether menopause required medical attention, and even at the end of the twentieth century, many of them still concluded that it did not. Despite the economic and cultural barriers that discouraged some women from viewing menopause in medical terms, many who did call on their physicians for help often brought with them clear expectations for the encounter. Having read about the promise of hormone therapy (or having learned about it from friends), they asked their physicians for prescriptions, their assertiveness leading many doctors to defer to their wishes, even when those wishes challenged the physicians' own clinical judgments. Further, women's demand for or acceptance of medical treatment did not imply a wholesale acceptance of medical rhetoric. Rather, women created their own interpretations of menopause, influenced (but not determined) by medical and popular characterizations of their changing bodies.

When writing about female agency, political minefields and conceptual pitfalls abound. Any given "choice," for example, can be read several ways. When a woman decides to take hormones, she may be hoping to relieve her hot flashes or to remain forever young; the decision itself looks the same, however the motivations differ. Further, acknowledging women's agency accords them at least partial responsibility for the choices they make: having internalized normative ideals of womanhood, women sometimes make choices that further their own oppression.[22] Feminist scholars cannot claim that women have agency only when they make choices we like. Patricia Kaufert and Sonja McKinlay tried this approach, applauding some women's active decisions to quit estrogen, while regarding others' reliance on hormones as a "passive" reaction to popular culture and the wily strategies of drug manufacturers.[23] But only by granting women power, while recognizing the constraints on that power, can historians legitimately argue that women influenced and created culture while they were simultaneously influenced by it.[24] Only female agency explains how women are able to construct meanings for their bodies different from the dominant medical model.[25] By recognizing that menopausal women are historical actors rather than historical pawns, this study explores women's choices while acknowledging the social pressures influencing those choices.

Although this history of menopause highlights women's agency and women's choices, I do not claim that their choices indicate *either* individual empowerment *or* cultural coercion. As historian Nancy Tomes has noted, health-care consumers should be understood to be "neither irrational, easily manipulated tools nor all powerful sovereign shoppers."[26] Further, I am not conflating women's individual choices with female empowerment. Rather, this work tries to understand the context in which women make their choices. How did menopausal women decide whether they needed medical attention? Why did they refuse or accept hormone treatment? What larger cultural conversations contributed to their choices? How did women interpret their choices? What options did they wish for but lack?

By exploring the intersections among women, medicine, and meno-pause, this history also aims to contribute to our understanding of medicalization in general and of the medicalization of menopause in par-ticular. The classic understanding of medicalization refers to the "process whereby more and more of everyday life has come under medical domin-ion, influence and control."[27] Critics of this process have concentrated most intensely on the medicalization of behaviors (addiction, homosexu-ality, hyperactivity) and of "natural" physiological events (childbirth, sexu-ality, reproduction), characterizing increased medical presence in these realms as a form of social control.[28] Scholars of menopause have enthusias-tically entered this discussion, claiming that when physicians defined menopause as a disease or syndrome, women automatically assumed a pas-sive role and deferred to their physicians' authority. In 1983, Frances McCrea, for example, characterized the medicalization of menopause as a medical "imperialism" dominating the "passive and dependent" pa-tient.[29] More recently, sociologists Sharon Rostosky and Cheryl Travis have claimed that the increasing "medical authority in women's lives" disempowers women because "they turn their care over to their physi-cians."[30]

Over the course of the twentieth century, menopause has undoubtedly attracted increased medical attention, and an increasing number of wo-men have sought medical care and treatment at menopause. Nevertheless, it is a mistake to regard all women seeking hormones or reassurance from their physicians to be passive victims of the male medical industry. On the contrary, many women embraced medical treatment for menopause as a means of wielding control over their changing bodies. With an impulse parallel to that explored by Judith Walzer Leavitt in her account of child-birth in *Brought to Bed,* some women at menopause requested medical in-tervention.[31] Leavitt, in discussing twilight sleep, argues that women de-manded "their own right to control their own birthing experiences."[32] Twilight sleep (as induced by scopolamine and morphine) promised a safe and comfortable birth, and, despite their physicians' cautions, some Amer-ican women insisted on its use. (Ironically, the active choice of twilight sleep resulted in a passive birthing experience.) In the case of menopause, while some women undoubtedly reacted passively to their physicians' rec-ommendations, others created, embraced, and rejected medical rhetoric and therapies, seeking the best way to retain control of their bodies.[33]

Further, the history of menopause demonstrates that medicalization is not an endpoint but a process that responds over time to cultural pressures and technological developments. As the medical tools, players, and theories shift against a changing cultural backdrop, the content and reach of medicine similarly changes. Medicalization consequently changes its shape at different historical moments.

Finally, this book suggests that medicalization might be too blunt an instrument for characterizing medical involvement in menopause. Medicine as an institution encompasses a variety of actors. Pharmaceutical companies eagerly offer the latest and greatest wonder drugs. Patent drug peddlers tout a cure for every ill and an ill for every cure. Elite physicians publish in national journals, claiming and proclaiming expertise over all things bodily, and thereby extending medical authority if not always medical jurisdiction. Physicians, acting as public educators, write books and magazine articles that sometimes drum up business for their colleagues and sometimes help women to stay out of medical waiting rooms. General practitioners, who may or may not have read the medical literature, just want to make their patients feel better. All these overlapping parties contributed—and contribute—to the medicalization of menopause, but in different ways at different times.

This work also aims to contribute to the emerging interdisciplinary exploration of age and aging. Within the past ten years or so, historians and other social commentators have increasingly argued that age serves as a profound cultural, social, and political organizing principle.[34] Age, within the contexts of race, class, gender, and sexuality, both bestows privilege and attracts scorn. It builds community, and it begets division. By differentiating among women by age, as well as by race, class, and sexuality, we can see how gendered expectations (and the ability and willingness of women to meet them) are not static. The history of menopause demonstrates that the meaning of womanhood and the expectations of and for women change as women age.

Menopause is a physiological process, a transition from fertility to infertility, a marker of bodily aging. Significantly, however, menopause also represents a social process, in grappling with which both women and their physicians address complex questions on the meanings of womanhood and the private and public roles of women. This book explores continuity and change in the lived experience and the medical perception of menopause in the United States throughout the twentieth century. Its chapters, taken together, demonstrate that the discussion of menopause reflected, created, and supported broader cultural judgments about women and about the contours of appropriate medical practice.

ONE

"Menopause Is Not a Dangerous Time"

Medicine, Menopause, and the New Woman, 1897–1937

In 1897, Andrew F. Currier, a New York City physician, proposed to set the record straight. He claimed that too little had been written about menopause, and what physicians had written "handed down the hoary tradition, which has been current from time immemorial among both the laity and the profession, that the menopause is an experience fraught with peril and difficulty." In contrast, Currier insisted that "menopause is not a dangerous time or experience for the majority of women, any more than puberty is. . . . It is only the exceptional woman who has a hard time, and comes to the doctor to tell him about it. Upon this exceptional experience, the doctrine of the danger and serious character of menopause has been built up."[1]

As the first American physician to write a monograph discussing menopause, Currier passionately argued that the medical profession's understanding of menopause relied on outmoded ideas generated at mid-century and reproduced without question for the next forty years. As a result, physicians remained inexcusably ignorant of the true nature of menopause, and middle-aged women remained unnecessarily afraid of their "change of life." He offered his contribution as both a useful corrective and a needed stimulus for further study.

Currier was not the only physician to contemplate and assess the nature and meaning of menopause at the close of the nineteenth century and the opening of the twentieth. In the 1890s, American medical journals began to publish more than the occasional article about menopause.[2] By the turn of the twentieth century, physicians (and eventually a few lay writers)

14

increasingly offered their conclusions directly to menopausal women. Books, pamphlets, and articles in the periodical press taught women how to prepare themselves for the "change of life."

Several factors encouraged the increased medical attention paid to menopause in the 1890s and its intensification over the next thirty years. First, at the end of the nineteenth century, the medical profession, in part by becoming increasingly scientific, gained the cultural authority to offer counsel about all matters biological, even when those pronouncements were not directly related to illness or medical practice. Physicians were particularly eager to offer advice about the nature of women's bodies and the connection of those bodies to women's roles in society. Debates over women's education, the desirability of the bicycle, the dangers and depravity of birth control and abortion, and the biological consequences of female suffrage—all became legitimate arenas for medical expertise.[3] Second, the rise of gynecology in the 1870s and 1880s increased the medical attention on female bodies. Surgical gynecology, having made its reputation in part from ovariotomies, which induced menopause, forced gynecologists and general practitioners alike to consider the effects of menopause on their patients and led them to construct menopause as a harmless, "normal" process, whether it occurred "naturally" at fifty or "artificially" at thirty.[4] Third, the fledgling field of endocrinology, emerging in the 1890s, focused attention on the ductless glands, including the ovaries. One of the projects of endocrinological research included understanding the hormonal regulation of the menstrual cycle and the physiological changes associated with menopause. This research also led to the development of "organotherapy" for menopause. While organotherapy did not catch on widely during this period, its possible viability marked one of the dominant conversations within the medical literature on menopause.[5] Finally, women physicians, themselves often "of a certain age," bemoaned the paucity of information on menopause available to women and the popular and medical misconceptions that existed. Their efforts helped fill the gaps and encouraged more discussion.

Physicians articulated their views on menopause in two forums, one medical and the other popular. This chapter relies on medical journal articles and gynecology textbooks to illuminate the medical discussion.[6] More than two hundred physicians contributed to this discussion, representing a wide swath of the medical profession—gynecologists, internists, surgeons, endocrinologists, and general practitioners. Although some of these physicians were part of the medical elite, including those holding university professorships, others were self-proclaimed family doctors, who depended on private practice for support. Unlike the authors of medical literature, some writers of popular literature were allied with medical practices outside the "regular" or "allopathic" tradition. The information and advice offered by these physicians did not differ, however, from that of their regular counterparts. Further, by the 1910s, nonmedical writers occasionally contributed to the popular discussion of menopause.

Reexamining Menopause

Even as some doctors paid increasing attention to menopause at the end of the nineteenth century, it remained largely unimportant to most physicians throughout this period. Major gynecological textbooks of the period rarely devoted more than a paragraph to menopause, and *Index Medicus* failed to provide menopause its own subject heading until 1921.[7] Throughout this period, dysmenorrhea and amenorrhea received more attention from American medical journals than did menopause.[8] Physicians themselves noticed the dearth of information on the subject; indeed, many bemoaned its neglect.[9] Dr. Sara Greenfield, writing in the *Woman's Medical Journal,* captured the concerns of many physicians. She complained that major textbooks devoted only "two or three short paragraphs to the subject and dismiss it with the statement that it is a natural physiological phenomena which needs no special attention." She couldn't understand "why such an important period in a woman's life should be treated so lightly."[10]

Physicians also condemned the lack of information written for menopausal women themselves. Homeopathic physician Emma Drake complained in the introduction to her 1902 book, *What a Woman of Forty-Five Ought to Know,* that "in no line of literature, perhaps, is a book so much needed as in the line of the present volume, because few books have ever been written upon this subject, and the few have not been addressed to women, but to the medical profession."[11] The neglect of menopause by the medical community endured throughout the early decades of the twentieth century, causing one commentator to note the "great paucity" of information on menopause as late as 1936.[12]

Because menopause failed to attract the attention it deserved, some physicians viewed menopausal medicine as a chance to build a private practice or a research reputation. A 1904 article, for example, argued that the neglect of menopause by the medical profession provided a golden vocational opportunity, considering the "number of prospective patients."[13] But physicians apparently failed to fill this professional niche; as late as 1932, doctors continued to see menopausal medicine as a rich, but unexplored, area in which to make a career.[14] So even as physicians devoted increasing attention to menopause, it remained a subject partially on the medical margins, perhaps because most physicians did not consider menopause a medical problem.

The leading authority on menopause in the English-speaking world (and perhaps in Germany and France) for much of the second half of the nineteenth century was Edward J. Tilt, an English-born, French-educated physician. In 1851, he published a small guide for women titled *On the Preservation of the Health of Women at Critical Periods of Life*. In 1857, an enlarged version of his text appeared, this time directed to the medical profession, under the title *The Change of Life in Health and Disease*.[15] This text went through two more English editions and several printings. It was published in the United States for the first time in 1871.[16] In his often-cited work, Tilt characterized menopause as a "critical period" for a woman, an epoch of "real trouble, anxiety and danger; for in the manner in which she crosses this broad Rubicon will depend whether the twenty or thirty years of after-life will be passed in tranquil happiness, or will be embittered by an endless succession of infirmities."[17]

By the 1890s, some physicians continued to refer to menopause as a critical period, but this view was slowly supplanted by a kinder, gentler menopause. Most early-twentieth-century commentators acknowledged that menopause represented an important milestone in a woman's life, but they denied that it was fraught with danger.[18] One physician, for example, remarked that menopausal changes "come about as gently as the falling of the autumn leaves" and maintained that the menses "fold their tents, like the Arabs, and as silently steal away." Others maintained that most women did not suffer at all during menopause.[19] An often-cited British article by the Medical Women's Federation supported this position, claiming that nine of ten women "carried on their daily routine without a single interruption due to menopausal symptoms."[20]

Medical Recommendations

The medical commentary on menopause agreed that, while menopause itself posed no health problems, women should nevertheless practice good health habits throughout their lives to ward off any potential problems.

Kate Campbell Hurd-Mead, for example, maintained that in order to meet the challenges of menopause, a woman "needs treatment before she is born, continual watching and teaching while she is growing, and great care when she becomes a mother, as well as good advice when she has reached the menopause." Health and fitness activist Bernarr MacFadden added that "if the physical condition has been kept at the highest point, the transition should be made easily and without any marked physical disturbance."[21] These comments indicate the importance of clean living over medical treatment in avoiding menopausal difficulties.

Women who failed to look after their health while young, however, might encounter, through their own carelessness, some difficulties at menopause. Many physicians conceded that to the "unprepared," "ignorant," or "irresponsible woman," menopause remained a "critical period."[22] A luxurious lifestyle was often indicted as a corrupting influence on the health of all women, and the cumulative effect of years of affluent living particularly threatened women at middle age. Physicians consistently employed an economic metaphor to warn women of the dangers caused by an indulgent life. One physician cautioned that "luxury draws heavy bills on the constitution, which must be eventually paid . . . with heavy and compound interest."[23] Emma Drake, similarly, warned her readers that menopause would be easily traversed if not for the "many debts to pay for the indiscretions of our foremothers, and so many entitled by our own neglects and carelessness. Nature is inexorable, and demands to the full all that belongs to her credit, and we perforce must pay."[24]

That physicians condemned luxurious living is not surprising. Physicians have long maintained that luxury contributes to disease in general and menopausal suffering in particular.[25] In the early twentieth century, however, the argument seemed to gain greater currency.

Although most doctors insisted that menopause was not in itself a cause for alarm, they nevertheless conceded that middle age heralded the onset of many illnesses, including cancer. In order to discover any lurking difficulties, physicians urged menopausal women to visit their doctors.[26] Physicians did not claim that women were more prone to problems at middle age than were men; rather, they regarded menopause as a physiological reminder of the passing years and of the need for preventive care. They emphasized medical attention not to treat menopause itself, but to differentiate between the normal and therefore harmless symptoms of menopause and the pathological and dangerous signs of serious disease. Physicians insisted that menopause itself posed no danger, but they believed that dangerous afflictions might arise at menopause and might even be masked by it. As a result, menopause marked the occasion for medical observation, but only to allow physicians to look for pathology that menopause might hide.

Among the possible pathological symptoms, physicians regarded hemorrhage to be the most serious. Doctors implored their patients to consider abnormally heavy bleeding at menopause as a sign of ill health because it often served as the first sign of cancer. Anna Galbraith, fellow of the New York Academy of Medicine, for example, warned her readers that it was "most erroneous and fatal" to consider copious bleeding at menopause normal. She maintained that abnormally heavy bleeding warranted immediate medical care. Physicians regularly recounted the tragic cases of women who died or suffered unnecessarily because they neglected to seek help for hemorrhage or other abnormal symptoms, thus "condemning" themselves "to months and years of frequently avoidable, miserable and hopeless invalidism."[27] Significantly, however, physicians did not claim that these women fell ill from untreated menopause; rather, they felt these women suffered from the effects of untreated diseases occurring at the time of menopause.

Despite physicians' belief that all women should submit to a medical exam at menopause, doctors frequently complained that menopausal women generally failed to show up. Physicians feared that misplaced female modesty contributed to women's reluctance to seek medical care. To rectify the situation, physicians often used scare tactics in their popular works to propel women into their doctors' offices for a complete internal exam. One physician, for example, warned his readers in 1934 that "false modesty may cost years of suffering." The medical literature likewise reminded physicians of the need to be thorough, despite women's possible protests.[28]

But physicians did not hold women solely responsible for neglecting their health. Doctors also blamed their colleagues for discouraging women's medical visits, routinely scolding other doctors for dismissing the concerns and complaints of menopausal women. Too often, they held, physicians merely told these women that their troubles were due to "the change of life" and then sent them home to wait it out. Alabama physician James Lewis Ellis complained, for example, that "the tendency is to relegate all the complaints at this time to the great limbo of patient suffering because it is nature adjusting the system to the change."[29] Gynecologist George Shoemaker in 1901 similarly feared that a misunderstanding of the nuances of menopause led physicians to overlook any abnormalities "as though [they] were all in the due course of nature."[30] Very little appears to have changed thirty years later, when another physician noted that women's complaints at menopause are "very often disregarded by the physician."[31] These physicians insisted that dismissing all women's concerns at middle age as harmless symptoms of menopause sentenced women to unnecessary suffering and premature death. Such an attitude threatened women's health, both by failing to diagnose serious illness and by discouraging women from seeking medical attention.[32]

Although they generally encouraged medical exams for menopausal women, many physicians also believed that medicine had very little to offer these patients beyond reassurance and a prescription for healthy habits. At the beginning of the century, physicians believed, not surprisingly, that "trust and confidence" were more valuable "than all the therapeutic agents under the sun."[33] As late as 1935, however, Johns Hopkins professor of gynecology Emil Novak maintained that physicians "earn their fees better through education and prevention than by writing out a prescription."[34] Many doctors maintained that their first duty to their menopausal patients was to ease their apprehensions. Both the medical and popular literature agreed that many women approached "the change" filled with dread, believing that menopause marked the passing of youth and the beginning of physical suffering. Woods Hutchinson complained, for example, that in the popular imagination menopause had been "distorted" from a "natural, physiologic, healthful process, an honorable discharge from one of the heaviest duties of life" into "one of the most critical and dangerous experiences."[35] Another physician similarly expressed his frustration that misinformation about the "terrible train of consequences" led women to dread menopause unnecessarily.[36]

So potent was this alleged fear of menopause that physicians worried that apprehension itself made women ill. In 1923, gynecologist William Robinson captured the concern of many of his colleagues: "Many of the dangers and diseases of the menopause are of our own making. Fear is a demon of most pernicious and most potent malignancy. It creates the things which it is feared it may create."[37] Another gynecologist agreed, maintaining that some women actually "induce quite independently of any actual menopause the very symptoms which they fear."[38]

Since apprehension and ignorance led to suffering, physicians claimed that reassurance and information could palliate many of menopausal women's difficulties. Physicians generally believed that an explanation of the physiological changes of menopause coupled with a description of the most common symptoms could alleviate a great deal of suffering. New York City gynecologist Herman F. Strongin noted that if menopause were "properly understood by the woman herself . . . anxiety, together with actual dangers, might be largely eliminated."[39] Other physicians claimed that women merely needed reassurance that their experiences were "normal" and that their symptoms did not represent disease.[40]

These physicians stopped short of claiming that a woman's problems at menopause were "all in her head." Rather, they gave credence to the notion that cultural messages and personal expectations influenced the response to physiological processes. As a result, physicians had an incentive to both talk with and listen to their patients, seeing them not as symptoms to be treated but as people to be educated.

Further reflecting the emphasis on advice and information, physicians generally agreed that their menopausal patients should acquire and maintain healthy habits. Physicians urged their patients to get lots of rest and daily exercise in the fresh air. They advised women to eat a moderate diet, avoid alcoholic beverages, and shun tight-fitting clothes.[41] Many physicians also recommended a change of scenery at menopause to divert women's minds from the details of domestic life.[42] A few doctors even suggested a visit to a "sanitorium" [*sic*] in severe cases.[43] Notably, this prescription for healthy living differed little from the regimen encouraged for all people, regardless of age, sex, or complaint.

Organotherapy

Unlike physicians in the nineteenth century, doctors during the early twentieth century had a new therapeutic tool to help ease a woman's journey through menopause—organotherapy. Organotherapy, also known as ovarian therapy, was the precursor to modern hormone replacement therapies. The emergence of organotherapy as a treatment for menopause arose from the fascination with "internal secretions," the mysterious and elusive substances assumed to exist in the endocrine glands of both men and women. Although the internal secretion from the thyroid was isolated in 1891, the existence of internal secretions in ovaries and testes remained speculative until the 1920s. Estrogen, for example, was not isolated until 1929, and progesterone was not isolated until 1932.[44] Even though the existence of hormones remained speculative, some scientists eagerly promoted their therapeutic use. French-born physiologist Charles-Edouard Brown-Séquard sparked the field by injecting himself in 1889 with extracts from guinea pig and dog testes; he reported renewed vigor as a consequence. The therapeutic enterprise developed along two paths. One sought to capitalize on the "rejuvenation" possibilities of organotherapy, a course dismissed as "quackery" by many physicians. Other researchers were encouraged by the therapeutic promise of internal secretions. By the first decade of the twentieth century, the field of "sex endocrinology" had been firmly established.[45]

Organotherapy during much of this period was crude at best. Until the 1930s, clinicians had at their disposal three methods of administration. At the beginning of the century, fresh ovaries were ground up and fed to menopausal patients. Gradually, this method fell out of favor, and physicians increasingly relied on the desiccated ovaries of farm animals, such as ewes, cows, and mares. According to one source, the most effective ovaries were harvested "during the time of [the animals'] full sexual maturity."[46] The most advanced method relied on "ovarian extracts," but even by the late 1920s, the extraction process had not been standardized.

The first use of ovarian therapy for gynecological disturbances occurred in Berlin in 1898, when fresh cow ovaries were fed to a young woman who had had her ovaries removed and was suffering from severe vasomotor symptoms. As early as 1899, *The Merck Manual of the Materia Medica* offered Ovariin, dried cow ovaries, for menopausal disorders.[47] By 1910, researchers in the United States had begun to report the use of ovarian preparations to "combat the insufficiency or absence of the ovarian function at the time of menopause."[48] By 1920, at least three companies were manufacturing ovarian extracts.[49] It was not until 1934 that Ayerst produced and marketed Emmenin in the United States, the first orally active estrogen. Made from the urine of pregnant Canadian women, Emmenin's cost as well as production problems threatened its viability.[50]

Although one historian has argued that physicians enthusiastically embraced hormones early in the twentieth century,[51] the evidence indicates that most physicians remained skeptical about their worth into the 1930s. Some physicians objected to organotherapy because the methods of administration were so difficult. Indeed, it was unclear whether ovarian extracts even contained the "active principle" that endocrinologists claimed resided within the ovary.[52] Looking back on the period in question, Novak concluded that the "various organ extracts were inert, or at best, that they contained only negligible quantities of ovarian hormones."[53] Other physicians objected on practical grounds, insisting that ovarian therapy had not been proven effective in relieving menopausal symptoms. In a response to a query, the editor of the *Journal of the American Medical Association* (*JAMA*) maintained that as "rational as ovarian therapy may theoretically appear . . . the actual results are rarely striking and often nil to the careful observer."[54] Still other physicians admitted that ovarian therapy sometimes helped menopausal women, but only as a "psychotherapeutic agent."[55] Endocrinologist Roy Hoskins, for example, reported in 1933 that some researchers reported "brilliant success" with ovarian preparations, but he admitted that the treatment worked even when the therapeutic materials lacked potency.[56] A few doctors similarly noted that ovarian extracts proved no more helpful in relieving menopausal symptoms than saline injections or other placebos.[57]

Several physicians claimed that ovarian therapy could help some women who suffered from especially distressing symptoms, but these physicians warned their colleagues that the effects were exceedingly variable.[58] Hurd-Mead, for example, admitted that while ovarian extracts were helpful in "special cases, . . . the dried extracts of the ductless glands have not taken the place in the treatment of the diseases of menopause that enthusiasts at first claimed for them."[59] Another physician noted that the initial excitement about organotherapy was followed by disappointment. He continued to regard it, however, as "a very valuable but not infallible" treatment for menopause.[60]

Despite these objections, some physicians, both gynecologists and general practitioners, did recommend hormonal therapy, sometimes enthusiastically. Howard Masters, for example, who would later gain fame as a sex researcher, maintained in 1923 that "organotherapy is of great value and should be used in those cases experiencing any difficulty." John Upshur agreed, claiming that the use of ovarian extracts had been "very satisfactory." Another physician, generally skeptical about the value of ovarian therapy, nevertheless viewed it as a "near-specific" in treating hot flashes.[61]

Even physicians who supported ovarian therapy, however, did so cautiously, insisting that most women did not need pharmaceutical therapy.[62] The views of the eminent gynecologist Emil Novak are instructive. In a 1922 medical journal article, Novak reviewed the efficacy of ovarian therapy for gynecological difficulties. While he concluded that ovarian therapy had not proved effective for disorders such as dysmenorrhea, sterility, or morning sickness, he believed that for the "vasomotor symptoms" of menopause—hot flashes in particular—ovarian extracts could be helpful. The "purely subjective" nature of the symptoms, however, left him unwilling to guess whether ovarian preparations worked physiologically or psychologically. Nevertheless, he claimed that "unless I have been greatly deceived, I have seen genuinely good results from organotherapy" in treating menopause.[63] But in Novak's popular work, *The Woman Asks the Doctor,* he insisted that "a large proportion of women go through menopause with scarcely a ripple and need no medical treatment whatsoever." He acknowledged, however, that in a minority of cases, "the administration of certain 'glandular' ovarian substances . . . often give[s] great if not complete relief from the symptoms."[64] His remarks demonstrate that even physicians who embraced hormone therapies did not encourage them for all menopausal women.

Most physicians who accepted the value of ovarian therapy (or at least conceded its promise) viewed it as part of a broader strategy that included "nerve tonics," rest, and travel.[65] Howard Aronson, for example, reminded his colleagues in 1936 that they should treat "the patient as a whole, not merely writing out a prescription for bromides or placebos, nor . . . solely treating her ovaries and uterus." He admitted that hormone therapy had its place but added that "treatment should aim at keeping the weight down [and] keeping the patient occupied."[66]

The wide divergence of opinion on organotherapy prompted one physician to remark in 1927 that the field of ovarian treatment during this period was "in a state of confusion and flat contradiction."[67] While some only saw conflict, others saw hope. One optimistic doctor mused that "at present reputable scientists are plucking at the weedy growth of gland therapy hopeful of removing from obscurity a few vigorous plants that may continue to thrive in the fertile soil of truth."[68] In 1931, the editor of *JAMA* agreed that while the present ovarian preparations had no therapeutic value, the "brilliant work" being done in endocrinology "promises to yield much of practical value . . . in the not far distant future."[69]

That physicians failed to embrace menopause as a particular medical concern suggests that it escaped the trends that characterized much of "scientific medicine" between 1897 and 1937. New technological gadgets, laboratory tests, and surgical procedures had little to offer menopausal women. Even as new pharmaceutical options became available, however, many physicians still resisted changing their traditional approach to menopause.[70]

Suppositories, Pills, and Tonics

Although physicians did not generally adopt organotherapy in this period, other "medical" practitioners readily filled the therapeutic bill, offering treatments outside a doctors' purview. In particular, patent drugs promised women relief from symptoms without ever leaving the home. The patent medicine market, unlike the doctor's black bag, was full of therapeutic options. Doan's Kidney Pills, The Famous Specific Orange Blossom, Lydia Pinkham's Vegetable Compound, and the Miller Company's Home Treatment were among the many suppositories, tonics, and pills guaranteed to relieve the "peculiar symptoms" of the change of life.

Patent medicine, costing just pennies a dose, appealed to women, rich and poor, for many reasons. First, patent medicines were associated with general female complaints. It is not unreasonable to assume that women who chose Lydia Pinkham's Vegetable Compound for menstrual cramps used what they found in their medicine cabinets for the change of life. Second, while physicians assured women that their symptoms would eventually pass, patent medicine explicitly challenged the position that women should stoically conceal their suffering. An advertisement for Vitae-Ore Vitae suppositories, for example, cautioned women against falling into the trap of seeing female trouble as the price of being a woman. Instead, the ad claimed that women who "procrastinate" merely invite disease to become established. Patent medicine advertisements both validated women's menopausal discomforts and exploited them to sell their products.[71] Third, patent drug sellers traded on female modesty to encourage women to buy their products.[72] By ordering Dr. Pierce's Special Prescription or the Wine of Cardui women could avoid the probing questions and eyes of male physicians. Further, the patent drug manufacturers exploited women's expected responsibilities to her home and family. Ads for Vitae-Ore Vitae suppositories, for example, emphasized that women can't be ill "without casting a shadow over the home." Using tactics that anticipated the marketing of hormones in the 1960s, this manufacturer also suggested that an otherwise attentive husband might eventually tire of an enfeebled wife and look elsewhere for the "high spirits, the physical vigor, and the entertaining vivacity" that was no longer available at home.[73] Finally, patent medicine advertisements acted as both medical advisor and confiding girlfriend. Advertisements routinely included testimonials from women who had suffered at menopause with a variety of symptoms but had found relief by using the product being advertised. While these statements were as likely to be fictional as not, the descriptions of sleepless nights, drenching hot flashes, uncontrollable mood swings, and alarmingly irregular periods certainly matched the experiences of some of the readers. By printing the addresses of the correspondent, advertisers encouraged women to believe that other women—some living right down the street from them— had secured relief from their menopausal symptoms.

Perhaps these products worked as well or better than the physicians' reassurance or bits of ewe's ovary to relieve menopausal discomforts. Whether they succeeded at relieving constipation, easing an aching head, or taking the edge off nervousness and anxiety, patent medicines probably did make women feel better. If nothing else, the alcohol content in some treatments provided a sedative effect some women probably welcomed. In some ways, the nonspecific, wide-ranging "symptoms" of menopause fit perfectly with the nonspecific, wide-ranging claims of the patent medicine manufacturers.

Menopause and the New Woman

The medical and popular literature in the early twentieth century suggested that menopause was not merely a bundle of symptoms and physiological changes but also a physical marker of a social transition. Physicians admitted that as women confronted their waning fertility, they also reassessed their social niche. Doctors joined menopausal women in considering the fate of women after their bodies forced them to retire from their most vaunted vocation—motherhood.

Medical commentators assessed the social role of menopausal women against the backdrop of far-reaching changes in women's place in American society. Beginning in the 1890s, for example, the popular media began noticing—with alarm and admiration—the "New Woman." The New Woman was white, college-educated, usually single, and committed to female self-determination. Between 1890 and 1910, female college enrollment tripled, and, alarmingly, these women typically remained single. In 1915, for example, only 39 percent of the graduates from the women's colleges married.[74] The New Woman, however, was not responsible for all the changes in women's roles during this period. Her more conservative sisters likewise expanded women's traditional role beyond the domestic sphere. These less radical women founded settlement houses, joined women's clubs, and gained prominence in labor unions, thereby increasing women's presence in public and economic life.[75]

Evidence suggests that the New Woman's increased power and involvement in civic affairs affected the way physicians, both male and female, viewed their menopausal patients. It would be too simplistic to claim that male doctors' discussions of menopausal women merely reflected their discomfort with female empowerment, although clearly this was occasionally the case.[76] More significantly, many physicians who discussed menopause supported women's increased power and visibility and claimed that middle-aged women were poised to take advantage of their expanded social opportunities.

Historian Carroll Smith-Rosenberg has argued that physicians in the nineteenth century used menopause and menarche as opportunities to warn women against trying to escape from the domestic role.[77] In the early twentieth century, physicians reacted somewhat differently. While doctors continued to recommend activities consistent with dominant models of womanhood, physicians nevertheless conceded that menopause released women from the most constraining demands of domesticity. Consequently, some physicians applauded women's increased opportunities and urged menopausal women to create lives beyond their homes.

After Babies and Bassinets

Between 1897 and 1937, physicians generally claimed that normal menopause held no physical dangers, but they nevertheless maintained that the "change of life" represented both a social and physical milestone, for it meant the passing of the childbearing capacity. Medical writers, however, debated the significance of this turning point. The discussion reflected differing understandings of women's most valuable contributions to society. In the beginning of the century, some male physicians claimed that menopause represented the beginning of old age and that women could look forward only to an inevitable decline. With menopause, these doctors maintained, women left their most important function behind them.[78] According to one physician, the menopausal woman "exchanges the fullness of sexual power for a condition of sexual atrophy. She realizes that . . . the highest function of her existence is departing."[79] Another physician vividly described in 1910 the prospects of the menopausal woman: "A woman's life may be compared to that of a tree. It springs up from the seed, grows beautiful and shapely, bears fruit for a time and then her productive years are over." This doctor admitted, however, that she remains "an ornament and blessing in the home."[80] In a similar vein, internist George Richter declared that menopause terminated the physiological basis "upon which the life of a woman, as a woman is based, and which constitutes the right and privilege of the female to be supported by the male."[81] Mincing no words, one physician claimed, "the female ceases to be a woman" at menopause.[82]

But the majority of medical commentators on menopause believed that such assessments grossly overstated the physical significance of menopause. Woods Hutchinson, for example, maintained that "the years of greatest power and usefulness in a woman's life, both in her family and outside of it, are often precisely those following the fall of the curtain upon the drama of reproductive life."[83] Sociologist Ernest R. Groves, author of popular marriage manuals, agreed with the medical assessment, scoffing at the notion that women existed "primarily for the perpetuity of the human race" and that after menopause women become "physiologically superfluous."[84] He argued that "such an interpretation of woman's life utterly fails to do justice to the social career of the modern woman as an individual and greatly exaggerates the physiological significance of the climacteric."[85] These authors used the prospects of menopausal women to promote their view that women rightly deserved a public life, a life that their mothers rarely had, but one that was becoming increasingly available to some women in the United States.

It is unclear how individual women regarded menopause during this period, but many women might have welcomed the end of reproductive life for at least two reasons. First, the falling birthrate over the course of the nineteenth and twentieth centuries indicates that most women had been taking active steps to prevent pregnancy long before they reached menopause.[86] Indeed, by 1900, women were typically in their mid-thirties when their last child started school and fifty-five when their last child married.[87] As a result, for many women, menopause allowed sexual encounters without the concomitant concern about contraception and unwanted pregnancies. Second, for some women, the menstrual cycle itself created its own turbulence. Acknowledging women's difficulties with menstruation, physicians and other commentators frequently contrasted menopause with the stormy episodes of puberty, childbearing, and menstruation and noted that after menopause women could find relief "in the unruffled waters of the harbor beyond the reach of sexual storms."[88] Similarly, W. Londes Peple noted that menopause was "the autumn of life when the harvesting is done . . . and not the blustering equinox with its sudden desolating storms."[89]

Limitless Opportunities

In addition to recognizing the physical benefits of menopause, physicians commonly promoted the social and intellectual benefits of life beyond the domestic sphere, claiming that menopause marked the foundation of limitless opportunities for women who had deferred professional ambition to care for their homes and families. Physicians viewed menopause and the release from domestic obligations as an opening to explore new interests and engage public life more fully.[90]

Physicians, joined by nonmedical health writers, encouraged women to regard menopause as a well-earned chance to enjoy the fruits of their labors. In 1934, for example, Sarah Trent congratulated the menopausal woman for having fulfilled her "duty . . . for the race" and urged her to seize the middle years to "live for yourself." Marriage counselors Gladys Groves and Robert Ross likewise heralded middle age as the time to learn "to be liked for herself alone," rather than for her sex.[91] These commentators recognized women's dual role in a society that was increasingly acknowledging women's wide-ranging contributions. Although most physicians did not downplay the importance of motherhood, they acknowledged that women's aspirations and aptitudes extended beyond the home. For a woman who had deferred her social or intellectual pursuits, physicians depicted the years after menopause as a "period of larger freedom . . . when she may take up and perfect some of the ambitions of her earlier years."[92]

To demonstrate this, the popular literature regularly described the accomplishments of older women. Emma Drake, for example, urged women over forty to find inspiration in the stories of temperance worker Frances Willard and lyricist Julia Ward Howe, whose greatest achievements came only in middle age. Not surprisingly, the list of middle-aged achievers grew longer throughout this period. By 1934, Trent was able to devote an entire chapter to the accomplishments of older women.[93]

Medical writers explicitly attributed the rosy outlook for life after menopause to increased opportunities for women. They claimed that the "changes in women's valuation" had created a climate that encouraged female participation in the public sphere. Many of them, particularly after 1930, celebrated "an end of the double standard" and the broadened opportunities for women. Psychiatrist W. Béran Wolfe, for example, enthusiastically favored the "emancipation of women," declaring that the "history of man's cruelty to women is one of the darkest chapters in the history of human kind." Henry Coe, president of the American Gynecological Society, believed that the New Woman represented "distinct progress," and insisted that the only impediment to her achievements was the lack of a "New Man." Several medical writers further noted that the recent "emancipation" of women particularly helped women over forty by providing outlets for women's newly found free time.[94]

Maternal Obligations and Community Housekeeping

Although many physicians approved of increased opportunities for women, they did not similarly excuse women from their maternal obligations.
Wolfe, for example, claimed in 1935 that women should not abandon
family life for the rewards of a career. He warned, "The unmarried woman
who has sacrificed everything for fame, for money, for prestige, finds very
often, when she has attained the goals of her childhood, that they are
empty fictions without meaning and without reality. Professional prestige
or business acumen, nay even money in the bank, have a curious way of
being small comfort on a cold night."[95] Wolfe's comments indicate the
limits of women's emancipation. Physicians supported women's increased
presence in public life, but not at the expense of family obligations.

Although many physicians and other health writers applauded women's
increased opportunities, they retained a gendered idea of the kind of activities they deemed appropriate. Physicians continued to promote motherhood as the ultimate vocation for women, even for menopausal women.
Emphasizing both the value of productive work and of mothering, physicians, both male and female, generally urged women to transfer the skills
that they used in running their homes to a broader "community housekeeping," applying their domestic skills of caring for others to the task of
looking after the health and welfare of their communities. These authors
urged women to take up social causes, particularly those addressing the
"welfare of others." This literature assured women that, even if their families no longer needed their immediate attention, they were "still mothers
in the truest and most comprehensive meaning of the word." The menopausal woman was urged to serve the world through her "universal motherhood." By promoting community housekeeping for postmenopausal
women, physicians encouraged women's participation in public life without challenging the primacy of motherhood and domesticity for younger
women.[96]

Physicians generally did not depict this community work as a way to
keep menopausal women busy and therefore out of their offices. Rather,
doctors and other health writers acknowledged the valuable contributions
of older women. Herman Strongin noted, for example, that "the cultural
life of America draws its support in overwhelming measure from the ranks
of women about this age. They are the dominant element in social relief,
women's clubs, and civic movements."[97] Edith Lowry similarly touted
the value of older women's contributions. She claimed that because older

women had added community housekeeping to their domestic tasks "many communities have undergone a thorough house-cleaning." But, she added, "the majority are just waiting for some experienced housekeepers to begin their work." She included the programs of the Children's Bureau, reforms in public health, and improvements in tenement housing as a few of the noteworthy accomplishments of women over forty.[98]

But community housekeeping was not just a task assigned to women by sympathetic men. Indeed, community housekeeping or "maternalist politics" was a strategy used by women to claim increased access to life outside the home. Activist women in the 1880s and beyond saw their authority over issues of care, nuturance, and morality as their key to expanded realms of usefulness.[99] As a result, maternalism "extolled the private virtues of domesticity while [it] simultaneously legitimated women's public relationships to politics and the state, to community, workplace, and marketplace."[100]

Women's use of a domestic strategy to gain increased political power should be read as part of progressive era reforms, optimistically based on the belief that social problems could be solved by "experts." In solving domestic social problems, older women who spent their lives governing their own domestic realm provided valuable expertise. During the first third of the twentieth century, as American politics became more concerned about care-taking, menopausal and postmenopausal women increasingly took up political causes, having talents "of the kind the world stands most in need."[101]

Women's efforts to secure the vote provides a key example of the deployment of the maternalist ideology. Until roughly 1915, suffragists fought for the vote by wielding rights rhetoric, claiming that women as humans deserved the same privileges as men. This strategy had very limited success. Opponents of suffrage for women viewed it as a movement to put female self-interest above duty to family and community. They balked at the notion that a woman would primarily stand as an individual rather than as a wife and mother. After 1915, however, prosuffrage activists tried a different approach. Rather than insisting on equality with men, they maintained that women's differences from men warranted women's suffrage. In particular, activists promoted a woman's nurturing character as a moral benefit to society. The maternal suffrage argument promoted a model of womanhood that appeared far less threatening to both men and women; as a result, it was far more successful in gaining political ground.[102]

Physicians concerned with the welfare of menopausal women between 1897 and 1937 embraced maternalist rhetoric as they considered what it meant for women to lose their fertility. Most physicians and other medical writers did not claim that menopausal women were used up, spent. Instead, these authors employed maternal rhetoric—the very rhetoric that threatened to brand menopausal women as obsolete and that helped women secure the vote—to argue that the country still needed older women's domestic skills. Indeed, after childbearing was completed, they argued, women could expand their contributions and increase their social value by mothering the nation.

Women Physicians Confront Menopause

In 1912, fifty-four-year-old obstetrician Angenette Parry complained that "the menopause is held up to women all through their lives as a bugaboo, a period to be dreaded, a period of inevitable horror and inevitable incapacity." She urged her colleagues to "do some genuine missionary work by seeking to rid our sisters of these unwholesome and troublesome thoughts."[103] Compare Parry's concerns with the characterization of menopause by Joseph Tenenbaum in his 1929 marriage guide. While Tenenbaum admitted that some women sail easily through menopause, he maintained that "the majority have a stormy sea to traverse; no wonder they become seasick; they experience the seasickness of menopause! They are torn between forces which they can neither control nor evade. . . . One must wonder at the brutality of egoistic nature that shows so little pity."[104]

Contrasting the opinions of male physicians with those of female physicians between 1897 and 1937 further illuminates medical assessments of menopause. Focusing on the sex of the physicians brings into relief at least three issues. First, it reviews the question of whether women doctors provided a different strategy in the practice of medicine or whether their medical training and professional ambitions blurred gender-based distinctions. Second, this comparison gauges how women physicians regarded female bodies—their own bodies—in terms of their political and professional liability. Finally, it examines how women physicians reacted to the paradoxical coincidence of the rise of the New Woman and her increased power, on the one hand, and the decline in the number and opportunities for women physicians, on the other.

In her book, *Sympathy and Science: Women Physicians in American Medicine,* Regina Morantz-Sanchez asks whether women physicians differed from their male counterparts either in their practice of medicine or their theoretical foundations. She concludes that, generally, women physicians' practice and opinions "reflected professional and scientific trends" rather than a gendered approach to medicine.[105] Morantz-Sanchez admits, however, that women physicians regarded menopause more positively than did male doctors.[106] The evidence suggests that, indeed, the dominant medical models for understanding and treating menopause and the strategies championed by women physicians generally overlapped. Despite the widespread agreement, however, women physicians differed, albeit subtly, from their male counterparts on several interpretations of menopause. Paying special attention to the nuances of language highlights differing agendas between male and female physicians, even when agreement existed on the surface.

Twenty of the roughly two hundred physicians writing about menopause between 1897 and 1937 were women. Fifteen of these women physicians practiced "regular" medicine while the five others professed sectarian allegiances. Like their male counterparts, some of the women physicians wrote primarily for a medical audience while others focused on a lay readership. Seventy-five percent of the women were definitely over forty at the time they wrote about menopause, and given their graduation dates from medical school, this percentage may be as high as 90 percent. Perhaps their personal experiences as menopausal women or eventual menopausal women led these physicians to help shape the popular and medical representations of menopause.

Along with personal concerns, the professional interests of women physicians also contributed to their assessment of menopause. Women physicians increased in number and influence during the second half of the nineteenth century, peaking in the first decade of the twentieth century. In some cities, such as Boston and Minneapolis, women comprised almost 20 percent of the physicians in 1900. By 1910, there were more than nine thousand women physicians practicing in the United States, representing 6 percent of all physicians. During the same period, women remained virtually absent in the other professions. In 1905, for example, there were only two hundred women lawyers in the entire country. Despite their strong beginning, however, the bright promise of women physicians remained largely unfulfilled. Once trained, for example, female physicians found they had few places to go. In 1921, only 8 percent of hospitals awarded internships to women. By 1905, all but three of the women's medical colleges had closed, and the opportunities for coeducation had decreased; in 1905, only 4 percent of all medical school graduates were women, falling below 3 percent by 1915. As a result, between 1910 and 1920, the number of women physicians fell, both in absolute numbers and as a percentage of the whole. After 1920, the percentage of women in the profession did not reach 5 percent again until 1950.[107] This decline in the prospects for women physicians provides a backdrop for understanding the professional stakes involved in women physicians' judgments of menopause.

As their prospects began to slip away, women physicians faced continued arguments against female education. Toward the end of the nineteenth century, when increasing numbers of women entered medical schools, a few influential male physicians argued that education, to say nothing of medical school, endangered women's health. The argument generally maintained that mental exertion taxed the energies that young women needed for the proper development of their reproductive functions. By the twentieth century, the prevalence of these arguments had decreased, but they had not disappeared. Eminent psychologist G. Stanley Hall, for example, claimed in 1903 that "the first danger to woman is over-brainwork. It affects that part of her organism which is sacred to heredity."[108] In 1905, physician John Upshur likewise decried increased education for girls and women because it funnels critical "nervous stimulus" away from their physical development. As a result, he claimed, an educated woman "leaves school, highly cultured, but a physical wreck," "unfitted" for motherhood and vulnerable to the trials of menopause.[109] The persistence of these arguments reminded women physicians that their biology continued to threaten their professional advancement.[110]

In the early twentieth century, medical language about menopause expressed cultural norms regarding older women, generally portraying the aging female body as a mere shell of its former self, no longer able to fulfill its function either as a sexual partner or as a reproductive vessel. Typically, male physicians described menopause as a "senile degeneration of the sexual organs," a process in which the ovaries and external genitalia "shrink" and "shrivel." One physician maintained that "the uterus atrophies until it is a mere hard remnant," and another noted that the breasts and vulva "degenerate." Physicians commonly contrasted menopause with puberty, during which life's potential bursts forth with all its promise. While puberty represents possibilities, both biological and social, menopause represents the "negative phase of a positive sexual wave."[111] Gynecologist William J. Robinson, in his 1925 book *The Menopause or Change of Life,* described menopause as "a period of withering, shrinking and closing-up," in which the vagina, particularly in "old maids" becomes so narrow that it makes intercourse painful or impossible. In addition, he noted that the "pubis looks moth-eaten," and that "the breasts begin to shrink and wither, hang[ing] down like two empty sacs." Not only did the ovaries atrophy, according to many male doctors, they also began to "dysfunction." An author of an influential gynecology textbook, for example, described menopause as "the exhaustion of the primordial follicles in the ovary," causing the "internal secretion of the ovaries [to] fail."[112]

It might be argued that menopause is indeed a period of decay and that these doctors were not describing women's loss of appeal and usefulness but rather the biological facts. To challenge this argument, the descriptions of female physicians are helpful. Admittedly, a few women physicians, particularly those writing at the beginning of the century, did describe menopause as "degeneration" and regression.[113] Sara E. Greenfield, for example, claimed that in menopause "the genital organs are assuming for the second time the infantile form."[114] But by the end of the first decade of the twentieth century, as the future of women physicians was beginning to appear less secure, some women physicians used language less overtly negative. Surgeon Mary Rushmore noted in her 1911 *Woman's Medical Journal* article that the "ovaries and the uterus become quite small." Rather than highlight the failure of the reproductive organs, she claimed that at menopause they "gradually cease."[115] Similarly, physician Edith Lowry described in 1919 the "changes" in the genital organs and the "suppression" of the internal secretions. In her description, the organs shrank; they did not shrivel.[116]

While male physicians generally focused on the inability of menopausal women's reproductive organs to fulfill their generative function, leaving the women both physiologically and symbolically barren, women physicians characterized the physiological process as transformative rather than degenerative. Male physicians emphasized menopause as a decline, but women physicians stressed instead the "readjustment" of the body to another, equally productive—if not reproductive—phase. These subtle differences in language suggest an attempt by those whose bodies would presumably undergo menopause to cast its progression in less negative terms.

Male and female physicians similarly diverged subtly on the significance of menopause for women. In downgrading menopause from critical to serious, women physicians swam with the tide of medical consensus. But the tone women physicians employed denotes a general impatience with the idea of considering female bodies particularly volatile. Homeopathic physician Emma Drake, for example, denied an earlier characterization that menopause involved "coming to a terrible Rubicon through which if we are enabled to pass without being engulfed, or at least physically exhausted, we are indeed to be congratulated."[117] In contrast, she maintained, menopause should have no more pronounced effect upon well women than the change from childhood to puberty. Physician Clelia Mosher, trained at Johns Hopkins, was outraged by gloomy characterizations of menopause and maintained that sexism colored some physicians' views. She noted that "it is interesting to know such statements are made nowadays almost exclusively by the old time chivalrous type of man who believes woman inferior mentally as well as physically, and who . . . labels woman as tolled off by a divine Providence for reproductive purposes only."[118] Mosher shared with other women physicians an awareness that male characterizations of female bodies could emerge from and contribute to political discussions of women's role in society. By rebutting negative appraisals of menopause, Mosher and other women physicians engaged in both the medical and the political debate about the nature of women's bodies.

Women and men physicians also differed in their perceptions of the physicians' role in menopause. The nautical metaphors that fill the literature are particularly helpful for understanding how physicians envisioned their relationship to menopausal patients. In a common scenario, the family doctor serves as pilot, guiding the menopausal woman through the storm. A male general practitioner in 1902, for example, phrased the relationship this way: "Like the skillful pilot who guides his craft over the rocks of a dangerous sea, so must the conscientious, scientific doctor safely direct the woman over the stormy and perilous ocean—The Menopause." Another male physician believed that doctors "chart the channel and plant the danger signals that the ship may pass in safety."[119]

Women physicians also employed nautical metaphors, but they interpreted the role of the physician differently. While many women doctors downplayed the role of the physician in menopause altogether,[120] others offered an alternative vision. Lowry, for example, argued that while women steered their own ships, physicians could provide valuable aid. "If a person were to cross a deep lake and had any doubts regarding the worthiness of the vessel provided, she would be very foolish if she did not have a trained boat-repairer examine the vessel and correct any weak places. It is just as important for the woman about to cross this period of her life to go to a trained repairer of bodies (a physician) and have him correct any weak places."[121]

While male physicians tended to see doctors at the helm, navigating through troubled waters, women physicians relegated their own profession to an important but undeniably supporting role as compared to the menopausal woman herself. In less metaphoric terms, whereas male physicians generally urged all women to visit their doctors as a matter of course, women physicians more frequently advised medical attention only if abnormal symptoms occurred.[122]

Physicians admitted that even women in good health might experience discomforting symptoms, both mental and physical. Women physicians, consistent with their view of women as pilots of their own ships, urged women to avoid blowing these symptoms out of proportion. They insisted that "suffering or its absence is . . . within their own control." With this in mind, Drake claimed that a woman's best defense was to "establish a habit of looking on the bright side." Others encouraged any woman approaching menopause to "hold oneself well in hand," claiming that the body should be "dominated by the intellect." Rushmore maintained in 1911 that the "way to escape the annoyances of this period . . . was to have trained the nerves from childhood to self-control and quietness." Anna Galbraith took the message of self-control further by claiming that "if the majority of women suffer, it is very often their own fault."[123] By challenging the notion that women were at the mercy of their bodies, these female physicians found themselves blaming women for their own misery.

Contrast this message of self-control and responsibility with the advice of male physicians. While they agreed that apprehension of menopause could exacerbate symptoms, male physicians believed that medical advice and reassurance, rather than female control, would ease the difficulties. Indeed, many male physicians maintained that women should not be held accountable for their behaviors because their actions were not within their control. Gynecologist James King, for example, recommended that "man should . . . view with kindly forbearance the futile effort of woman to overcome by her will the very powers that shape and control her mental processes." Sociologist Groves, echoing the position of many male physicians, maintained that women's symptoms during menopause "are no more to be thought of as faults or failures of self-control than is seasickness during a channel passage."[124]

These differences reflect the contrasting social positions between male and female physicians. As women, female physicians confronted arguments claiming that their own bodies made them unfit for certain jobs. As women physicians, they saw their position within the medical profession dissolving, both in terms of absolute numbers and in terms of professional opportunities. As aging women, they rejected the notion that their usefulness was behind them. Drawing their opinions about menopause from all of these identities, they rejected the image of the emotionally fragile woman controlled by her biology. Women doctors urged self-control as a way of testifying that women's psyches were more powerful than their physiology.

To help women cope with menopause, female physicians emphasized the importance of preparing for postmenopausal life by actively pursuing interests outside the home. "Mothers as a rule are too unselfish" and too devoted to their homes and children, claimed Drake in 1902. She therefore urged these women to cultivate outside interests.[125] Other women physicians claimed that women who "put all [their] eggs in one basket" stumbled at menopause, unable to make a smooth transition to life without small children and domestic demands.[126] These women physicians justified their advice by claiming that professional women suffered very little at menopause.[127] Stanford physician Martha Dyment, for example, maintained that women needed only "good hygiene and an absorbing occupation" to live through menopause unscathed.[128] Acknowledging the value of life beyond the domestic sphere, another woman physician claimed, bucking the general medical trend, that perhaps single women fared better after menopause than did wives and mothers, because they had never become preoccupied with home and family.[129]

Although women physicians celebrated the achievements won by the New Woman, they argued that society must continue to increase the social and political opportunities for women. While admitting the advances women had made, Lowry nevertheless argued that older women remained America's most "shamefully wasted" natural resource.[130] To rectify the situation, Galbraith demanded that the disturbances of menopause "must cause serious consideration of the physiologic necessity for a definite occupation for the daughters as well as for the sons of the rich."[131] Mosher argued that "equal suffrage, like many of the economic and philanthropic opportunities now open to women," would help middle-aged women cope with the changes of menopause. She noted that too often women arrived at menopause without intellectual or social interests. Women's suffrage, she argued, would bring civic concerns into the home for discussion by "mother and daughters as well as the father and sons." This created a "passive interest in politics" that would continue until a woman's family responsibilities subsided. As a result, she concluded, "'votes for women' becomes not only a safeguard to the woman of middle age, a help in preserving the integrity of the family, but a protection to the community from the menace of the unoccupied middle aged woman. It becomes economically an asset in the productive use of the force and intelligence otherwise wasted in doctor's bills, sanatorium treatment, or too often expended in dangerous fads."[132]

These women physicians explicitly connected the physical and mental symptoms of menopause with the social and political opportunities for women. They maintained that as long as women were most valued for their roles as wives and mothers their lives after the daily domestic demands ceased would be filled with mental and physical complaints. Women physicians were not the only doctors who applauded women's newly won achievements, but they stood apart from male medical writers in demanding further advancements as a way to prevent menopausal discomforts.[133]

Women physicians' rejection of the most negative descriptions of menopause and their insistence that women could and should control their reactions to the physical and emotional upheavals of menopause indicates their concern that female bodies could be wielded as a weapon to thwart women's aspirations. This consciousness led women physicians to revise the most egregious portrayals of menopause. They urged women to prevent their bodies from being used against them by using their minds to "steer their bodily course."[134] But they insisted that increased political and professional opportunities were likewise needed to assure women of a comfortable passage through menopause.

All in all, the medical assessment of menopause between 1897 and 1937 suggested that physicians worried little about the biological consequences of menopause and that its sequelae posed few problems to most women. When we examine physicians' concerns about the psychological impact of menopause, however, a significantly darker image emerges.

TWO

"Endocrine Perverts" and "Derailed Menopausics"

Gender Transgressions and Mental Disturbances, 1897–1937

In 1918, health and fitness crusader Bernarr MacFadden noted that menopausal women experience a pervasive "instability of the nerves." He added that these women are "apt to lose their power of judgment and their power to think clearly; they become restless, hesitating, indecisive, moody and depressed. They sleep badly, are troubled with distressing dreams and may evidence fear that they are going insane."[1] Earlier in the century, a physician described the same phenomena more succinctly: at menopause, he said, "everything is changed, the woman is not herself."[2]

As physicians came to explore the nature of menopause and the experience of menopausal women, nervous and emotional symptoms attracted intense scrutiny. The nature of these symptoms varied, but they were often described by the catch-word "nervousness." They included depression, irritability, fatigue, anxiety, hysteria, melancholy, and despondency. In rare cases, "nervousness" gave way to more profound mental disorders, such as involutional melancholia, dementia, and psychosis.[3] These afflictions differed in severity rather than kind; irritability might progress into psychosis, moodiness into melancholia. Most physicians claimed, however, that the only women who became truly insane at menopause were those with a previously established neurotic constitution; worry about insanity, however, might itself lead to emotional distress.

As described in Chapter 1, when doctors addressed the physiological transition of menopause, they often heralded women's increased social opportunities, responding in part to the efforts of the New Woman. Many physicians writing about mental difficulties, however, revealed an underly-

40

ing anxiety about women's changing social role. Significantly, the same physicians welcomed women's enlarged cultural niche while worrying about its cost to women, womanhood, and the larger social fabric. Although this contrast may appear paradoxical, it coincides with early twentieth-century expectations of women. As long as middle-aged women remained sufficiently feminine, doctors encouraged them to enter public life. But as soon as women's menopausal symptoms presented behaviors that challenged normative gender roles, many physicians warned against crossing social boundaries.

The doctors considering the nervous symptoms of menopause included many of the same gynecologists, endocrinologists, and general practitioners who were concerned with the physical symptoms. They were joined, however, by a new set of contributors: neurologists, psychiatrists, and alienists. Their unique client base and interpretive models gave them a slightly different perspective on menopause. Their perspective, concerned particularly with pathology and informed by psychoanalysis, became more central to the discussion of mental symptoms over the course of the period.

Historians have employed several models to understand the relationship among physicians, women, and mental difficulties. Some have argued that the diagnosis and treatment of mental instability in women provided male physicians with an opportunity to control and victimize their "helpless" women patients.[4] In contrast, other historians have claimed that women gained power, albeit limited, through their mental illness, arguing that mental illness provided women a "voice" when they were otherwise silent.[5] More recently, Elizabeth Lunbeck and Nancy M. Theriot have shown how debates among health and welfare professionals and female patients and their families together shaped the fractured and contentious discussion of women and mental illness.[6]

In order to understand the mental aspects of menopause and their treatment in this period, we must appreciate how deeply social changes in the role of women influenced physicians' thoughts about their menopausal patients. Medical perceptions of women's mental and emotional changes at menopause reflected prevailing cultural standards of femininity and social expectations of women, and the medical views of menopause changed in relation to social and political events affecting women's lives.

The connection between the mental symptoms of menopause and the changing social visibility of women, especially middle-aged women, is seen in both the "risk profile" of the mentally disturbed patient and in the content of the mental symptoms themselves. Neither the risk profile nor the diagnostic behaviors remained stable between 1897 and 1937. Before 1920, delicate, middle- and upper-class women were identified as especially prone to menopausal instability. After about 1920, physicians warned that women who challenged gender prescriptions—in particular, single, "masculine," and "sexually aberrant" women—were most prone to emotional problems at menopause. A similar shift occurred with regard to the symptoms of mental perturbation. Only after 1920 or so did physicians regard "masculine" and "hypersexual" behaviors as *evidence* of mental instability. Selfishness, however, marked the menopausal woman throughout this period.

The overlap between the presenting symptoms of menopausal disorder and the risk profile for menopausal imbalance is striking, raising the chicken-egg dilemma: were menopausal mental difficulties caused by the rebellion against gender constraints, or was the rebellion itself evidence of mental difficulties? For the physicians and other health writers who explored the mental effects of menopause, this was not a problem. They were able to separate—in theory—behaviors that put women at risk for mental disorders from the mental disturbances themselves. In reality, however, physicians often blurred the distinction.

The Mind-Body Connection

By the beginning of the twentieth century, physicians writing on menopause attributed mental disorders to changes within women's bodies. Two competing models provided scientific justification for linking female reproduction and mental instability. Some physicians relied on the concept of reflex sympathy or arc, developed by British neurologist Marshall Hall in 1847 and popularized by William James in the 1890s.[7] Imagined much like a telegraph wire, the reflex arc explained how a defect or disease in one part of the body led to symptoms and disease in quite another. In the case of women, the reflex arc typically connected diseased reproductive organs to other parts of their bodies, but most importantly, to their brains. As a result, a diseased (or declining) ovary could easily result in a disordered, unstable mind. Anna Galbraith, fellow of the New York Academy of Medicine, for example, invoked reflex sympathy when she attributed mental disorders to women's reproductive organs, in an example typical of this model. Galbraith claimed in 1904 that the "strong reaction of the sexual organs on the central ganglia is the principal cause of mental disease . . . sometimes sufficiently severe to lead to insanity and suicide." She also claimed that the menopausal upheaval of the reproductive system might cause "permanent derangement of the mental and moral faculties."[8]

Although the concept of reflex sympathy endured into the twentieth century, by the late 1800s it was already competing with an endocrinological model. Indeed, a few physicians explicitly saw hormonal explanations for the nervous symptoms of menopause as a substitute for the "doctrine of 'reflex nervous disorders.'" By the 1920s, reflex theory had virtually disappeared from the discussion of menopause, but some physicians warned against replacing one all-encompassing model with another, fearing that hormones had become a modern incarnation of the reflex theory.[9]

Physicians accepted the hormonal model for understanding menopausal symptoms partly because it provided a possible treatment. By the turn of the century, physicians debated the importance of ovarian secretions in causing menopause and their efficacy in relieving symptoms (see Chapter 1).[10] Initially claiming that ovarian secretions were primarily successful in treating hot flashes and genital atrophy, by 1930 some physicians were recommending these secretions (with a great deal of debate) as a treatment for the mental symptoms of menopause.[11]

Not all explanations for the mental effects of menopause, however, rose from physiological causes. Indeed, physicians also worried that apprehensive women might create their own mental and emotional problems. Psychiatrist Mary O'Malley, for example, claimed in 1925 that "many of the nervous and mental symptoms" could be avoided by "proper instruction on what to expect."[12] Stanford University physician Clelia Duel Mosher agreed, noting that the typical woman looks forward to menopause "with dread, expecting to be incapacitated or perhaps insane. Thus her own nervous anticipation tends to increase whatever incapacity she may have to suffer."[13]

Finally, many physicians acknowledged that social factors affected women's emotional state at menopause. These doctors acknowledged that menopause coincided with many possible personal and familial changes. These events could include the death of a husband, a child's wedding, a family break-up, or a financial loss. Such events could precipitate a depression or a psychotic episode in a susceptible person.[14]

The Fragile Wife and the Mannish Spinster

Between 1897 and roughly 1920, physicians generally believed that most women who suffered from mental breakdowns at menopause had preexisting nervous constitutions.[15] Not surprisingly, this assessment was linked to social status. Medical practitioners identified paragons of middle- and upper-class femininity by their delicate, unstable nerves and their fragile constitutions, maintaining that these women suffered more from mental disorders during the menopause "than their less fortunate sisters" because of their "more sensitively organized nervous system."[16] In addition to fragile nerves, physicians blamed indulgent lifestyles that encouraged self-absorption rather than useful work. They claimed that poor women were too busy "eking out a living at service, at the washtub, in the factory, or on the farm" to suffer from nervous prostration.[17] One physician claimed that the only women who suffered from nervous ailments at menopause were those with the "time and leisure to think about them, and that relatively few are seen in the dispensaries."[18] In addition to delicate women, physicians maintained that married women were more prone to nervous difficulties at menopause than their single counterparts. Doctors explained this, in part, by claiming that married women's nerves were exhausted from the burdens of childbearing and child rearing.[19]

Before 1920, then, many physicians claimed that the women who best fit the feminine ideal—delicate, fragile women who were also wives and mothers—were most prone to suffer nervous disorders. After about 1920, however, the profile of those women whom physicians considered most vulnerable to mental difficulties began to change. Although class-based characterizations did not entirely disappear,[20] physicians became increasingly concerned with three overlapping categories of women at risk: they saw single, sexually aberrant, and masculine women as most vulnerable to mental tribulation.

In the beginning of the century, physicians acknowledged that bearing and raising a large family might fatigue women's emotional and mental control. Gradually, however, single women emerged as the women most at risk for nervous disorders. In 1918, for example, Illinois alienists Frank Norbury and Albert Dollear admitted that while menopausal insanity more frequently attacked married women, "widows and single women who have been active in business or professional life are quite prone to this disorder."[21] By the early 1920s, medical opinion coalesced around the notion that unmarried and childless women were more likely to suffer.[22] In 1923, physician and birth-control advocate William Robinson, for example, presented five case studies representing the spectrum of menopausal symptoms. The first three cases, portraying the least severe symptoms, were married women. He chose two single women to depict the most severe manifestations of menopausal mental disturbance. Of these two women, one became "melancholic" and committed suicide, and the other became "intensely erotic" and "violently insane" and was committed to an asylum.[23] Other physicians more explicitly claimed that single women, because they had been unable to fulfill women's highest calling, suffered more acutely from mental turmoil. In 1934, alienist Norbury remarked "How different is the mental outlook for the normal reproductive mother with her children than the barren wife or the barren spinster, when they approach or enter the menopause. To them, age with its declining possibilities for motherhood as a fulfillment of woman's destiny, becomes the source of constant irritation at her social-psychological level."[24]

Physicians did not, however, doom all single women to mental torment at menopause. Although gynecologist Robinson cataloged in 1923 the various special dangers unmarried women faced at menopause, he also offered them a slim ray of hope. He acknowledged that some unmarried women could move through menopause without mental turmoil, but the price of "serenity" was high. He described the case of a "highly cultured and educated virgin of forty-five." She sailed placidly through menopause because her "femininity never meant anything to her . . . and now she put her sex life beyond an iron door and threw away the key."[25] Robinson indicated that women must choose between careers and sexual fulfillment. Single women became threatening only when they insisted on sexual activities without marriage.

In addition to single women, physicians often believed that women with aberrant or inadequate sexualities appeared vulnerable to mental difficulties during menopause. Indeed, physicians frequently maintained that sexual difficulties constituted the core of most mental problems. One form of sexual inadequacy was "immature sexuality," which included the inability to connect sexually with men. In a 1932 study of four women whom they considered representative of mental problems in the menopause, New York psychiatrists Gerald Jameison and James Wall considered two of the women to be sexually frigid, a third to be lacking in "fully developed . . . adult sexuality," and the fourth "never reached a heterosexual level."[26] Neurologist W. A. Jones employed similar language to describe one of his "nervous" patients. Because she was childless ("as so many of these women are,") Jones concluded that she was also "sexually unfit or sexually unprepared, or sexually asleep. She does not believe in the sexual life and does not want any one else to believe in it. She is a selfish old thing."[27] Although these physicians avoided blaming their patients' mental illnesses exclusively on their sexual histories, they believed sexual maladjustment contributed to their mental difficulties.

In addition to single and sexually abnormal women, physicians often warned that "masculine" women, who deviated from gender expectations in both appearance and behavior, were similarly vulnerable to mental disorders. The authors of a 1931 study of psychosis at menopause, for example, claimed that women of an athletic or "robust" build or those "showing conspicuous intersexual traits" were more likely to suffer from psychosis at menopause.[28] Psychiatrist A. B. Brill claimed that women who "found it hard to give up masculinity" weathered adolescence least well. He maintained that these women "did not wish to become women; they really wanted to be men. At menopause the same conflict again comes up. The desire to be a man is revived, but it is thwarted by the cognition of its futility."[29]

Political Women at Risk

Why this shift of concern from appropriately gendered women to gender transgressive women? The image of the aging masculine woman reflected a more widespread anxiety that developed in the late teens and 1920s about the masculinizing of American women. This concern emerged from several related trends. First, the theories of Sigmund Freud were gaining a following in the United States psychiatric community in the late 1910s. Freud's American followers (and the more casually affiliated dabblers) engaged with Freud's theories of sexuality and psychosexual development (or at least with the language of those theories) because they explained a wide variety of behaviors and provided an idiom with which to articulate widespread social anxieties.[30]

Second, by 1920, physicians and other social commentators suggested that the nation was on the brink of a "marriage crisis," sparked in part by the behaviors of the so-called "New Woman." By this time, the vocational, matrimonial, and reproductive choices of the New Woman had been the subject of sustained and critical discussion in the popular, scientific, and medical literature. In particular, these women's disregard for marriage, coupled with the general society's rising divorce rate (the divorce rate doubled between 1900 and 1920), led many to fear for the future of marriage as traditionally conceived.[31]

To avert social disaster and to accommodate women's increased access to economic opportunity and birth control, social commentators reconsidered the basis for marriage. Recognizing the changes in middle- and upper-class women's lives, there emerged the "companionate marriage," promoting a partnership between husband and wife based on friendship and sexual intimacy. Indeed, nonprocreative sex served as the centerpiece of the newly imagined marriages, which acknowledged female passion and promoted sex for pleasure rather than reproduction. In addition, the companionate marriage supported women's interests outside the home. This more egalitarian model of marriage left women with little rationale for avoiding matrimony; indeed, during the 1920s, marriage rates for college-educated women increasingly reflected those of the rest of society.[32]

The companionate marriage, while validating women's sexual passion within the confines of marriage, did not similarly relax sanctions against sexual relations outside of wedlock. Instead, it more narrowly defined women's acceptable sexual expression by intensifying pressure on women both to relate sexually to men and to confine sexual behavior to marriage. As a result, abnormal sexuality came to include frigidity, sexual relations between women, and all sexual relationships outside of marriage. Significantly, single women could fall into any or all of these categories, and physicians increasingly worried that they would.[33]

Disapproval of women's increasing presence in public life in the years leading up to 1920 provides a third explanation for the medical attention to the mental hazards of gender transgression. In the beginning decades of the twentieth century, some middle- and upper-class women marshaled their allegedly "domestic" skills for the social good by working with settlement houses, women's clubs, and labor unions. In addition, some of these women demanded a place within government. The creation in 1912 of the Children's Bureau, established within the federal bureaucracy to look after the health and welfare of women and children, reflects the increasing success and visibility of their efforts.

But not everyone was comfortable with women's increasing presence in political life. Discomfort with this "politicized domesticity" culminated in the debates surrounding the Sheppard-Towner Maternity and Infancy Protection Act during the period 1918 to 1921. These debates provide a snapshot of the anxieties many physicians felt when they confronted powerful, single, middle-aged women working to shape public policy.[34]

The Sheppard-Towner Act addressed the high infant and maternal mortality rates plaguing the nation in the 1910s by providing federal matching funds to states willing to develop programs to combat the problem. It funded prenatal and child health clinics, visiting nurse programs, midwife training, and general health education programs. Promoting the "welfare and hygiene of maternity and infancy,"[35] the act mobilized American women like no other issue except suffrage.[36] Sheppard-Towner received broad-based support, garnering patronage from diverse groups such as the Daughters of the American Revolution, the League of Women Voters, and the National Association of Colored Women.[37] Designed by Children's Bureau Chief, Julia Lathrop, the campaign for Sheppard-Towner was visibly—and threateningly—led by single women of roughly menopausal or postmenopausal age.[38]

Opponents of the controversial act resisted the increased government involvement in domestic affairs, claiming that it smacked of Communism. Many physicians, in particular, viewed Sheppard-Towner as a government takeover of responsibilities rightly belonging to private practioners. They also maintained that unmarried, childless women should not create policy about motherhood. Motherhood, these physicians argued, was both instinctive and natural, not something childless women could teach. In an attempt to defeat the legislation by discrediting its proponents, an *Illinois Medical Journal* editorial characterized these "spinsters" as "endocrine perverts" and "derailed menopausics."[39] These unstable, "mannish," indeed unnatural, women could not be trusted to create social policy.[40]

The example of Sheppard-Towner is telling for two reasons. The epithets wielded to discredit its middle-aged supporters referred to the characteristics—unmarried, sexually aberrant, and masculine—that physicians warned made women vulnerable to mental instability. (*Sexually aberrant* and *masculine* also described, in part, the symptoms of mental disorder at menopause.) In addition, the rhetoric surrounding Sheppard-Towner explicitly maps onto women's bodies physicians' concerns about these women's newly won independence and power. The changes in women's lives highlighted by the concept of the New Woman along with her right to vote and her increased influence in political affairs influenced medical opinions about middle-aged women. In the example of Sheppard-Towner, physicians deployed these medical assessments to undercut women's public aspirations. Even when the physicians' intentions were less transparent, the medical literature often warned women of the dangers of transgressing the traditional feminine role.

The campaign for women's suffrage, gaining momentum throughout the century and capturing victory in 1920, supplies another explanation for the changed risk profile for menopausal instability. Suffrage obviously gave women the vote, legitimizing their participation in the public sphere, but it also provided a visible marker of middle-class women's increasing presence beyond the home. In response to the suffrage movement, some physicians and other commentators expressed concern about the deleterious effects of suffrage on women and womanhood.

The campaign for suffrage raised concerns in particular that women were losing their femininity. One physician wondered, for example, whether "modern life, with its double burden upon the woman," had transformed normal women into "flat-chested, bony-jawed, hair-bobbed and hair faced women" who looked and behaved like men.[41] Other commentators expressed unease about how these developments might affect American families. One physician and lecturer on sexual matters, for example, worried that women's rights might diminish the "primitive sex instinct" that attracts the sexes to each other, thus discouraging marriage. To ensure the stability of society, he claimed that man must remain a "strong, virile, forceful provider and defender, and woman a quiet, conservative home maker and willing bearer of offspring."[42]

One of the most virulent condemnations of the "woman movement" and of the women who led it came from physiology professor William Sedgwick. In an article on the biological fallacy of the feminist movement, Sedgwick cited menopause as evidence that women were physiologically unstable. He also challenged the womanhood of feminists.

> It is not surprising that it seems to be these very masculine women, these mistakes of nature, aided and abetted by their counterparts, the feminine men, who are largely responsible for the feminist movement. . . . But what is surprising . . . is that these "half-women" should achieve a certain leadership over many normal women, women who have all the instinctive, ineradicable feelings of wifehood and motherhood. [43]

These warnings about the masculinizing effects of increased social and political power only occasionally came from the same physicians who warned about mental instability at menopause. But by similarly highlighting the risks of rejecting traditional feminine values, physicians participated in the larger cultural discussion about women's proper place.

Diagnosing Mental Disturbance

Gender expectations did not only affect the development of a risk profile for menopausal patients; they also influenced how physicians interpreted mental and emotional distress during menopause. In particular, descriptions of menopausal nervous difficulties highlight the centrality of gendered expectations of female sexuality and domestic behavior. Physicians' descriptions of the mental symptoms of menopause are telling on two fronts. They indicate that some women keenly experienced the symbolic significance of menopause and viewed it as a moment for considering their futures and their pasts. Further, physicians' descriptions of emotional imbalance illustrate the effect of gender roles on their determinations of the mental health or illness of their patients. In particular, physicians concluded they had an emotionally disturbed woman on their hands if the patient exhibited what they deemed masculine tendencies, aberrant sexualities, or selfish behaviors. The first two of these became symptoms of mental disorder at the same time they became part of the risk profile; physicians associated mental disturbance with selfishness throughout this period.

Bearded Ladies and Betting Women

Physicians between 1897 and 1937 described menopause as a masculinizing process, leaving women, if not more male, certainly less female. Sylvanus Stall claimed in 1901 that menopause made women more physically masculine in the contours of the body and the distribution of hair. Indeed, he claimed that the hair on menopausal women's faces grew so thick that it "somewhat resembles the beard of a man."[44] This interpretation was clearly connected to the notion that hormones endowed bodies with both masculinity and femininity.[45] According to endocrinologist Samuel Bandler, the "internal secretions" were responsible for the physical differences between men and women and also the "differences in tastes and emotions."[46] After about 1918, physicians continued to note the physical masculinizing effects of menopause, but they also claimed that menopause changed women's psyches toward things masculine. Internist George Richter, for example, noted in 1917 that at menopause, "the secondary signs of femininity wither, the voice deepens, the psyche tends towards the interests of man which, in some instances, may be the cause of divorces after several decades of married life."[47] Prosser Picot noted with some alarm that a menopausal woman might "assume an aggressiveness that she had never previously possessed."[48]

Although they always viewed the masculinizing psychic effects of menopause as undesirable, physicians did not always claim that masculine behaviors indicated mental disorder. Occasionally, however, physicians explicitly linked masculine behavior and disordered mental states. James Segall, for example, claimed in 1934 that at menopause "women lose much of the particular quality that gave them their general characteristic of femaleness, and serves to bring about definite changes in the glandular makeup, reflected in the physical, and more particularly in the nervous system, and constitute problems that press for solution upon hundreds of thousands of our people. And yet which frequently respond to proper psychological and endocrine treatments."[49] In other words, the withdrawal of the feminine hormones created nervous symptoms that needed psychological or hormonal treatment. New York psychiatrists Jameison and Wall described one of their mentally disturbed patients, who acted like "the man of the house," betting on the horses and playing poker. One indication of her recovery was her return to a more nurturing role when her husband suffered a stroke.[50] These explicit connections invite speculation that physicians more generally believed that masculine tendencies were not merely an inevitable effect of menopause but rather a pathological symptom of mental disorder.

Scheming Seductresses

Before 1920, many commentators noted the effect menopause had upon a woman's sexual desire. Indeed, many physicians, particularly those favoring sexual continence, a movement already losing favor by the beginning of the twentieth century, claimed that at menopause a woman lost all her sexual desire.[51] Because these physicians believed that women naturally lost their libido at menopause, they similarly warned women that it might be dangerous to indulge in sexual intercourse during this period.[52] William Walling warned married couples in 1904 to refrain from frequent intercourse after menopause "no less for her own sake than that of her husband." Walling reminded his readers of the "medical maxim" that "every time [a man] delivers himself to this indulgence he casts a shovelful of earth upon his coffin."[53] Other physicians assured women that they could continue to enjoy a fulfilling sexual life—perhaps more fulfilling because the fear of unwanted pregnancy had disappeared.[54] A few physicians admitted, however, that some women may experience an increased libido. While some physicians worried about this increase—such as the doctor who warned that a menopausal woman might solicit lovers "to satisfy her amativeness"[55]—elevated sexual drive was not generally considered a sign of mental imbalance. Indeed, an increased libido, when it was a problem at all, was considered a *physical* not a *psychological* problem.[56]

After 1920, the belief that a woman's sexuality continued after menopause gained greater currency among physicians.[57] At the same time, however, physicians linked a wide variety of psychological problems to an aberrant sexuality, a catch-all phrase that included frigidity, promiscuity, and lewd fantasies. Underscoring this point, endocrinologist Edward Podolsky commented in 1934 on "the close relationship that exists between sexual maladjustment and nervousness." He and other physicians agreed that "most of the nervous ailments of women are to a large degree due to frustration of normal sexual desire."[58] These physicians obviously relied on Freud for the theoretical connection between sex and mental problems. It was only around 1920, however, that physicians deployed Freudian theory so intensely against menopausal women, because only then did Freud's ideas resonate with larger cultural anxieties in the United States.

Although physicians warned women throughout this period about gratifying an abnormally strong libido, after 1920 the number of physicians offering warnings increased, and the possible consequences they cited grew more dire. In his 1923 book, *The Menopause or Change of Life; Its Dangers and Disorders, Their Prevention and Treatment,* gynecologist, sex educator, and birth-control advocate William Robinson, presented a series of case studies of menopausal women and their "bizarre" behaviors. His work combined sketches of women who suffered from mental conditions with descriptions of their behaviors. Highly sexualized behaviors among menopausal women figured prominently. Robinson insisted, for example, that incidences of increased desire at menopause should be carefully guarded against because "coitus is a flame that feeds upon what it consumes." In "abnormal" cases, he maintained, the situation was even more severe, and "sexual relations must be unequivocally forbidden," because the path to nymphomania was easily encountered.[59] Endocrinologist Podolsky agreed, claiming in 1934 that an increase in desire should be "corrected at once in order to avoid later and more serious complications."[60] Another physician noted that some women suffer occasional "attacks" of increased libido leading them to marry younger men. He lamented the sad end to many of these cases. "The final outcome is jealousy and misery—In such cases, psychoanalysis will reveal important facts."[61]

Several types of sexual behaviors at menopause concerned physicians. An Oklahoma psychiatrist, for example, included among the symptoms of the "mental syndrome accompanying the menopause" insomnia, phobias, "self-pity," and "sexual impotency, frigidity, nymphomania and inversions."[62] Another physician noted that "erotomania may be the first sign of an unstable psychic balance and the patient may be doomed to a life of invalidism."[63] These physicians then linked a wide range of sexual behaviors to mental imbalance.

Physicians noticed with particular horror the promiscuous encounters that otherwise "normal" women might undertake at menopause. Because physicians began to regard sexual promiscuity as a sign of mental imbalance, and because menopausal women formed an identifiable group, their behaviors alarmed the community, earning the menopausal epoch the designation, "The Dangerous Age."[64] Joseph Tenenbaum vividly described the situation in 1929. "Menopausal women abandon right living for new unchartered roads of dangerous adventure. Stout believers of morality may suddenly become sex mad. The former church devotee may now turn out to be a devilish Bacchante."[65] Robinson painted a similar scene. He described a single woman whose "libido became so strong and uncontrollable that she became scandalously dissolute. At first she tried to conceal her transactions, but afterwards she threw all prudence to the winds, and rather advertised the fact that she was to be had by anybody who wanted her."[66]

In some cases, physicians focused not on promiscuous behaviors, but on promiscuous imaginings. In their 1932 study of "paranoid" menopausal women, G. H. Stevenson and S. R. Montgomery focused on the sexual adventures and fantasies of their patients. According to these physicians, a representative patient "eagerly . . . tells of the sexual outrages she has endured, of the sexual demands made upon her by her brute of a husband, of the many offers of marriage that she has had in the past few years, and of the many men who have desired to possess her."[67] Robinson also focused on the sexual fantasies of menopausal women. In a chapter dedicated to "menopause and the persecution of men," he claimed that "both priests and physicians are often annoyed and endangered by [the sexual fantasies] of unmarried women in the climacteric."[68] He outlined several cases where single women, overwhelmed by their sexual desires, imagined liaisons, suitors, and seductions. He offered as an example a description of a woman who accused her doctor of sexual assault. According to Robinson, "the woman had a coarse face; she looked slouchy and slovenly, fat and stodgy; she had no more of a waistline than a barrel."[69] To Robinson's relief, the judge dismissed the woman's case against the doctor, and she was sent to a private sanitarium. (Robinson didn't consider that her claim of harassment might have been true.)

While most physicians worried about promiscuity or fantasies of promiscuity, a few physicians claimed that menopausal women might also turn to other women for sexual gratification. Podolsky noted in 1934 that sexual "abnormality" was one of the "great dangers of the menopause" and that he "often sees in women, bored or unhappily married, a retrogression to homosexuality at or near menopause." He urged physicians to prevent women from "wandering off into strange sex channels" by teaching them to "sublimate their sexual desires" into creative ventures.[70] Robinson agreed that "cases in which conscious, hidden or marked homosexuality breaks forth openly and actively during the menopause are not infrequent."[71] Unlike Podolsky, however, Robinson did not regard this behavior as a particular problem.[72] This fairly bland reaction to lesbianism reinforces recent historical scholarship that argues that the medical profession was deeply divided over the nature and significance of homosexuality in the 1920s and 1930s. While some physicians continued to condemn homosexuality as an abomination and only a few physicians accepted homosexuality as a completely neutral category, many regarded homosexuality sympathetically.[73]

Physicians explained these wide-ranging aberrant behaviors in a number of ways. Physicians generally saw them as signs of a desperate and pitiful last grasp at motherhood, a "final flare of the dying generative flame."[74] This desire was thought to be most intense for single or childless women. According to Robinson, "old maids . . . are passionately eager to hold onto life, perhaps to capture or recapture some romance . . . before the candle finally goes out."[75] Sociologist Grace Loucks Elliott offered a similar interpretation in 1936. She claimed that a single woman's "fear of a closing door tends to urge her on to the kind of adventure, which may endanger other values she has spent her life in building up."[76]

Other physicians and psychiatrists blamed the sudden perverse behaviors on a lifetime of repression. Minnesota neurologist W. A. Jones's descriptions of psychotic menopausal patients "who suffer from . . . sexual perversion" are illustrative. He claimed that these women harbored unsatisfied but "normal instincts, . . . desires and longings." He maintained that when these women, "approach the climacteric, they throw discretion to the winds and permit themselves to emerge in butterfly costume and satisfy their long pent-up desires." Although it is unclear what made Jones define these women as pathological, he insisted that such cases were not uncommon because, he said, there were a "great many disappointed women in the world."[77]

Selfish Wives and Neglectful Mothers

Physicians' perceived connection among female masculinization, aberrant sexuality, and mental disturbances intensified around 1918 as debates over suffrage and the Sheppard-Towner Act escalated. Another manifestation of menopausal imbalance—selfishness—concerned physicians throughout this period. Mentally disturbed women, they believed, exhibited various selfish behaviors. In particular, physicians saw these women as self-centered, given to inappropriate introspection, careless in their domestic duties, and burdensome to their families. Consistent with this array of symptoms of selfishness, physicians had a ready solution: they encouraged women to resist dwelling on themselves.

Some physicians considered menopausal women's alleged self-centeredness as shocking. In 1900, for example, Lyman Sperry noted that at menopause, women's "thoughts center on themselves."[78] Later in the period, William Fielding noted that "there is a tendency at the change of life for the woman to become self-conscious and self-centered—that is, everything conceivable is considered as relating to herself, the pivotal center."[79] Jameison and Wall used a patient's own words to pass on the same judgment. After a psychotic episode, their patient described the experience as a "frightful condition of self-concentration and monumental selfishness."[80]

A few behaviors were not explicitly labeled selfish, but their characteristics can be read as a repudiation of selflessness. Physicians were alarmed by the stubborn, irritable, and querulous ways of menopausal patients. Physicians described these women variously as peevish, fretful, discontented, grumbling, and marked by "envy, ill-will, avarice . . . [and] restlessness."[81] Although physicians did not explicitly identify these behaviors as selfish, they attracted medical approbation from their colleagues by contrasting them sharply with such traditional female characteristics of selflessness as deference, compliance, and docility.

Physicians believed that self-absorption at menopause led women to reassess the value and significance of their lives. Psychiatrist Frank Norbury bemoaned in 1918 the self-pity that characterized several of his menopausal patients. To his dismay, he found middle-aged women taking as their credo, "I am deprived. I have had little out of life. I am a slave to my home and my family." The complaints of a minister's wife particularly disturbed him: "I am a slave to my husband's congregation, as well as to him and my family," she cried. "I will get nothing out of life except a place to sleep, something to eat." He notes that such women "sink into . . . repulsive egoism."[82] Other psychiatrists described a woman who complained that while her husband had remained young through his social and professional contacts, "she has aged raising her family and staying constantly at home. She compares herself to a worn out old horse, not receiving the respect and care due to such an animal."[83] These physicians believed that to express such dismay and dissatisfaction with the role of middle-class womanhood was in itself inappropriate and pathological. Moreover, these examples show that women viewed menopause as a catalyst for reconsidering their lives. Too often, perhaps, menopausal women discovered that a life spent sacrificing their own interests and ambitions to the needs of their families left them angry and disappointed when the demands of family waned.

In the detailed case descriptions provided by some physicians, the ability of menopausal women to perform domestic tasks indicated whether a woman had fallen ill and likewise whether she had regained her mental balance. Emma Drake, for example, claimed in 1902 that far too many menopausal women demonstrated the "neglect of family and the substitution of personal inattention for thoughtfulness, for neatness of appearance and for the exhibition of proper domestic concern."[84] In 1932, psychiatrists Karl Bowman and Lauretta Bender included an inability to keep house as a symptom of the neurosis of one of their patients. After treatment, the patient became "pleasant" and "agreeable." Further, "she never complained and kept things to herself. She stayed at home, was a good housekeeper and was extremely religious."[85] John Upshur also noted that after treatment the menopausal woman regained the ability and inclination to "confront the duties and responsibilities of domestic life and to find joy and comfort indescribable in administering to the comfort or contributing to the happiness of those around her."[86] The concern about domesticity dramatically illustrates the connection between a diagnosis of mental problems and expectations of gender. When a woman who cheerfully cooked and cleaned for her family for twenty-five years suddenly refused to wield the broom or stir the stew, physicians saw a mentally troubled woman. Physicians then gauged the efficacy of the treatment by whether the patient willingly returned to the confines of domesticity.

Because menopausal women focused on their own problems and neglected their domestic obligations, physicians and other health writers claimed that they were a burden to their families and perhaps to the society at large. Alienists Norbury and Dollear claimed, for example, that "the woman is, in her own mind, a martyr, and her endeavor is to make everyone else acknowledge her right to be so recognized."[87] Although not a physician, Bernarr MacFadden also claimed in 1918 that menopausal women's "thoughts center about themselves and every pain is aggravated by their apprehensive imaginings. Thus they make their own lives a much greater burden than is at all necessary."[88]

In particular, physicians and others worried that women took pleasure in "broadcasting" their menopausal troubles. Commentators soundly scolded women who used menopause to gain attention and "to wring sympathy from their non-understanding friends and families."[89] Edith Lowry encouraged her readers to "never affirm or repeat about your health what you do not wish to be true. . . . Do not fall into the habit of making every conversation with your acquaintances an 'organ-recital.'"[90]

To combat selfishness, physicians pleaded with women to forget their own troubles and return to securing the welfare of others. Anna Galbraith, for example, claimed that "any mental occupation that will take the woman out of herself is the best possible safeguard against a state of introspection which conjures up a host of evil fantasies, and which is the first step in the downward road to a fixed and permanent melancholia."[91] Joseph Greer agreed. He encouraged menopausal women to "not let the mind . . . dwell too continuously upon self."[92]

That physicians throughout this period considered selfishness in various guises a symptom of menopause and a marker of mental disturbance reflects, perhaps, the social unease created by the New Woman.[93] Throughout her life-course, the New Woman promoted female self-determination and autonomy. This emphasis made many social commentators uneasy, even those who applauded women's increasing public opportunities. Writer Margaret Deland, for example, in her 1910 article "The Change in the Feminine Ideal," noted that the New Woman championed a shift from female selflessness to a feminist individualism, trading her primary obligation to help others for a life dedicated to personal ambition and individual achievement. Although Deland applauded female self-determination, she nevertheless viewed this new selfishness as a threat to the family. She cautioned against abandoning one's duty to society in the pursuit of personal fulfillment.[94] The fear that the New Woman had abandoned the feminine characteristic of selflessness was mapped onto menopausal women's bodies as soon as the New Woman emerged.

THREE

"Consider the Patient as a Woman and Not a Group of Glands"

Women, Menopause, and the Medical Encounter, 1938–1962

In 1947, a middle-aged Smith College alumna was preparing for a "long and difficult journey." Although she had noticed a decreased, but more frequent, menstrual flow and some fatigue, only her need for a clean bill of health led her to call on a doctor. Her first doctor insisted that she needed "deep x-ray therapy" before he would provide a favorable medical report. The treatments, which presumably disabled her ovaries, made her feel a bit nauseated, dizzy, and generally unwell. After the initial symptoms subsided, she began experiencing frequent hot flashes. Her doctor suggested that she take small doses of a relatively new synthetic estrogen, diethylstilbestrol (DES). DES did not eliminate her hot flashes so in the midst of her travels, she visited a second physician who urged her to switch from the synthetic DES to another new estrogen, Premarin. Her flushes continued, and because they were sometimes quite intense, she sought out the advice of a third doctor. He suggested that taking hormones "slowed up nature's process of readjustment," and he recommended that she give them up. She tried to follow his advice, but she found herself, in 1950, occasionally resorting to Premarin because her hot flashes continued.[1]

This account of medical involvement with menopause should not be read as typical. Nevertheless, it illustrates several issues that characterize the medical encounter between doctors and menopausal patients between 1938 and 1962. It shows, for example, the central role of hormone replacement therapy in the treatment of menopause during this era. It also demonstrates the absence of medical consensus about which kind of kind of estrogen was best or whether replacement estrogens should be used at all. Further, it suggests that many women were disinclined to seek medical care just because they were entering menopause. Finally, this example shows that the bodies of menopausal women bore the consequences of medical interventions and debates.

New biomedical developments provide an important backdrop for this woman's experience. Although hormone treatments for menopause had been available in one form or another for most of the twentieth century, the late 1930s and early 1940s mark the development of two new estrogenic preparations that significantly changed the therapeutic landscape for menopausal patients. In 1938, an English biochemist, Charles Dodds, developed the synthetic hormone diethylstilbestrol (DES). Although DES eventually gained notoriety for its use to prevent miscarriage, it was first prescribed for menopausal women.[2] DES, unlike many estrogen treatments that preceded it, was cheap, efficacious, and widely available. Unfortunately, it also made many women intolerably nauseated.[3] Although the FDA did not approve DES until 1941, physicians anticipated its potential importance almost immediately after its invention. In 1942, on the heels of synthetic estrogen, researchers at Ayerst, McKenna, and Harrison, a Montreal-based drug company, developed an estrogen extract from the urine of pregnant mares. This product, known as conjugated estrogen and sold most familiarly under the brand name Premarin, had all the benefits of DES with none of its potential side effects.

The development of cheap, widely available, and effective hormonal treatments provided physicians with expanded treatment options for their menopausal patients. As described in Chapter 1, hormone treatments were not new to this era, but their visibility increased markedly with the development of conjugated and synthetic estrogen. Drug companies began aggressively advertising estrogen replacement therapies (ERT) to doctors in medical journals and through drug salesmen, known as detail men. Women's magazines featured articles on the medical marvels of female hormones. Confronted with ad campaigns pushing estrogenic compounds on the one hand and menopausal women who wanted them on the other, physicians were forced to consider the role of ERT in the treatment of their menopausal patients. Be they elite physicians at prestigious medical schools, suburban doctors with middle-class patients, or rural general practitioners, physicians had to decide how they would treat menopause.

The role of medicine in menopause altered profoundly between 1938 and 1962 with the development of the newly formulated hormone treatments, resulting in equally substantial changes in the nature of the office visit between menopausal women and their physicians. The available documentation allows two angles of approach to understanding the nature of and changes in this medical encounter: the medical *model* for the treatment of menopause as described in the published medical literature and medical *practice* as experienced by menopausal women (and their physicians). Explored together, these sometimes contradictory perspectives illuminate both the construction of menopause and the practice of medicine in the 1940s and 1950s.

The medical literature vividly demonstrates that physicians did not hail replacement hormones as a therapeutic panacea for menopausal patients. Instead, physicians, at least the physicians who wrote about menopause, regarded estrogen therapy with caution, insisting that reassurance about symptoms remained the treatment of choice in most cases. Hormones, these physicians claimed, should be reserved for the few patients with severe and unrelenting symptoms.

The reluctance on the part of published physicians to rely primarily on a pharmaceutical solution reveals a great deal about how they understood the menopausal transition. As this chapter shows, physicians understood that menopause marked both a physiological and a social transition in women's lives. Personal finances, marital health, and intellectual interests might all affect how a women anticipated and experienced her waning fertility. As a result, physicians publishing in the medical literature generally insisted that the difficulties of menopause could best be addressed by considering a patient's social circumstances. These physicians insisted that the patient must be treated as a whole person within a social setting; her problems should not be reduced to the fluctuations of her glands. This suggests that historians may have overstated the extent to which twentieth-century therapeutics increasingly reduced patients to their symptoms.[4]

Further, although acknowledging that some women's menopausal symptoms warranted treatment, most publishing physicians refused to construct menopause as a pathological process that *required* treatment; they refused to define it as a disease. The effort to describe menopause as a natural transition while admitting that its symptoms could make women feel quite ill forced a tricky semantic dance. Sociologist Susan Bell has argued that the medical language of menopause, including references to "symptoms" and a "menopausal syndrome," demonstrated medical acceptance of a disease model of menopause during this period.[5] In contrast, the evidence suggests that some physicians self-consciously used the language of "symptoms" to separate the physiological process of menopause from its occasionally unpleasant manifestations. This allowed physicians to argue that while severe menopausal *symptoms* might warrant medical intervention, menopause itself remained a natural transition.

Medical orthodoxy between 1938 and 1962, as expressed in the medical journals of the period, does not seem to have responded to the new synthetic and conjugated hormones by changing to any extent the treatment and perception of menopause. But the views promoted in the medical literature represent only a narrow segment of the views held by medical professionals. In reading the medical literature alongside the popular literature and by looking at archival records detailing menopausal women's experiences, a different conclusion about prevailing treatments emerges. Indeed, it was precisely during this period of medical conservatism that women routinely began using estrogen therapy to ease their menopausal symptoms. Ignoring, or at least revising the recommendations in the medical literature, many physicians apparently readily prescribed hormones to their patients, who, just as readily, accepted them. Comparing the medical literature with glimpses of medical practice suggests that the influence of hormone therapies on the medical understanding and personal experience of menopause eludes simple characterization.

But the exploration of the medical encounter in the 1940s and 1950s does not merely illuminate the medical and cultural construction of menopause. It also indicates that menopause and its pharmaceutical treatment posed challenging professional questions for the practice of medicine more generally. What does doctoring entail in an era of so-called miracle drugs? Can physicians treat symptoms without thereby "creating" a disease? Who should make decisions about patients' treatment: the patients who must live with the consequences or the physicians who claimed cultural authority over bodily concerns? Does the ability to provide relief of symptoms create an obligation to offer that relief? When writing medical articles about the appropriate treatment for menopause, when considering the best course of action for a woman with hot flashes, physicians were also considering these larger professional issues. Menopause and its treatments urged physicians to recognize that they too were in the midst of a cultural and professional transition.

Three types of evidence reveal what happened when a menopausal woman met with her physician for advice, reassurance, or treatment during this period: the medical literature, popular literature, and women's testimonies, available primarily through survey results. The medical literature—literature written for a medical audience—characterizes the advice physicians offered one another on the treatment of menopausal patients.[6] The authors of this medical literature do not, of course, represent the entire medical profession. Indeed, most of these physicians were among the professional elite. Roughly 80 percent of the doctors writing for journals on this topic were "specialists," for example, meaning they had passed an examination in their professional niche at a time when only 25 percent of all physicians did so. The majority of these specialists were obstetrician/gynecologists, but endocrinologists were also well represented. Further, at least 60 percent of these physicians held university positions. As a result, the views promoted in this medical literature do not necessarily capture the beliefs and the practices of most physicians then treating menopausal women. Nevertheless, the published medical literature identifies, according to leading doctors, the critical medical issues with respect to menopause and menopausal patients.

The articles in the medical literature during this period offered three, somewhat overlapping, approaches to menopause and its treatment: medical musings, retrospective analysis, and therapeutic research. The majority of the literature on menopause during this period fell into the first category. In this genre, physicians described their opinions on and approaches to menopause and tried to persuade their colleagues to adopt their positions. Occasionally, these physicians would illustrate their opinion with a few case studies. Writers presenting retrospective analysis offered conclusions based on their clinical practice. In an example typical of this approach, C. L. Buxton reported on ninety-one menopausal patients referred to the endocrine clinic of Sloan Hospital for Women in New York City, describing the variety of symptoms the women presented and their responses to various treatments. Such articles often included a literature review to help situate their findings within current medical knowledge. Few articles followed the third path, presentation of research results. Virtually all articles in this category described the effect of estrogenic preparations on various menopausal symptoms or the efficacy of one hormonal treatment relative to another.[7]

Popular literature provides a distinct perspective on the relationship between physicians and their patients. Written primarily by doctors, these public messages were promulgated to reassure women about the changes in their bodies. The category includes books about menopause, women's health guides, and articles from general interest and women's magazines.

Finally, women's testimony of their own experiences illuminates their relationships with their physicians. The most useful of the two primary sources for these is a 1950 questionnaire circulated by Dorothy Hamilton Brush and Hester Hoffman. Graduates of Smith College in 1917, Hoffman and Brush hoped to write a book on menopause and turned for information primarily to their Smith classmates, who were at the time of the survey typically fifty-five, most having been born in 1895. The sociological work of Ida Davidoff and Marjorie Platt provides a second point of access into women's experiences. In 1957, Davidoff and Platt interviewed fifty women to understand how the women's movement affected them as their children left home. The women interviewed lived with their husbands, had never worked permanently or full-time while raising their children, and had seen their last child leave home at least a year earlier. The average age of these women was fifty-four at the time of their first interview.[8]

Neither the Davidoff nor the Brush samples provide a cross section of American women during this period. Certainly both groups were better educated than most women. All the Davidoff women and more than 80 percent of the Brush women, for example, earned college degrees. Given the demographics of Smith College at the time, their families of origin were most likely upper middle class, white, and Protestant. Nevertheless, as relatively privileged white women, the women in both samples represent those women most likely to seek medical advice and treatment in non-emergency situations. As a result, these women were among those most likely to visit their doctors at menopause and thus can illuminate the encounter between medicine and menopausal women between 1938 and 1962.

Why Women Sought Medical Care at Menopause

Although this chapter focuses on the medical encounter between doctors and their menopausal patients, it is important to realize that most women in this era did not routinely visit their physicians at menopause. Throughout this period, physicians maintained that few menopausal women (a typical estimate was 10 to 15 percent) needed or sought medical care.[9] Several factors may have discouraged women from consulting a physician, the most important of which was that both the medical and popular literature maintained that the majority of women did not experience symptoms severe enough to warrant medical assistance.[10]

The cost of medical care deterred some women who might have wanted to see a physician. During this period, most people did not have health insurance that covered doctors' visits.[11] As a result, a nonemergency medical visit would have been out of reach for many women. At least one of the women in the Brush study had wanted to see a doctor, but she could not afford it. She lamented that even though her symptoms had worried her, she had not seen a physician "soon enough." "I was scared that I had heart trouble or was having a nervous breakdown and I didn't have the money to go to the doctor."[12] In addition, for many single women and some married women, a trip to the doctor may have represented lost wages.

Although most women did not visit their physicians at menopause, they may still have sought "medical" treatments. Patent medicines remained a viable alternative to physician care during this period. In 1949, for example, nonprescription drugs accounted for more than 40 percent of all medicines sold.[13] Proprietary medicines often targeted menopausal women. One advertisement for Lydia Pinkham's Vegetable Compound asked women "Is your age betrayed by hot flashes. Do you suffer from cranky high-strung feelings—all due to the functional middle age period peculiar to women?"[14] These advertisements, frequently placed in periodicals and newspapers targeting working-class or rural populations, occasionally offered free samples to lure women into trying their product. The popular literature targeting a middle-class audience warned, however, about the dangers of self-medication. In a typical example, physician James Scott advised ominously, "Don't try to treat yourself; you may not get away with it."[15] These warnings reflected physicians' ongoing attempts to discredit patent medicines and gain ultimate control over pharmaceutical interventions.[16] Despite these cautions, the enduring patent medicine industry indicates that many women, particularly those with limited economic resources, may have continued to rely on over-the-counter remedies for relief during menopause despite the emergence of new hormone preparations.

The circumstances bringing women into contact with their physicians at menopause varied greatly. Some women visited their physicians at middle age as part of a preventive care regimen. Throughout the century, physicians had urged middle-aged women to seek regular medical attention and, in 1922, the American Medical Association (AMA) officially recommended periodic physical examinations for all healthy people.[17] The popular literature encouraged menopausal women to secure a thorough medical examination *before* they experienced any menopausal symptoms. Medical writers insisted that as "one approaches forty, it is important to have frequent examinations by a good gynecologist."[18] Significantly, however, physicians generally believed that, although women should see a physician at middle age, "the primary reason is not the climacterium; it is general health."[19]

Some of the women in the Davidoff sample illustrate that their contact with the medical profession was not necessarily prompted by menopausal discomforts. Mary Rathbone, for example, remarked that her gynecologist raised the issue of menopause during a routine exam. Other women similarly claimed that they learned about menopause and their connection to it during unrelated visits to their doctors.[20] These women, however, were probably not typical. Although the popular literature recommended that women secure regular preventive care, most did not. According to a 1954–1955 California study, only 10 percent of medical visits constituted "health supervision." More significantly, fewer people between the ages of forty-five and sixty-four received routine examinations than in any other age group.[21]

Some women sought medical attention at menopause because they wanted reassurance that their experiences were normal, not because those experiences were troubling. Ada Cooper, for example, "consulted a doctor once just to check [her] own conclusions" that she had reached menopause and that her experience was normal.[22] These women, then, used their physicians to verify their own hunches rather than to acquire medical treatment.

Hysterectomy forged the connection between medicine and menopause for many women. Roughly 20 percent of both the Davidoff and Brush women underwent hysterectomies before they reached menopause. Although some of these women retained their ovaries and therefore continued estrogen production, most of them probably experienced "artificial" menopause.[23] But as one woman's experience showed, even a hysterectomy did not guarantee sustained medical involvement. In 1941, a San Francisco woman wrote the Children's Bureau seeking advice and reassurance. When she was twenty-nine, she had had a hysterectomy, during which her doctor removed both ovaries. She complained that her doctor, "a very busy surgeon, considers the case closed with the actual operation completed and gives me no further information about what to expect, than that there will be no more periods." She claimed that the "hot flushes" gave her a "very vague feeling that something strange [was] happening." She wondered how long the symptoms would last and how menopause would affect her health and sex life. She was also unsure whether her nausea and "jittery nerves" were "normal."[24] This woman's experience shows that even women whose menopause was medically induced did not necessarily receive sustained support from their physicians.

The dramatic experiences of friends and families persuaded some women to consult a physician at menopause. The experiences of their mothers seem to have been particularly compelling. Although most of the women in both the Brush and Davidoff samples claimed that their mothers took menopause "in stride," a few said their mothers had suffered.[25] Mary Rathbone noted that her "extremely high strung" mother had shut herself in the bathroom during menopause, and her mother's doctor finally prescribed medicine "to quiet her." When she herself reached menopause, Rathbone turned to her own physician.[26] Mildred Lewis claimed that because menopause had been the "indirect cause of [her] mother's death, [she] was determined to have medical aid if needed."[27]

Finally, women visited their physicians at menopause because they experienced menopausal symptoms and wanted relief. The medical literature on menopause and the testimony of menopausal women depict a wide range of physical and emotional difficulties at menopause. On the physical side, physicians and menopausal women alike viewed the hot flash as the representative menopausal symptom. Other frequently listed symptoms included menstrual irregularities, headaches, heart palpitations, vertigo, insomnia, and vaginal dryness.

In addition to the physical symptoms of menopause, women often turned to their doctors to relieve the mental or emotional consequences of menopause. These included nervousness, irritability, weepiness, fatigue, depression, and anxiety. Stanford University gynecologist Charles Fluhmann described the myriad mental afflictions that might befall women at menopause. The menopausal woman, he claimed, might "become irritable, apprehensive, impatient, unreasonable, inattentive to personal appearance, tire easily, develop a loss of memory and have prolonged crying spells."[28] Seeking relief from these "nervous" symptoms, women turned to their physicians for advice or treatment.

By accident or by intention, for reassurance or for treatment, many women (but not most) called upon a doctor at menopause. What kind of treatment did they receive? Because so many different circumstances brought women to their physicians and because the medical profession itself was not monolithic, women encountered a wide variety of medical scenarios. The medical profession's own model for the treatment of menopause emerges from a reading of the medical literature.

The Medical Encounter: Therapeutic Restraint

Physicians writing in the medical literature overwhelmingly promoted pharmaceutical restraint in treating menopause, insisting that hormone therapy should be a treatment of last resort, given only to the few women who exhibited a specific set of symptoms. Rather than rushing into hormone treatments, physicians called for a three-tiered treatment regimen. They maintained that menopause should be treated with education and reassurance, supplemented, if necessary, with sedatives; only if the woman's symptoms did not abate, should hormones be prescribed.[29]

Physicians advised their colleagues to diagnose menopause carefully before proceeding with treatment. As they had earlier in the century, many physicians complained that others in the profession frequently attributed every ache and pain, every episode of nervousness, to menopause. They bemoaned the tendency to "hold the menopause responsible for all the disturbances encountered at this period."[30] Many physicians believed that their colleagues too easily accepted a woman's own mistaken diagnosis of her symptoms. Emil Novak, professor of gynecology at Johns Hopkins School of Medicine, for example, claimed that even well-informed women were apt to blame every twinge that occurred in middle age to menopause. He blamed other doctors for fostering such nonsense by agreeing too easily with such explanations.[31] To prevent misdiagnosis, published physicians insisted that all middle-aged women provide a thorough medical history and receive a careful physical exam.[32]

After securing a firm diagnosis, physicians writing in the medical literature urged their colleagues, as noted above, to treat their menopausal patients first with education and reassurance. Because they believed that many women suffered at menopause primarily because they believed a great deal of misinformation, physicians advocated an informal type of psychotherapy aimed at relieving ignorance and apprehension. Physicians blamed other women and, to a lesser degree, the lay press for women's distorted perceptions. Columbia University professor of gynecology Robert Frank, for example, claimed that many women turn to their doctors "because they are disquieted by their gossipy friends as well as by the articles they read in the newspapers or magazines."[33] Bridge parties were apparently hotbeds of menopausal misinformation. Another professor of obstetrics and gynecology at Columbia complained that physicians were routinely visited by women, "who from reading the lay literature or from listening to the conversation of their companions round the tea or bridge table, get an exaggerated picture of the ills and troubles that may befall them at this time." He insisted that an important component of the physicians' treatment must be to "correct . . . the distorted ideas she may have acquired."[34]

Another physician's opinion on menopausal misinformation revealed a more significant attitude about women in general. Willard R. Cooke, chair of obstetrics and gynecology at the University of Texas, claimed that the "greatest obstacle to the successful management and to the satisfactory outcome of the case is the patients' female friends and relatives." He insisted that physicians must convince "the patient that what she has been told, and will continually be told, is based upon ignorance and is wholly false. The great majority of women are eager to give vent to the innate primitive hatred of every female for every other female. . . . The practice of gynecics would be truly utopian if women would keep their noses out of every other woman's uterus."[35]

Cooke's startling imagery and sneering attitude certainly feeds the claim that physicians harbored a great deal of animosity toward their female patients.[36] Overt examples of misogyny such as his were infrequent in the medical literature, however, and even his comments are difficult to interpret. We cannot assume that his scornful regard for womankind necessarily led to mistreatment. Indeed, his concern for his individual female patients led to his frustration with women as a group. Nevertheless, the larger characterization of women as gossipy, vengeful creatures with too much time on their hands may have encouraged physicians to see their female patients as hypochondriacs, suffering not from the trials of menopause but from the influence of interfering friends and relations.

Because some women feared the possible physical transformations of menopause, most physicians believed that a straightforward description of the physiological changes would greatly assuage women's apprehensions. Physicians urged their colleagues to explain the physiology of menopause, to discuss with women what they might experience, and to emphasize that symptoms would eventually diminish on their own.[37] Physicians believed that once women were armed with knowledge, even the hot flashes would "diminish in importance and cease to be troublesome."[38]

Many physicians understood, however, that women's anxieties about menopause did not necessarily disappear after a physiology lecture. Before assuring women that menopause was normal and insisting that the symptoms would eventually subside, physicians needed to establish themselves as trusted advisors and confidants. Patients needed to believe that their doctors cared about them, not just about their symptoms. As some medical authors put it, patients must be convinced of the doctors' "earnest desire to help."[39] Indeed, one gynecologist warned that offering reassurance too soon after meeting with a patient is the "equivalent of belittling a patient's symptoms."[40]

Careful listening provided an easy and effective path to winning a patient's trust while simultaneously achieving therapeutic ends. Specialists and generalists alike agreed that women found relief through unburdening themselves. A Beverly Hills doctor claimed, for example, that the patient often "gets considerable relief from the mere telling of her story."[41] Another physician similarly insisted that "a sympathetic listener is like a safety valve which lets off a dangerous head of steam."[42]

While admitting that listening required time, the medical literature insisted that it was crucial. A physician weighing in on matters menopausal urged physicians to "take all the time necessary. The more time spent with the patient at her first visit the better. It takes time plus sympathetic understanding and reassurance to create the state of mind essential for management of these patients."[43] Cooke, having already displayed his misogynistic attitudes, revealed his ambivalence about the importance of listening and his condescension toward his patients.

> Tiresome, uninformative, and time consuming as it is, letting the patient tell her own story as the first item puts the patient at ease and creates the impression that the doctor is really interested in her as an individual. Further, one obtains in this way the best general concept of the most salient features of symptomology. The reception of this story must be attentive—and at this point it is really necessary for the doctor to become an actor for a time, concealing his boredom under an air of friendly interest.[44]

Cooke's comment conjures up an image of a distracted physician looking at his watch and yawning as his patient describes her very real and perhaps very distressing symptoms. It certainly highlights the condescension with which some physicians viewed their female patients. Conceivably, this remark reveals less about gender relations and more about physicians' (at least this physician's) attitudes toward their patients more generally. It is difficult to imagine, however, a physician treating a male patient by feigning interest in his story.

His comments also suggest that, while some physicians pretended to listen, they were not actively hearing what their patients had to say. Indeed, the posturing may have been more common than the sincere engagement with patients' concerns. But we should not read the discussion of listening too cynically. Even Cooke argued that patients' narratives of their own experiences provided information of great use to the doctor. The medical emphasis on listening, therefore, allows us to imagine a negotiation between physicians and their female patients wherein women wielded a great deal of power. By insisting that doctors should listen to their patients, physicians affirmed that, for better therapeutic results, women and their experiences should be taken seriously.

As demonstrated in Chapter 1, the deployment of reassurance as a treatment for menopause was not new to this era. Its importance for this period, however, lies in its resilience in the wake of an increasingly powerful pharmaceutical arsenal. Although hormones provided an effective treatment for some menopausal symptoms, physicians did not relinquish reassurance and education as the treatment of first choice. They apparently believed that in the practice of medicine, more was owed to patients than merely attending to their symptoms. The medical discussion of menopause indicates that physicians, specialists and generalists alike, saw their role as comprehensive. The treatment of menopause required medical providers to be confidants, counselors, educators, and, only if necessary, prescribers.

Significantly, by resisting hormone therapy for all cases of menopause, physicians avoided reducing women to their biology. Instead, they promoted the widespread belief that "the menopause is neither psychic nor organic but a combination of the two."[45] The persistence of reassurance as the first treatment choice illustrates physicians' willingness to "consider the patient as a woman and not a group of glands."[46]

The insistence that menopausal women be treated as people rather than as symptoms suggests a reconsideration of the often repeated claim that twentieth-century medicine rejected caring, reassurance, and education as central features of medical practice in favor of scientific diagnostics and treatments.[47] Indeed, in the case of menopause, it is precisely the medical elite—the specialists and the medical school professors—who championed, at least in part, "old-fashioned" healing practices that required no lab tests or pharmaceutical preparations.

By the "old-fashioned" practice of listening, doctors learned from their patients that menopause was not merely a physiological transition and that women's concerns at menopause extended far beyond the changes taking place in their bodies. Physicians discovered that many women feared both the possible physical and emotional changes of menopause and the possible economic and familial upheavals of middle age.

One of the factors that women allegedly feared was the loss of attractiveness. Gynecologist Frank claimed that women unnecessarily dreaded menopause "because they expect to lose their attractiveness (with appearance of wrinkles, gray hair, flabbiness, hirsutism), sex allure, physical vigor and shapeliness."[48] Another doctor acknowledged that women fear that they will "become less attractive sexually, and that their sex life will be disturbed."[49] Physicians insisted that this fear was unwarranted, but they believed that the apprehension was rampant.

Physicians also acknowledged that menopause had symbolic significance for many women because it marked the end of fertility. Many doctors understood that menopause encouraged women to take stock of their lives, evaluating both the accomplishments of their past and their plans for the future. Occasionally, this psychic inventory led to shattering results. Psychiatrist Esther Richards described the situation. "The look back upon the life behind is not always pleasant. Disappointed hopes, unrealized ambitions, self-comparisons and deprecations chase each other like fall clouds over the mountains and valleys of the journey thus far traveled."[50] After evaluating both her past and her future, one woman concluded that "I seem like a monster squatted on my own horizon."[51]

While some women suffered because of psychic realizations and recriminations, physicians understood that other women suffered at the demands of day-to-day living. Generalists and specialists alike recognized that household transitions posed potential problems for women at menopause. Children moved out, parents moved in, and marriages fractured. One physician claimed that menopausal stress might be caused "when the patient became engaged, when the mother-in-law came to live in the household, when the son went overseas, and when the husband started noticing the blonde next door."[52] Gynecologists Douglas Cannell and Arthur Squires described the confluence of events that converged on one of their patients at menopause. She was a "well-groomed" woman whose life had been healthy and "fairly happy." Her first hot flashes coincided with a series of family crises. Her husband had a heart attack, was forced to his bed for six weeks, and never completely recovered. Her daughter brought her husband and new baby back home because they could not find a place of their own, and the patient regarded them as "unwelcome guests." Then, her favorite son contracted tuberculosis and "had to go to the sanatorium." The patient was overwhelmed by her problems, "never having had serious responsibility before; she could see no way out and began to feel hopeless and utterly exhausted with weeping spells; she feared she might become insane." She endured bouts of depression for two years after her last menstrual cycle. Squires and Cannell concluded that "the menopause came at an inconvenient time in this woman's life, but plays a relatively small role in her sickness."[53]

Physicians also understood that middle age did not always guarantee a stable or adequate income and that poverty, or the fear of poverty, could contribute to women's anxiety at menopause. Two San Francisco physicians, for example, claimed that one of their patients suffered at menopause in part because she had to care for her ill husband while "living in a trailer alongside noisy traffic."[54] After she was able to move and her husband recovered, her menopausal symptoms improved. These physicians understood that psychotherapy was inadequate to solve all their patients' social problems. One physician, for example, believed that the true solution to menopausal problems "would be to modify our economic system as to assure at least a modest degree of security for all."[55] In lieu of a reconstruction of market capitalism, physicians believed that advice, reassurance, and a sympathetic ear could help women face and cope with their situations.[56]

Occasionally, physicians noted, perhaps with some derision, that women at menopause were also influenced by the concerns of the larger body politic. Edmund Novak, son of Emil Novak, for example, claimed that, in addition to domestic problems, women were also worried about "the atomic bomb, or whether the Dodgers will win the pennant."[57] Although this comment belittled women's anxiety as misplaced (as well as ascribing to them an inability to differentiate national risks from National League contests), as domestic caretakers they were often encouraged to bear the consequences of events well beyond their control. A 1942 *Good Housekeeping* article urged women to avoid worrying about things outside their purview. An advertisement for Lysol on the same page, however, showed women "What to do—in air raids—in first aid—with incendiary bombs."[58]

Physicians' medical writings on menopause often demonstrate a realization that medicine must address all the potential sites of trouble when treating and advising menopausal patients, including their social setting and emotional stability. Did this mean that physicians considered most menopausal symptoms figments, if not of women's imagination, at least of their misplaced anxiety? Did doctors consider their patients' menopausal

troubles to be "all in their heads"? Without justifying physicians' condescension, surely some women did suffer because of what they feared might
happen. Considering that at least one woman implicated menopause in
her mother's death, the apprehension could be overwhelming. Further,
physicians understood menopause as a cultural symbol of women's changing roles, a marker of actual transformations within women's homes, and a
physiological transition in women's bodies.

It is possible that relying on the psychological etiology of menopausal
symptoms led physicians to treat their patients with a dismissive pat on the
knee and an equally dismissive "there, there, dear." But in theory at least,
the integration of social and physical components can be interpreted as
empowering rather than patronizing. This holistic approach affirmed a
woman's right to understand the workings of her own body. It encouraged physicians to both talk and listen to their patients rather than hastily
writing a prescription. Further, it acknowledged that women's bodies do
not exist apart from their social circumstances; published physicians discouraged their colleagues from treating physical symptoms without addressing the social causes of those symptoms.

Despite the deliberate sensitivity to the social factors affecting women
at menopause, physicians writing in medical journals routinely tried to
soothe away women's reactions to outside concerns. Nearly all physicians
who offered advice to their colleagues recommended "mild" sedation—
typically fifteen milligrams of phenobarbital, three times daily—as a useful
tool in the treatment of menopausal patients.[59] Aware of the addictive potential of barbiturates, most physicians recommended sedation only as
short-term therapy to temporarily ease the anxiety and nervousness many
women experienced. Harry Friedlander, for example, employed sedatives
to "assist with the period of mental reorientation." He reported that one
of his patients, who had had a history of nervousness in her youth, felt
"useless" at menopause. Friedlander prescribed phenobarbital, which provided a "sense of well-being." Concluding that it had eased her anxiety, he
discontinued the prescription after several weeks.[60]

Medical consensus held that sedation served several purposes. First, it
eased the nervous symptoms so many women experienced. By taking the
edge off anxiety, physicians claimed that sedation allowed women to better
cope with the difficult social and physiological changes they were experiencing. Second, sedatives helped menopausal women get a good night's
sleep. Either because of anxiety or hot flashes, many women complained
that sleep regularly eluded them. Insomnia begat fatigue which begat irri-

tability which begat. . . . By providing rest, physicians believed sedatives could help women better adapt to their changed situations.[61] Finally, some physicians claimed that sedatives could relieve the physical as well as the emotional symptoms of menopause. One physician claimed, for example, that 50 percent of his patients were "completely relieved of all symptoms by . . . sedation therapy."[62]

It is tempting to interpret the use of sedatives as a form of social control, an attempt to keep women quiet and docile during a period marked by irritability and complaints.[63] Perhaps this is part of the explanation. It is also tempting to regard sedative use as the smoking gun proving that physicians did not take their menopausal patients' complaints seriously. Again, some women probably did perceive (perhaps rightly) that a prescription for sedatives was a dismissal, a statement that their troubles were all in their heads. Neither of these interpretations, however, adequately captures the possible motivations behind sedative use; several other explanations similarly fit the circumstances. Surely some physicians did prescribe sedatives to pacify a querulous patient or to ease a husband's irritation. However, other motivations recommended the use of sedatives.

First, physicians viewed sedatives as a way to avoid over-medication. Led by their conviction that menopause itself did not require treatment, physicians viewed the indiscriminate use of hormones as overly intrusive. Sedatives, by focusing directly on symptom relief rather than systemic reconfiguration, appeared the more prudent course. Second, many women experienced nervous symptoms brought on by physical adjustments, social changes, and personal evaluations, and they sought relief. Rather than dismissing those symptoms, physicians employed sedatives as a way to take those concerns seriously. Because many physicians did not believe that hormones relieved emotional difficulties,[64] physicians prescribed their best solution for the symptoms that troubled women most. Finally, the use of sedatives can be read as resistance to reducing women to the fluctuations of their glands. Physicians realized that menopausal difficulties emerged in part from middle-aged women's inadequately defined social niche; medicine had no cure to offer for the dilemma of being a middle-aged woman, but physicians could relieve some of the apprehension that coincided with that position. Sedatives provided some relief as women learned to adjust to changes in their physical and social status. By resisting the use of hormones, physicians acknowledged that the emotional problems of menopause were not caused by a woman's innate "femaleness" but rather by her role as an aging female.

Only if reassurance and sedatives failed did most published physicians recommend hormone treatments for menopausal patients.[65] Even then, physicians proposed strict guidelines for hormone treatments.[66] The majority of physicians insisted that only a very few women needed hormonal treatment. Physicians typically claimed that only 10 percent of women seeking medical attention at menopause required hormone therapy, and a few insisted that the number was closer to 5 percent.[67] Most physicians agreed with Emil Novak, who claimed that, in general, "it seems better to let nature take its course except in those cases and at that those times when symptoms become very troublesome."[68] Doctors generally concurred that physicians should prescribe hormones only for those women whose symptoms were incapacitating rather than simply inconvenient.

Severe symptoms were necessary but not sufficient to warrant hormone therapy. Physicians generally agreed that only symptoms clearly connected to decreased levels of estrogen should be hormonally treated. Most physicians claimed that hot flashes and night sweats were the only symptoms helped by hormones.[69] Some conceded, however, that hormones might indirectly affect nervousness. If, for example, a woman suffered from severe hot flashes that wakened her several times a night, she might consequently suffer from sleep deprivation and therefore irritability. In this scenario, if her vasomotor symptoms were controlled, her irritability might also recede.

For the most part, physicians writing in the medical literature emphasized the palliation of severe symptoms as the guiding rationale for hormone treatment; they explicitly argued (as if in opposition to another view) that hormones could not reverse or prevent menopause. Edwin Hamblen, chief of reproductive endocrinology at Duke University, for example, argued that hormone therapy should "mitigate severe symptoms" and make menopause "less rocky." He dismissed as "irrational" the notion that estrogen therapy could prevent menopause and likened it to foolish attempts to "prevent old age itself."[70] Consequently, most physicians argued that doctors should not strive for "total replacement" of hormones or to reestablish a premenopausal hormonal balance.[71]

Because hormones were indicated for symptom relief, the overwhelming majority of physicians insisted that estrogen be seen as a "temporary crutch" rather than a long-term treatment. Indeed, because they believed that hormone therapy prolonged the body's ultimate adjustment to diminished estrogen, physicians agreed that women should remain on hormones for the shortest possible time. In making the case for short-term treatment, one physician insisted that hormones worked at cross-purposes to "nature's efforts" and insisted that women accept the "endocrinological readjustment that must come sooner or later."[72] Ultimately, he argued, a woman must allow her body to complete its plan.

Concern about hormone dependence also convinced some members of the medical profession to recommend a limited duration for estrogen treatments. The director of the Sloan Hospital for Women in New York City, for example, warned: "Estrogens are habit forming drugs and patients should be warned accordingly."[73] Other doctors agreed, noting that many women "who have been taking [hormones] for several years for various and sundry complaints" become vehemently "unwilling to stop taking the drug."[74]

In addition to believing that hormone treatments were unnecessary, many physicians prescribed hormones cautiously because of their carcinogenic potential. By 1940, more than a dozen scientific papers had been published showing that both synthetic and natural estrogens were capable of causing cancer in female animals, particularly mice and rats.[75] Other researchers expressed fears about the carcinogenic effects of estrogenic compounds on women's breasts and uteri.[76] The fear was great enough for Edgar Allen, one of the pioneers of endocrinology, to condemn the "indiscriminate" use of estrogen therapy in menopausal women.[77] This threat became even more menacing in 1947, when Columbia University gynecologist Saul Gusberg linked estrogen to cancer of the endometrium, leading him to conclude that physicians over-prescribed estrogens to postmenopausal women. "The relatively low cost of stilbestrol [synthetic estrogen] and the ease of administration have made its general use promiscuous."[78]

Authors of medical articles disagreed about whether estrogen therapy caused cancer in menopausal women. Only a very few physicians found the evidence of a link between estrogen and cancer persuasive. Endocrinologist Hamblen was definitely in the minority. Although he did not condemn the use of hormone treatments in all cases, he believed that the cancer risk was real and that introduction of DES into the market potentially endangered women. He feared that synthetic hormones, because of their price and their oral administration, "constitute[d] a definite hazard" creating "ideal circumstances . . . for the production of carcinoma."[79] At the other end of the spectrum, some physicians claimed that hormone therapy for menopause posed no threat. In his 1956 literature review, Joseph Rogers of Tufts University asserted that the concern about the connection between cancer and hormone therapy "does not seem justified."[80] Most physicians stood somewhere between Hamblen and Rogers, denying that estrogen treatments caused cancer but agreeing that medical uncertainty called for a conservative approach. Gertrude Jones illustrates the typical position. In 1949, she claimed that "although there is no proof that estrogenic substances are carcinogenic in themselves," she was persuaded that cancer did occur more frequently in women with high estrogen levels. As a result, she recommended that hormones be prescribed for short-term use only.[81] Similar concerns led most doctors to regard a family history of cancer as a contraindication for hormone use.[82]

Elite physicians, then, had several pragmatic reasons for regarding hormone treatments cautiously. The resistance to hormones may have also had a more theoretical foundation for some physicians. Some elite physicians resisted any effort to regard menopause as anything but a natural physiological transition. Hamblen decried in 1940 the notion that menopause was pathological, insisting that if menopause was a disease, "life itself has indeed become a disease."[83] A gynecologist agreed, insisting that "menopause is an integral part of the process of aging; in no sense can it be regarded as a disease."[84] Making the same point slightly differently, a few physicians distinguished between treating menopause and treating its concomitant symptoms. University of California physician Minnie Goldberg, for example, argued that "it is not the menopause per se which requires treatment but the distressing symptoms thereof."[85]

Physicians clearly believed that a significant distinction should be made between menopause and its symptoms. Although a few sociologists have argued that the reference to symptoms itself points to a medical belief in the underlying pathology of menopause,[86] this position obscures several points that emerge only if we take the separation seriously. First, the separation allowed the menopausal patient to remain at the center of the decision to treat menopause. If menopause itself required treatment, then presumably all menopausal women, regardless of their experiences, would need medical intervention. By gauging the need for therapy on the severity of symptoms—a wholly subjective measure—women's perceptions of their own bodies mattered. Second, it reflects physicians' resistance to labeling female aging as pathological. By self-consciously focusing on symptoms, menopause itself remained safe from medical onslaught. Only when the menopausal transition became difficult was medical intervention warranted. Finally, and perhaps with very different implications, the separation of menopause and menopausal symptoms validated medicine's presence in the lives of healthy women. Disease was not necessary for medical involvement.

Perhaps the same motivation led to the widespread rejection of the Pap smear as a valuable test to determine who needed estrogen therapy. The Pap smear, developed in 1935 by George Papanicolaou and Ephraim Shorr, provided objective evidence both of the need for estrogen treatment and of the efficacy of the therapy. During a woman's fertile years, the cells lining her vagina are generally large and flat and include only a few leukocytes. During menopause, her vaginal cells become smaller and flatter and leukocytes dominate. A vaginal smear could have been used to determine who was physiologically menopausal and thus warranted treatment. In other words, this test provided an objective gauge of the need for and efficacy of treatment quite apart from a patient's "subjective" needs.[87] Indeed, in theory, it allowed physicians to distinguish between "the true ovarian insufficiency symptoms" and a patient's experience of menopausal symptoms.[88]

In general, when they discussed the role of the Pap smear at all (which they did only rarely), physicians denied its clinical appeal; only the symptoms, as experienced by women themselves, needed treatment. This refusal to embrace the smear for this purpose demonstrates most physicians' refusal to see menopause itself as pathological. If they had seen menopause itself as a condition needing treatment, a Pap smear would have been employed to provide clear evidence of diminished estrogen levels, thus justifying a prescription for hormones. The underlying physiology was instead seen by most publishing physicians as normal. Emil Novak, for example, reminded his colleagues that because there was no correlation between the smear and symptom relief, the smear had little role to play in the therapeutics of menopause. Another doctor agreed that listening to "what the patient said of herself" remained far more important than any "objective" test.[89] Goldberg reminded her colleagues that "the degree of suffering is the yardstick by which the need for relief should be measured."[90] The general indifference toward the test, coupled with the prominence of symptom relief as the therapeutic goal, demonstrates that women's experiences of their bodies mattered to physicians.[91] As Goldberg put it, "we are primarily concerned with relieving distress rather than normalizing the vaginal smear."[92] This indicates that, in contrast to the dominant characterization of twentieth-century therapeutics (and in contrast to the nineteenth-century conflation of women with their reproductive organs), twentieth-century physicians resisted separating women's symptoms from their experiences of those symptoms.

The Therapeutic Vanguard

Although almost all physicians publishing in the 1940s regarded hormone therapy as the last option for treating particularly stubborn symptoms, by the 1950s a few doctors were urging a more liberal use of hormone therapy. Robert Greenblatt, chairman of the Department of Endocrinology at the Medical College of Georgia, for example, admitted in 1952 that a few women might get by with reassurance or sedation, but, he insisted, "the large majority with distressing symptoms need replacement therapy."[93] The chair of obstetrics and gynecology at the University of Colorado School of Medicine agreed, noting that while 75 percent of menopausal women experienced no trouble, those with vasomotor symptoms were best treated with estrogen. Even he, however, reminded his colleagues that the "counseling the physician can give his patient" remained more important to the patient's overall outlook than estrogen alone.[94]

Consistent with the emerging acceptance of a more central place for estrogen therapy, a handful of physicians began in the mid-1950s to promote its unlimited use. The probable origin of this approach was the work of Fuller Albright and his colleagues at Harvard Medical School and Massachusetts General Hospital. In a 1941 *JAMA* article, Albright claimed that the "postmenopausal state" was the most significant factor in osteoporosis and that estrogen therapy helped bones retain calcium.[95] Following the implications of their mentor's work, Albright's students Philip Henneman and Stanley Wallach believed that long-term use of estrogens was important to halt the progression of postmenopausal osteoporosis.[96] Making bolder claims than had their teacher, Henneman and Wallach also suggested that estrogen therapy benefitted women's "emotional stability, sleep patterns and sense of energy," constituting an "important dividend of estrogen therapy." This dividend alone provided "sufficient reason for the general use of prolonged estrogen replacement of the postmenopausal woman."[97]

Other researchers made similar claims about the ability of long-term estrogen therapy to reduce coronary atherosclerosis in postmenopausal women. As early as 1953, researchers claimed that women's increased incidence of heart disease after menopause was due to decreased estrogen, and, by 1954, researchers claimed that estrogen therapy decreased the incidence of heart disease. This led to the recommendation for long-term hormone use to prevent heart disease.[98]

By the 1950s, physicians began making bolder claims regarding the benefits of long-term hormone use. In 1954, E. Kost Shelton, Clinical

Professor of Medicine at the University of California at Los Angeles and proprietor of the Shelton Clinic, claimed that limiting the duration of estrogen therapy cheated women. In establishing his case, Shelton described both the ravages of menopause and the rejuvenation afforded by hormones, focusing on the aspects that potentially affected a woman's ability to attract and hold a mate. He warned that menopause frequently transformed a woman into a "shell of the former alluring woman." In the past, older women "had fulfilled their destiny as seed-pods and were willing to dry up and blow away. However, the grandmother of today is, or should be, an entirely different person. She no longer willingly relinquishes the husband of her youth to the designing widow down the street. . . . [B]y clever cosmetology, greater social freedom and smarter raiment she can hold her place with women twenty years her junior—that is, provided she remains in some degree physiologically intact."[99] He vehemently rebutted the argument that because menopause was natural, it should be allowed to progress without intervention. He pointed to the apparent fallacies of such a position. "The final argument that the menopause is a natural phenomenon and should not be tampered with, is to me the most vapid of all. It is reminiscent of the outworn arguments against anesthesia . . . against everything progressive in life. . . . The very person who argues that menopause is a natural phenomenon fights nature everyday. He pasteurizes his milk, boils his instruments, vaccinates his stock and his children . . . makes new elements and splits the atom." He further argued that, while other treatments for menopause alleviated symptoms, "they will not postpone the aging process. Estrogen will."[100]

Although Shelton's position remained on the medical fringe, he attracted followers. William H. Masters, who later gained fame as a sex researcher, advocated hormone treatment for all "neutral gender" adults, defined as women past menopause and men past steroid production. He argued that medicine had erstwhile failed to address the needs of this group, and he saw long-term hormone treatment as a way to rectify the slight. He believed that physicians "can no longer ignore the responsibility of effectively supporting our aging population."[101] Allan C. Barnes, chairman of obstetrics and gynecology at Johns Hopkins University, agreed. In his often cited 1962 article "Is Menopause a Disease?" he noted the impending tide of women who would "outlive" their ovaries. He warned that unless this "deficiency" was remedied, these women would experience decades of unnecessary and rapid physical decline.[102]

These advocates of long-term hormone use held several things in common. First, they viewed the *ability* to treat women with hormones as an *obligation* to do so. They claimed that conscientious physicians must provide their patients with this pharmaceutical fountain of youth, arguing that doctors owed it to the aging population. Second, hormone supporters denied that natural or universal processes were necessarily desirable. Death was natural, they argued, yet physicians spent their lives plotting their patients' escape from its throes. Finally, with the exception of Barnes, these doctors stressed the cosmetic benefits of hormone therapy. These physicians assumed women feared becoming less "womanly" and losing their attractiveness.

This position on hormone use did not represent common medical thought, even in the 1950s. The rhetoric of Shelton, Masters, and others, however, foreshadowed a trend that would intensify throughout the 1960s. Despite the emerging claims for and research on the benefits of long-term estrogen therapy in treating osteoporosis and atherosclerosis and the more radical claims that hormones could delay aging itself, most published physicians between 1938 and 1962 remained cautious about their use.

In general then, the medical sources paint a portrait of medical restraint. They suggest a clinical encounter in which physicians listened to their patients' complaints and offered advice and reassurance. Women in these imagined settings were not reduced to their symptoms but were treated as people. Menopause, too, was treated as a complex social and biological transition and not reduced to the consequences of ovarian failure. Physicians, although generally valuing hormones as useful medicine, nevertheless discouraged their widespread use, recommending instead mild sedatives to ease women through their physical and social discomforts. The medical literature suggests that when physicians did prescribe hormones, they did so as a short-term attempt to palliate symptoms rather than as a strategy to forestall or prevent the long-term effects of estrogen depletion.

And yet the intensity of this conservative advice and its very repetition suggest an attempt by the medical elite to correct some aspect of current practice. Indeed, the medical literature itself, combined with other forms of evidence, intimates that not all physicians exercised therapeutic restraint when it came to their menopausal patients. Perhaps some physicians, and some menopausal women, regarded hormone therapy as a safe and effective treatment for the variety of ills plaguing women at middle age.

The Medical Encounter: The Hormonal Fix

Somewhat obscured within the larger message of medical caution, expressions of dismay at the indiscriminate and perhaps dangerous use of hormones also appear in the medical literature throughout the 1940s and 1950s. Some physicians worried that hormones were being over-prescribed for middle-aged women and condemned widespread use of estrogen as therapeutic abuse rooted in shoddy diagnostics.[103] In 1948, for example, a Philadelphia gynecologist complained: "Too often when a patient in the fifth decade of her life presents herself to her physician for advice, she is told that her symptoms are due to the 'menopause,' is treated with some hormone preparation and often is not even examined. It is too easy for the busy or undiscriminating physicians to place patients at this age in the category of 'going through the menopause' on 'hormone pills' without adequate investigation."[104]

A few physicians feared that the economic benefits of hormones discouraged careful diagnosis and therapeutic restraint. Gynecologist Chloe Fry, for example, warned that estrogen therapy had "become a lucrative racket" in medicine and that it encouraged physicians to forgo the "time consuming practice" of diagnosis."[105] The indiscriminate use of hormones endangered women, a few doctors scolded. Without specifying the risks, these doctors insisted that unnecessary hormone therapy posed "a distinct menace" to women.[106]

Survey evidence suggests that physicians were right to be concerned. A 1941 survey of one hundred women indicated that roughly 28 percent of all postmenopausal women had received some kind of medication at menopause, either hormones or sedatives.[107] Further, more than 30 percent of both the Brush women (surveyed in 1950) and the Davidoff women (interviewed in 1957) received at least some hormone therapy.[108] All of these sources indicate that hormones were used more widely than the medical literature advised, suggesting that the model of therapeutic restraint was frequently ignored.[109]

How does the caution expressed in the medical literature fit with the widespread hormone use among women in a certain privileged demographic? As anthropologist Margaret Lock has noted, the therapeutic protocol advocated in the medical literature does not necessarily describe the behaviors and the decisions of physicians in the clinical setting. For a variety of reasons—some based on physicians' own experiences and others determined by the experiences of their patients—physicians developed strategies for caring for menopausal women quite different from those in the model proposed by the medical elite.[110]

Several factors contributed to the liberal use of hormones. First, the use of estrogens in this period must be understood within the context of a larger therapeutic revolution. In particular, the development of sulfa drugs and penicillin in the 1930s and 1940s led to the general belief that physicians and the drug therapies they controlled could cure disease with a bottle of pills. In the wake of these new "miracle drugs" and the accompanying increased faith in medicine, physicians were encouraged by drug manufacturers and patients alike to end a medical encounter by prescribing a drug.[111]

Capitalizing on their successes, drug companies began promoting their products in earnest, approaching physicians both through print advertisements in medical journals and through the newly emerged practice of detailing, direct sales visits to doctors. This changed approach to advertising reflects, in part, new regulations put in place to control the distribution of pharmaceuticals in the United States. In the wake of a drug tragedy that killed more than one hundred people, Congress enacted the Food, Drug and Cosmetic Act of 1938. This act required that all drugs be tested for safety, and it created the category of prescription drugs. Before this legislation, patients could in theory (if rarely in practice) obtain most drugs directly from their pharmacists. After 1938 (the same year that Dodds developed DES), drug companies advertised less often to consumers and more often to physicians. The shift was dramatic. In 1930, drug companies targeted roughly 90 percent of their advertising budget at consumers. By the early 1970s, direct-to-consumer drug advertising had fallen to roughly 20 percent of the advertising budget, most of which related to the continued marketing of over-the-counter medications.[112]

Menopausal hormone advertisements directed at physicians in the 1940s and 1950s promoted estrogen as the solution to a wide variety of complaints. Headaches, vaginitis, nervousness, hot flashes, and family discord were all allegedly cured by the administration of conjugated or synthetic estrogens. Combinations of tranquilizers (meprobamate) and estrogen guaranteed a menopausal "transition without tears" and advertisements for Premarin stressed its ability to secure "that feeling of well-being."[113] Advertisements also promoted menopausal estrogen as a therapy for the whole patient. Take, for example, a 1959 advertisement for Premarin. "When, because of the menopause, the psyche needs nursing—'Premarin' nurses. When hot flushes need suppressing, 'Premarin' suppresses. In short, when you want to treat the whole menopause (and how else is it to be treated?), let your choice be 'Premarin.'"[114] These ads presented hormone therapy as a way to meet the various needs of menopausal patients: physiological, sexual, or psychological. Surely some physicians faced with distressed patients recalled these ads when deciding on a therapeutic course.[115]

The significance of print advertisements, however, paled in comparison to the influence of detailing or direct sales to physicians. By 1961, the major drug houses spent almost 60 percent of their advertising dollars on detailing. Indeed, physicians in the 1950s were much more likely to learn about drug efficacy and advisability from a detail man than from a journal article.[116] Emil Novak in 1945 noted this trend with dismay when he accused his colleagues of too often following the advice of hormone manufacturers rather than reading the medical literature.[117]

But drug company tactics were only one source of the pressure physicians felt to prescribe hormones. Patients also demanded them. Again, hormones were not unique in this respect. Newspapers and magazines regularly heralded new medical breakthroughs in the treatment of disease. Cures for cancer, asthma, baldness: all seemed within reach by popping the top off a bottle of pills.[118] The promise of modern medicine encouraged patients to see their physician to secure a specific prescription rather than medical advice.[119] Indeed, physicians noted with exasperation that their patients came to them asking for tranquilizers for family strife and antibiotics for colds. Worried that patients would take their medical business elsewhere, however, physicians often gave in to their patients' demands.[120]

In the case of hormones, the evidence suggests that this pressure was intense. Physicians writing in both the medical and the popular literature complained that women sought medical care at menopause with the expressed purpose of receiving hormones. Gynecologist Joseph Rogers, for example, maintained that women "report to the physician asking for the 'change-of-life shots.'"[121] Other doctors, mostly gynecologists, complained that women "expect hormone treatment during the menopause and they like it because of the immediate relief it gives them." A professor of obstetrics and gynecology claimed in 1957 that women "actually beg the physician" for treatment that would "prevent the development of any of the troublesome symptoms."[122]

Sometimes husbands, rather than their menopausal wives, demanded that hormone treatment be made available. Obstetrician and gynecologist Frederic Loomis, for example, urged husbands to guide their irritating wives to doctors for treatment. As a 1950 *Better Homes and Gardens* article suggests, "long-suffering" husbands were sometimes the impetus behind a visit to the doctor and a demand for hormone shots.[123] (A more thorough examination of the family response to menopause appears in

Chapter 5.) The image of an impatient husband waiting in the car while his wife secures a prescription complicates our understanding of patient demand. While most women probably sought hormones to help themselves feel better, others may have been driven to hormone use to make their husbands feel better about their wives.

Some physicians protested that women's expectations were completely unreasonable. Abner Weisman felt compelled to remind women that there was "no fountain of youth." He claimed that far too many aging women try to "cling to their youth by the use of hormones or anything else that offers hope." He worried that some women believed that "perennial youth" could be purchased "at the cosmetic counter or at the doctor's office." Another physician similarly protested the unrealistic demands of his patients. He claimed that many women, having been misled by their friends, believed aging could be postponed by using hormones.[124]

While most doctors seemed to view patient demand as a challenge to their authority, a few welcomed women's input. Minnie Goldberg, perhaps not coincidentally a female physician, viewed women's demands in a different light. She noted with approval that menopausal women, "enlightened by our uninhibited press, and by the reports of their hormonally treated sisters, insist on more than reassurance and explanations of facts long known to them. They want relief and they are entitled to it." Note that Goldberg did not advocate hormones for all menopausal women. She believed that reassurance and sedation played an important role in the medical treatment of menopause. Still she argued that women were not mistaken in diagnosing their own suffering and that suffering women could best be treated, at least sometimes, with estrogens.[125]

Despite physicians' dismay at women's demand for hormones, a look at the popular literature makes women's fascination with the treatment understandable. Enthusiasm in the popular literature for the available medical marvel of hormone therapy may have propelled some women to their physicians.[126] The literature heralded hormone treatments as "one of the most brilliant accomplishments of modern medicine."[127] Journalist Maxine Davis proclaimed that because "modern medical science has swept away the cobwebs of superstition" women no longer needed to "suffer from the change of life."[128] Declaring the march of medical progress nothing short of divine, Albert Maisel promoted the "medical miracles" brought by hormone therapy, claiming that it saved at least "half a million women every year . . . from . . . terror and illness."[129] This literature highlighted the horrors experienced by past generations who endured the trials of menopause without medical assistance. University of Wisconsin endocrinologist Elmer Sevringhaus, for example, insisted that the triumph of medical research allowed the present generation of middle-aged women to escape the physical and mental discomforts endured by their grandmothers.[130]

Although most of the popular literature emphasized that only a few women needed therapy, some medical writers indicated that hormone therapy held promise for many, if not all, women. Helen Haberman, for example, wrote in 1941 that estrogen "could mitigate the suffering of millions of women."[131] Bernadine Bailey similarly reported enthusiastically on the benefits of hormones. She claimed that women on hormones experienced a "magical transformation" leading to a "thrilling new self confidence . . . greater energy and sense of well-being." She goaded her readers to seek out hormone therapy, dismissing women's resistance as wrongheaded and old-fashioned: "Like a well run train, put on the brakes gradually, via medical science's newest aid to women. . . . Don't be like the supposedly intelligent woman who [refused to take hormones] who said, 'Indeed I won't! Our grandmothers got along without those things, and I guess we can too.' But who wants to go back to the good all days of kerosene lamps, unpaved streets, wood-burning ranges, cotton-stockings—and the 'fearsome' forties."[132] A physician writing in the popular health magazine *Hygeia* similarly encouraged his readers to take advantage of scientific remedies. He insisted that resistance was both "foolhardy" and "dangerous."[133] Physician Miriam Lincoln likewise urged any woman with hot flashes to "go at once to her doctor, tell him her woes and get a supply of hormone medicine, for hormones cure the hot flashes like magic."[134]

These popular characterizations made it seem reasonable and progressive for women to seek medical relief at menopause. The modern woman should reject the plight of her grandmother, resist the role of martyr, and take control of her body and her health. Medical science made that control possible. Even when these authors claimed that most women would not need hormones, women with symptoms might have assumed that *their* symptoms required medical intervention.

The laudatory depictions of estrogen therapy impelled more than a few women to seek out the latest and greatest medical treatment. At the very least, some women sought out medical advice at menopause. Still, a 1941 report indicated that only 28 percent of the women surveyed sought medical care at menopause.[135] Women from both the Brush and Davidoff samples indicated that they found it appropriate to turn to medicine to alleviate their menopausal symptoms. Edith Filmore urged her counterparts to "consult a good doctor for physical ills and a psychiatrist if neces-sary."[136] Lydia Fanning remarked that she survived the menopause "by be-ing too busy and letting the doctor do the prescribing."[137]

Other women specifically embraced medical care because of the avail-ability of hormone treatments. For example, a Brush respondent taking DES claimed that "with all the things there are today to make you com-fortable . . . it is silly not to go to a doctor and get help."[138] Another woman similarly advised women to "go immediately to a doctor when symptoms appear—either mental, physical or emotional—A few pills or a shot or two can work wonders—and to me solves the whole problem of menopause." She urged other women to "be sensible and treat as any ache or pain."[139] Ada Cooper similarly advised menopausal women to "seek and accept the help of a good physician."[140]

Some women's demands for hormone therapy suggests that the medi-calization of menopause was not foisted on passive patients.[141] Women who turned to their doctors for assistance, who occasionally requested hormone treatments, accepted, embraced, and encouraged increased medical involvement in menopause.

Women's eagerness to take hormones and physicians' willingness to prescribe them does not mean that either group considered menopause pathological. As already demonstrated, physicians insisted that menopause was not a disease but a natural process. For the Brush and Davidoff re-spondents, too, hormonal treatment did not elevate menopause to the sta-tus of a disease; rather, it allowed women to diminish the significance of menopause in their lives. Two women who urged others to forget about menopause and to "think of it as little as possible," for example, were nev-ertheless themselves receiving hormones.[142] Similarly, Ella Davenport be-lieved that "medical progress" had allowed women to "take the meno-pause in stride."[143] Another Brush respondent, Hannah Martin, scolded women for exaggerating the significance of menopause. Her "nice pink pills" controlled her symptoms and allowed her to ignore menopause.[144] In this way, hormones did not encourage women to see menopause as pathological: it encouraged them to view it as inconsequential.

Nevertheless, comments from doctors and women alike indicate that some of the rhetoric extolling hormone therapy as a necessary replacement for declining estrogen had begun to be accepted by menopausal women in the 1950s. When one Smith graduate claimed that her doctor provided the "body elements lacking" she suggests that she believed her body was incomplete, perhaps inadequate, when lacking significant amounts of estrogen. A gynecologist sensed the same trend when he complained that women were demanding hormones because they liked the "feeling that a deficiency is being supplied, that a vital force is being restored as if by magic."[145] In subtle ways, perhaps, the language of "estrogen deficiency" was beginning to influence how menopausal women understood and experienced the changes in their bodies.

Although most of the Brush and Davidoff women seemed pleased with their physicians and their medical care, a few women were disappointed by the effects of hormone therapy. Jane Petit, for example, took hormones for awhile but "gave them up as a bad idea—an attitude now confirmed, I understand, by gynecologists."[146] Another woman "tried a few shots" but found that the "cold chills they induced were worse . . . than the hot flashes."[147] Ruth Mandelbaum received hormones from her doctor but, believing that "she took them too long," she changed doctors.[148]

Other women were frustrated by their physicians' unresponsive attitudes to their complaints about menopausal symptoms. Theresa Walters, for example, remembered incredulously that her doctor had told her to "grit your teeth and take it."[149] A participant in the Davidoff study wept as she recounted that her doctor had told her to "weather it by keeping very busy and laughing at self."[150] Beryl Stimsen, who advised women to visit their doctors for "reassurance," nevertheless failed to speak glowingly of the result. "From what I hear the average doctor is not too good in dealing with this particular phase of a woman's life. Perhaps gynecologists and obstetricians are wiser but I have heard of many cases when it seemed as if a little kindly advice would have helped immensely."[151] These examples demonstrate that, despite widespread faith in physicians and medical care in the 1950s, the specific experience of the medical encounter addressing menopause was sometimes, perhaps often, disappointing.

FOUR

"The Change Emancipates Women"

Menopause, Domesticity, and Liberation in the Popular Literature, 1938–1962

In 1949, endocrinologist Edwin Hamblen explained to women how they should understand the physical and social transition of the menopause. "The change of life," he wrote, separated two equally important and active phases of womanhood. The first phase was for "procreation and for the fulfillment of racial responsibilities." The era after menopause, however, provided a woman an opportunity for "the realization of her personal aims and aspirations. Released from her reproductive functions, woman . . . often enjoys greater health and more freedom of self expression. . . . These become her prime years of life." Hamblen's rosy depiction of the postmenopausal years offered hope and reassurance to women who might have been approaching middle age with apprehension or dread. He suggested that menopause marked the beginning of personal fulfillment and a focus on the self. Even as he promoted the liberating effects of menopause, however, he reinforced the notion that before menopause women were obligated to sacrifice personal ambitions to the needs of family and "race."[1]

Hamblen's comments illustrate a trend in the cultural prescriptions about menopause common between 1938 and 1962. Popular advice literature typically emphasized the liberating aspects of life beyond the reach of childbearing while reinforcing the reproductive obligations of middle-class women. As demonstrated in Chapter 3, discussions of hormone replacement therapy dominated the medical literature on menopause during this period. Although the popular health literature similarly heralded the benefits of hormones, it simultaneously raised issues unrelated to medicine and medical developments. Popular writers stressed that menopause, marking the end of fertility, produced both physical and social changes in women's lives. Popular health texts consequently offered advice about alleviating the discomforts of hot flashes and filling the hours of newly available free time.

The popular discussion of the physical consequences of menopause focused primarily on hot flashes, vaginal dryness, frayed nerves, and figure control. The consideration of the social consequences ventured further afield. These discussions engaged with questions about the very nature and meaning of womanhood. What did it mean to be a woman after forcible retirement from her presumed biologic career? What were her responsibilities within the home? What was her role outside it? What gendered expectations remained in effect as postmenopausal women assumed their new roles? How did women's postmenopausal roles reinforce gendered social roles for younger women?

In response to these and similar questions, the popular health literature emphasized the liberating aspects of menopause. Popular health writers recognized that by releasing women from their reproductive obligations, menopause allowed them to move beyond the demands of home and family. Indeed, many writers believed that menopause should be welcomed because it marked the beginning of physical and social rewards for women. The literature encouraged menopausal and postmenopausal women to resurrect long-dormant personal interests, to dedicate themselves to worthy causes, and to enjoy their "golden years." The various transformations of menopause provided a culturally sanctioned opportunity for women to expand their interests and influence.

Between 1938 and 1962, however, the freedom from gendered constraints was far from absolute. While menopause allowed women to expand their activities in significant ways, the popular literature of the period reminded middle-aged women of their continued obligation to act "womanly." Menopause allowed women to throw away both diaphragms and diapers, but gender continued to define and constrain their activities and behaviors. In particular, discussions of menopause typically reminded women of their continued domestic obligations, the value of self-denial, and the appropriateness of pursuing a role in community care-taking.

Further, by emphasizing the freedom gained at menopause, the popular literature simultaneously reinforced women's domestic duties during their fertile years. Popular health texts on menopause generally assumed that women devoted their premenopausal years to childbearing and homemaking. Indeed, magazine articles and self-help books warned their readers of the potentially dire consequences of refusing to fulfill these biological and social obligations. The emphasis on motherhood reminded middle-aged women of the costs of ignoring their biological calling, and in doing so, prescribed a life-course for all women. Women could follow their own dreams and interests outside the home, but only after they had fulfilled their domestic obligations.

Class and race assumptions undergirded the discussion of middle-aged womanhood in mid-twentieth-century America. When popular writers described how women's lives might change at menopause, they included only certain women. Popular accounts, for example, generally assumed that menopausal women, supported comfortably by a hard-working husband, did not work for wages. Instead, women described in such accounts devoted their time and energy to child rearing and housekeeping, with an occasional afternoon off for a round of bridge. While this profile probably captured the experiences of some white, middle-class women, it certainly did not describe the lives of most working-class women, both black and white.

The discussion of womanhood inspired by menopause did not, of course, emerge from a cultural vacuum. Women's social roles and the meaning of womanhood have never been absolute and have always required constant attention, maintenance, and adjustment. Despite the different circumstances brought on by the Depression, World War II, and postwar prosperity and global uncertainty, women's roles within the home and outside it remained a constant concern in the culture. The popular texts on menopause arose from this environment. Indeed, the bodies (and minds) of menopausal women served as a site for engaging larger cultural questions of women's roles.

Women and Domesticity

During the Depression and continuing into World War II, white women entered the workforce in unprecedented and ever-increasing numbers. During the Depression, the inability of many men to provide for their families forced some women, both married and single, into the workforce. During the labor shortages of the subsequent war years, war propaganda called upon women to fulfill their patriotic duty by embracing nontraditional jobs. Neither the Depression nor the war, however, led to a cultural acceptance of working women, particularly if they were white, particularly if they were married. Neither emergency loosened the hold of a domestic ideology that encouraged white women to devote their lives to their families and to value "dependence, submissiveness, and self-abnegation." Indeed, according to historian Nancy Woloch, the emergencies created by the Depression and the war did not weaken domesticity but rather "confirmed a shared conviction that in the best of times as in the worst of times woman's place was in the home."[2]

In the cold war years, domestic prescriptions intensified, perhaps as a reaction to women's wartime penetration into traditional male bastions.[3] In her book *Homeward Bound: American Families in the Cold War Era,* Elaine Tyler May characterizes the gender prescriptions during this period as "domestic containment." Within this model, women were expected to eschew careers and to gain happiness and satisfaction through their roles as wives and mothers.[4] Within marriage, traditional models of femininity reemerged, challenging the tenets of the more egalitarian (at least in theory) companionate marriage. As evidenced by several trends, some women eagerly embraced domesticity, racing to the altar young and in record numbers and birthing the demographic blip known as the baby boom. Other women aspired to such roles, but financial need or racial discrimination prevented it. (The divorce rate also surged briefly after the war, reflecting, perhaps, dissatisfaction with hasty wartime marriages.)[5] Further, surveys regularly indicated that "domesticated" women were happy with their choices. A 1955 *Life* magazine survey of housewives found that nine of ten women claimed that they liked and found personal satisfaction in housework, and a 1962 Gallup poll claimed that "few people are as happy as a housewife."[6]

But the popular media did not merely promote a life of Jello molds and Hoover vacuums. While "domestic containment" does characterize some of the popular rhetoric aimed at middle- and upper-class women in the postwar period, popular culture and the lived experience of women suggests a more complex gender ideology. As Joanne Meyerowitz has shown in her study of popular magazines between 1945 and 1962, women who pursued lives unbounded by domestic containment were regularly valorized. Women with demanding careers often appeared with approval and admiration in popular periodicals. While these articles frequently highlighted career women's concessions to domesticity and femininity, Meyerowitz argues that "they did not serve solely or even primarily as lessons in traditional gender roles."[7]

Further, American popular culture in the 1950s acknowledged that a life devoted solely to home and family did not always lead to happiness and fulfillment, even for the women with the economic means to secure such a life. Indeed, popular magazines in the postwar period readily admitted that marriage and motherhood, while central to the expectations of middle- and upper-class womanhood, could be frustrating, dull, and exhausting. Even before the war's end, women were voicing their dissatisfaction with lives dominated by washing, cooking, and ironing. Some texts encouraged a more complete embrace of domesticity as the solution to women's dissatisfaction with homemaking, but others highlighted the benefits and joys of professional careers. The popular media thus legitimated both domestic containment and professional achievement for women, sometimes in the same article. Consequently, popular magazines offered women more than one model of womanhood.[8]

Acknowledging that some women wanted (and other women were forced to seek out) something other than pot roast and patty-cake to fill their days, the popular media explored the legitimacy of wage-labor for women. While some sources urged women, particularly married, middle-class women, to devote themselves full-time to homemaking duties, as the war years receded, more and more popular articles demonstrated how women could juggle the responsibilities of both home and paid employment.[9] Organizations such as the National Manpower Council and the Commission on the Education of Women worked to bring more women into the labor force and to improve their lives while employed.[10]

And women, even middle-class white women, did venture beyond their front stoops for purposes other than PTA meetings and bridge parties. The trend toward increasing female employment, which had begun even before the Depression and had accelerated during World War II, did not diminish in the 1950s even in the face of a growing emphasis on domesticity. While many of the women who had never worked before the war did tend to return home after it, female employment continued to grow.[11] By 1950, compelled by basic financial need, the desire for a new washing machine, or a yearning for personal fulfillment, a third of all women worked (though only one-third of those worked full-time) and roughly 50 percent of working women were married, doubling the 1945 figure.[12] By 1960, 30.5 percent of wives worked for wages.[13]

Should a woman find personal fulfillment at home or in the workplace? Could a woman be a good mother and a valuable worker? These unresolved questions encouraged an explicit debate on (or at least discussion of) women's place and encouraged the consideration of the "dilemma" of the "modern woman."[14] Some pundits recognized, as Margaret Mead noted in 1946, that "modern" women, pulled by the call of both personal ambition and domestic life, felt "confused, uncertain and discontented with the present definition of women's place in America."[15] Glossy magazines, best-selling books, and academic journals all weighed in on women's biological purpose, psychological adjustment, and social roles. Some social commentators, led by psychiatrists and psychologists, urged women to embrace motherhood and the "feminine" ideals of passivity and dependence, rather than work outside the home. This view was articulated most famously by Ferdinand Lundberg and psychiatrist Marynia Farnham. In their best-selling 1947 book, *Modern Woman: The Lost Sex,* they described the gravity of the problem as they saw it, charging that "contemporary women in very large numbers are psychologically disordered" because they were tempted by "masculine strivings." Victimized by the false promises of feminism, these unfortunate women developed in the world outside the home the "characteristics of aggression, dominance, independence and power." Farnham and Lundberg insisted that women needed to be guided back to "satisfactions profoundly feminine" that could only be found within domestic life.[16] Other commentators, mostly women professionals, condemned such domestic ideology, however, claiming that it unfairly restricted women's achievements, costing women and society dearly. Sociologist Mirra Komarovsky, argued, for example, that domesticity left women open to "self-abased subjection to tyranny and a deterioration of personality." She and her fellow travelers urged instead self-reliance and personal fulfillment.[17]

The particular physiological and social situation of menopausal women was used as evidence by both sides of this debate. In general, this situation created an opening for ideological compromise within the larger cultural discussion. Acknowledging that full-time domesticity did not always provide everything women might want from life, popular health writers promoted menopause as the physiological escape route: middle-class women did not need to choose between home and career. Women could do it all, fulfill their biological obligations to reproduce and later pursue goals of a more personal bent. Further, because women should not reach middle age completely unprepared to pursue their wider ambitions, earlier steps toward exploring their interests were validated, if only slightly.

Expect Very Little Trouble

Before 1938, women looking for published information about the menopausal transition had limited options. While a few magazine articles in

Hygeia and the radical *Independent Woman* instructed women on how to cope with the "change of life," most discussion was limited to books bearing titles such as *What a Woman of Forty-Five Ought to Know* (1902) and *The Woman Asks the Doctor* (1935). Between 1938 and 1962, the sources of information available to women expanded significantly. Magazines, marriage manuals, family health guides, and public health pamphlets all carried advice about menopause. But publication on menopause did not occur evenly throughout this period. Although the development of conjugated and synthetic estrogens between 1938 and 1942 contributed to a spike in publications on menopause, the great majority of information was published only after World War II.

Although this literature addressed a lay audience, it was overwhelmingly medical in perspective. The authors were primarily physicians—usually gynecologists—but even when nurses, journalists, and other social commentators contributed to the genre, they relied heavily on medical sources and the results did not generally differ from what the physicians produced.

These sources targeted, at least for the most part, white, middle-class women who had the economic means and leisure time to make non-emergency personal health a priority. This audience also had the financial resources that enabled them (in theory at least) to abide by the cultural demands placed on women. But surely women outside this narrow demographic, anxious for reassurance and advice, also read these texts. These texts' construction of womanhood, both before menopause and after, was bounded by class and race.

The popular literature of the period generally prepared women for the physical effects of menopause by insisting that it was a natural event, much like menarche in reverse, that gave most women very little trouble.[18] Indeed, advice texts routinely insisted that 75 to 90 percent of all menopausal women experienced only minor inconvenience or no symptoms at all. Most authors agreed with health educator and popular writer Maxine Davis, who claimed in her 1951 book, *Facts about the Menopause,* that "the large majority of women can and do take the menopause as an incident of life and either notice it not at all or else shrug off its transient annoyances as indifferently as they do the sniffles."[19]

To allay their readers' fears, the popular health writers explained the physiological processes of menopause. The aging (or, in some cases, failing) ovary was identified as the cause of the physiological changes. According to these accounts, as ovaries gradually "wore out," they no longer produced much estrogen, though some writers pointedly insisted that the ovaries and adrenals continued to produce some. The pituitary responded to the decreased estrogen by vigorously producing more hormones, in a futile attempt to coax the ovary back into production. As one author put it, "the combination of a too persistent pituitary and progressively failing ovaries" led to a body out of balance.[20] But imbalance was only part of the problem. Decreased estrogen production also led to the withdrawal of the "distinctly feminine physical traits" and to changes in "all organs that characterized the female."[21] The ovaries and the uterus shrank, the lining of the vagina thinned, and the breasts "grew flabby." The decreased estrogen (and progesterone) disrupted the proliferation and shedding of the endometrium, leading to sporadic menstrual periods, sometimes scant, sometimes heavy; eventually, menstruation disappeared altogether. Despite the widespread changes caused by the declining ovary or the tenacious pituitary, the popular health writers generally insisted that women's bodies eventually did find a new equilibrium. Noting the systemic nature of these changes, physicians and other health writers did not claim that menopause passed without notice. Nevertheless, they encouraged women to see the physical twinges as irksome rather than serious.

Hot flashes (or flushes) for example, received particular attention, not because they were serious but because they could be disconcerting. For the most part, popular descriptions of the hot flash made it sound fairly benign: a feeling of warmth centered in the upper body that rapidly moved up into the neck and head. A few women authors, however, described the disruption these "quick flushes" could cause. Davis, for example, admitted that hot flashes sent many women rushing to the window in the middle of the night, "gasping for air." Miriam Lincoln, professor of medicine at Washington University, reassuringly claimed in 1950 that some hot flashes were "scarcely noticeable," but she also conceded that some women became "disoriented and confused" by their bodies' misfiring thermostat. "She is not only hot and uncomfortable, but also embarrassed and enraged." Lincoln asked her readers to sympathize with the plight of some women who wake up in the middle of the night with wet sheets, wet nightgowns, and wet (and presumably displeased) husbands.[22] These accounts make clear that hot flashes don't pose a serious health concern, but they also challenge the depiction of flushes as essentially harmless.

The hot flash received particular attention, but health writers acknowledged other physical symptoms of menopause as well. These included headaches, heart palpitations, numbness, dizziness, joint pain, frequent urination, weight gain, and an inability to concentrate. Again, the advice downplayed the significance of these symptoms and urged women to take them in stride. Popular texts frequently compared menopause to menstruation, reminding women that menstruation, clearly a natural process, also caused minor inconveniences. Women should consider menopausal twinges as no more significant than menstrual cramps.[23]

Nervousness and Irritability

While generally downplaying the physical effects of menopause for most women, physicians and other popular health writers nevertheless conceded that many menopausal women suffered emotionally. Medical writers routinely listed nervousness—a vague and fluid category that included irritability, anxiety, and weepiness—as a frequent companion of menopausal women. Physician Lincoln described the variety of nervous symptoms as ranging from a "suspicion that life is not as wonderful as formerly believed, through mild irritability, to tension that makes sleep elusive. The extreme of nervousness may bring periods of emotionalism when anger or tears appear without normal provocation."[24] In his 1947 article, "Why Nervousness at 45?" Harold Shryock described the plight of one of his "nervous" patients: "Her thoughts at night were so full of anxiety and followed each other in such rapid succession that it almost seemed as if she were listening to some alarming broadcast . . . Loss of sleep left her with such meager store of energy that it was hard to carry on."[25]

Medical experts and health writers disagreed about why menopause made women nervous. Some writers blamed menopause's emotional "symptoms" on its physiological changes. As popular health writer Madeline Gray put it, as various glands tried to compensate for the diminished supply of estrogen, the whole nervous system was thrown "out of balance." As a result, menopause could "shake you up from tip to toe." A physician compared menopause to cigarette withdrawal: Just as lack of nicotine made smokers testy, he claimed estrogen withdrawal similarly made menopausal women irritable.[26] More often, however, medical writers argued that apprehension rather than physiology caused the very symptoms and circumstances women dreaded. Physician Edward Stieglitz, for example, insisted in 1946 that "apprehension raised by old wives' tales, unwise physicians, and well-meaning confidants is a more potent source of turmoil than the physiologic" changes of menopause.[27] Davis described in 1948 how apprehension became a self-fulfilling prophecy. She told the story of a very successful businesswoman who dreaded the emotional and physical consequences of menopause. At the first signs of menstrual irregularity, her personal life fell apart, just as she had predicted: "One of her daughters ran away from Vassar to a gypsy marriage in a trailer home. She brooded over her suspicions of her husband and a synthetic redhead." Davis reproached this woman, claiming that it was not menopause but her fear of it that caused "the very destruction that she feared."[28] It is unclear how this woman's fear would have led her daughter to leave college, but this example illustrates how women were blamed for bringing their menopausal problems on themselves by their "irrational" fears.

The popular literature also claimed that menopausal women often overreacted to "trivial" concerns. Edwin Hamblen, director of the Duke Sex Endocrine Clinic, for example, noted that at menopause "small vexations, which in the past caused no worry," became difficult to ignore and kept "recurring to be turned over and over in the mind."[29] Another physician noted in 1952 that menopausal women were "easily excited" and likely to "become upset over trifles."[30] These examples invite speculation on the nature of the "trivial" vexations at issue. A husband might consider shoes left in the living room trivial; a teenage son might regard sandwich fixings left on the drainboard as trifling. For a menopausal woman (or any other woman for that matter) the cumulative effect of years spent moving shoes and wiping away crumbs might well warrant a fit of pique. Nevertheless, women were condemned for such outbursts, and presumably the shoes were again left in the living room.

Medical writers acknowledged that some women experienced emotional problems at menopause well beyond the occasional nervous twinge or irritable outburst. Some women, they conceded, suffered excruciating depression. Paul de Kruif, widely known at the time for his descriptions of microbe hunters, vividly described in 1948 "the melancholy that haunts many women in this condition, so that they lose interest in life, cry for no reason at all, lie awake at night with anxiety that something dreadful is going to happen, begin to believe that the world and even their dear ones are against them."[31] These women too were blamed for overreacting to what should be seen as an inevitable and normal moment in women's physiological lives.

While conceding that menopause sometimes led to frayed nerves and less frequently to debilitating depression, the popular literature rigorously denied the widespread lay belief that menopause frequently drove women crazy. Gynecologist Joseph Rety lamented in 1940 that menopausal insanity had become a "feminine superstition" with distressingly strong staying power. He insisted that real mental disorders at menopause were "extremely rare." Physician Stieglitz dismissed the myth of menopausal insanity as left over from "an age of medicine dominated by superstition and dogma." He reassured women that the "actual chances of a climacteric psychosis are decidedly less than the chances of being permanently and irreparably crippled on the way home from shopping."[32] Gray blamed the "afternoon bridge table" for the unwarranted apprehension. "The game is over, and coffee has not yet been served. There is time for leisurely gossip and talk." Such talk, she maintained, included alarming stories about acquaintances who lost their minds at menopause, leading to misplaced fear.[33] Other popular health writers tried to hedge their bets, denying that menopause caused insanity while noting that it might exacerbate already existing psychoses.[34] Popular writer Bernadine Bailey admitted in 1947 that some women might think that they are losing their minds, but she insisted that no woman goes crazy.[35] By the 1950s, the message was less equivocal: while women could develop mental illness at any age, menopause did not cause mental illness. Lawrence Galton, writing in *Better Homes and Gardens* in 1950, noted that involutional melancholia, the affliction most commonly attributed to menopause, was three times more common in men. Moreover, he maintained, when women were afflicted, menopause was completely uninvolved.[36]

In sum, women seeking information about menopause between 1938 and 1962 learned from the popular media that its physical consequences caused most women very little trouble. Mood swings, generalized nervousness, and even minor depression might unsettle many women, but these effects, too, were generally dismissed as minor inconveniences that would pass with time.

Amid the information about hot flashes and irritability were implicit but clear messages about who needed to be counseled about menopause and whose experiences and behaviors counted to the dominant culture. The menopausal women in these texts frequented bridge parties, spent leisure time shopping, and shuddered at the thought of a daughter living in a trailer. This suggests, of course, that these texts assumed a middle- or upper-class readership. But more significantly, they constructed the menopausal woman as a middle-class woman.

An Emptied Nest?

The popular texts did not limit their discussion of menopause to physiological and emotional reactions originating within women's bodies. They also described the many personal and familial changes that might exacerbate—but not cause—women's difficulties at menopause.[37] These included the rebellion of children as they entered their teens, illness in the family, and marital conflict and estrangement.[38]

Conflating the end of fertility with the end of motherhood, many health writers believed that women worried that their social and familial value disappeared at menopause.[39] One commentator claimed that many women feared the end of "their usefulness to society."[40] In 1951, health educator Davis described the situation more vividly: "Suddenly she, who was needed on all sides . . . finds that her job seems to be done. There are no more faces to wash, no more lessons to help with. . . . The darning basket is almost entirely empty and the house is always orderly. The days can stretch long and lonely."[41] Davis placed the onus of adapting to family changes on the menopausal woman and worried that, if she fails to find ways to remain useful, "she becomes a neurotic patient complaining to her doctor of all the symptoms she has ever heard of, and probably a lot more."[42] Stella Applebaum offered a similar analysis in 1953. She claimed that a menopausal woman's "dilemma lies in the fact that her 'lifetime' job (in the traditional view) is over" at the very time her husband's career is taking off. She claimed that women must learn to adapt to their "changing role as wife, mother and person."[43]

In addition to the problem of the empty nest, popular health writers acknowledged other potentially unsettling changes in household demographics. Writer Gray, for example, warned in 1951 about the need to adjust not only to shrinking families but also to growing ones. She noted that while one child might be moving out, others might be moving back in, bringing spouses and children along.[44] Other authors noted that adult children, especially women, often inherit responsibility for aging parents, both their own and their husband's.[45]

As household demographics frequently changed at middle age, so too did family finances. Reflecting the class assumptions underlying most of these texts, popular health writers frequently described menopause as a time of financial security and increased leisure opportunities.[46] These authors, reflecting, perhaps, the postwar economic boom, assumed that economic stability would allow middle-aged women to enjoy their post-menopausal years. A few commentators admitted, however, that middle age might yield economic hardship rather than financial bounty. Gray, for example, reminded readers of the possible "shock of the financial setbacks that often come at maturity," warning that a husband might have "to scheme hard to hold on to what financial security he has."[47] Other authors reminded readers that economic need might force women into securing jobs in their middle age.[48]

As these examples show, popular texts assumed that family fortunes rose and fell with the efforts of the husband. The sources implied both that women did not work for wages before menopause and that only economic need forced women into the labor market at middle age. Women who supported themselves or who contributed significantly to the economic support of others were largely absent from the popular discussion of menopause. These texts simultaneously described both the social and familial challenges of menopause and the gendered economic roles of women, further constructing the menopausal woman as married and middle class.

Loss and Reconversion

Disruptive hot flashes, sleepless nights, mouthy teenagers, and demanding mothers-in-law introduced real disturbances into the lives of many menopausal women. The popular literature, however, acknowledged that the symbolic significance of menopause also influenced women's reactions to it. Throughout this period, but particularly during the postwar baby boom, what did it mean for women to lose the ability to conceive? In 1948, physician Anna Kleegman Daniels highlighted the significance of the transition, describing menopause as "a period of reconversion from a reproductive or child-bearing body-economy, when woman reproduced the species, to a body-economy when she can no longer reproduce and bear children."[49]

This metaphor of menopause, inspired perhaps by the painful transition from a war-time economy to a peace-time economy, presages Emily Martin's analysis of the discourse surrounding menstruation and menopause. In her 1987 work, *The Woman in the Body*, Martin argues that cultural metaphors of menopause and menstruation fortify women's traditional reproductive roles. She claims that in these descriptions women's bodies serve as procreative factories, subject to work stoppages, breakdown, and, ultimately, obsolescence.[50] Yet while Daniels certainly suggested that women's ability to fulfill their original purpose disappeared at menopause, she resisted characterizing postmenopausal bodies as useless or outmoded. Instead, she believed that postmenopausal women, like the rest of the citizenry, needed to recreate themselves to meet the new demands of their changed roles.

A few popular health writers, mostly physicians, did claim that a woman's biology had only one purpose and that menopause marked the end of her biological and perhaps her social usefulness. These commentators generally believed that women's social role was tied inextricably to their biology; women were designed primarily to bear children. Because menopause marked the end of this ability, these physicians insisted that menopause necessarily prompted feelings of uncompensated loss. Physician Abner Weisman, for example, claimed in 1951 that "women were designed for one purpose and one purpose alone; that is the bearing of children to perpetuate the race." He therefore believed that women must mourn the passing of fertility. He insisted that women who felt "relieved" at menopause were subconsciously "devastated": her "body grieves," he declared.[51] Daniels agreed. She claimed that at menopause, a woman realizes "her biggest asset, her value to the species, her ability to produce 'young,' is gone, gone forever, never to return. No wonder she is depressed. No wonder she literally goes to pieces under this impact of biological doom."[52] Although Daniels believed that most women overstated the negative aspect of menopause, she nevertheless held that women had legitimate reasons for depression.

Miriam Lincoln recognized in 1950 that some women might balk at being characterized solely as baby-makers. She conceded, however, that biological destiny was inescapable.

> Complicated and beautifully engineered, a woman is as fine an instrument for her purpose as a Swiss watch or a jet-propelled airplane is for its use. Intricate and able, she is at the center of all human life. She arrives in the world a miniature creature with her body's life purpose clearly mapped out. . . . As emancipated women, in a wonderfully free land, we may not relish the idea that we are meant chiefly for the propagation of the human race. However, that seems to be the niche we are intended to occupy in the universal biologic plan.[53]

Women's physiology notwithstanding, however, Lincoln did not assume that women would grieve for their lost fecundity at menopause.

That the literature on menopause reinforced women's alleged biological destiny as mothers reflects one side of the postwar debate about the centrality of motherhood in middle-class women's lives. According to historian May, "motherhood was the ultimate fulfillment of female sexuality and the primary source of woman's identity" in the postwar period.[54] Popular culture, particularly movies and magazines, affirmed the maternal ideal. These messages reflected and reinforced the realities of some women's lives. Beginning during World War II and continuing through the 1950s, American couples were having children at an unprecedented rate, reversing a decline in fertility that had lasted for nearly two centuries. This turnabout cut across all social classes. In the 1950s, women bore, on average, 3.2 children, up from 2.4 in the 1930s.[55] An astounding 41 percent of all white women in 1955 claimed that it would be ideal to have four children.[56] Even during this baby boom, alarmists raised the specter of race suicide, reinforcing the need for middle- and upper-class white women to reproduce. The popular media claimed that the more education women attained, the fewer children they bore. In fact, the birthrate increased most sharply among the most educated women.[57] But significantly, women—particularly middle-class women—widely practiced birth control, especially after the first years of marriage.[58] By the time most women reached menopause, they had been actively preventing reproduction for years. The writers of the popular literature must have known that the loss of fertility at menopause was partly symbolic. The emphasis on fertility loss served to remind premenopausal women that although they could control the timing and frequency of pregnancy, contraceptives did not relieve them from the obligation to bear and raise children.

Menopause, Matrimony, and Motherhood

Because the obligation to reproduce loomed so centrally in women's identity, physicians expressed concern about the reaction to menopause of childless and unmarried women. Medical writers did not agree, however, on how single women fared as menopause approached. Some claimed that unmarried women had an easier time accepting the loss of fertility. Endocrinologist Hamblen, for example, believed in 1949 that "spinsters doubtlessly accept sexual aging with more readiness than most married women. To them, ovarian cycles and menstruation have had only a nuisance value." He also maintained that unmarried women had not lost themselves in the needs and demands of their families.[59] Other medical writers claimed that "old maids" suffered more at menopause than women "who have had many children."[60] Sociologist Laura Hutton maintained in 1950 that while unmarried women were not more troubled physically than were married women, the transition carried different psychological meanings for the two groups. She claimed that at menopause a married woman with children "has fulfilled her function as a wife and mother and her body now informs her that this task is finished." In contrast, a single woman has failed to complete her biological task and yet must abandon hope that she might one day become a mother. Hutton maintained that single women typically react with "disappointment and frustration in the recognition that all the wonderful provision made for the bearing of children has been allowed 'to fust in us unused.'"[61]

Gynecologist Weisman offered an even harsher theory in 1951. He maintained that single women experienced a more severe "nervous and emotional reaction" to menopause because their "primary woman functions have never been fulfilled, and the conscious and unconscious hopes of womankind are forever blasted when the menopause comes on." He conceded, however, that married women without children fare better, because "at least part of [their] sexual powers have been put to use."[62] In Weisman's interpretation, childless women suffer not merely from personal disappointment but from the wrath of a thwarted biological imperative.

Physicians showed very little sympathy for women who remained childless or unmarried. Lincoln, a married woman herself, warned that unmarried women had no one but themselves to blame for their grief. A woman who remained single "should blame her own mistakes of action or emotion, her own failure to experience at a proper time of life, those adventures she now feels imperative to the fulfillment of her purpose in life."[63] Gynecologist Harold Imerman agreed, condemning women who after "wasting their fruitful years, feel that they have been cheated."[64] While other physicians did not regard single women as pathological, they generally believed, as one physician noted, that marriage was undeniably more normal. Physician David Cauldwell, for example, best known for his popular pamphlets on transsexuals, did not contend that women must marry, but he believed that "the mated female, as well as the mated male, is invariably a happier and more normal person than the unmated."[65]

The general, though not universal, condemnation of single women and the valorization of marriage and motherhood—at least for white, middle-class women—provided a clear message to women of all ages. Female fulfillment, both social and individual, depended upon creating and tending to a nuclear family. Menopause, this literature warned, marked a biological point of no return. Women seeking to avoid the personal regret, social stigma, and, perhaps, physical discomfort of menopause needed to act while they still could. Only the rare commentator suggested that women who rejected married life experienced fewer changes (and thus less trouble) at the change of life.

But some authors understood that lives devoted solely to homemaking might in retrospect look unappealing to women. Reflecting the larger cultural awareness that some women did not find joy or fulfillment in seeing that their families' clothes looked their whitest white, some popular writers suspected that, when women assessed their lives at menopause, they occasionally concluded that much of their time had been squandered on mind-numbing, unappreciated tasks.[66] Feminist physician Lena Levine claimed that many women "look back on lives that have been fantastically empty, through no fault of their own. Millions of women discover, at the middle of their lives, that they have worn themselves out repeating dull and unrewarding activities, many of which are necessary to keep a normal life routine going."[67] Even some of the male authors admitted that women might come to "detest" the "daily grind" that constitutes much of homemaking.[68]

Presumably responding to such complaints about domesticity, popular health writers described menopause as a well-deserved reward to women for a life of service spent fulfilling their reproductive obligations. Obstetrician Frederic Loomis, for example, encouraged women to regard menopause as a time to "collect some of the rewards that the hard but happy years of sacrifice have stored up for her."[69] Journalist Galton agreed, claiming in 1950 that "menopause is actually a reward—Nature's way of freeing a woman from no-longer-needed childbearing functions and from any monthly inconvenience, liberating her for greater personal pleasure and accomplishment."[70] By positioning menopause as a reward, these authors acknowledged that domesticity demanded a great deal of women and that the rewards of homemaking did not always, by themselves, compensate for the sacrifices some women made. (Perhaps some years were harder than they were happy.) Surely not all (perhaps not even most) women who had children needed to be goaded into motherhood. Nevertheless, packaging menopause as a reward suggested a biological bribe to make the obligatory reproductive years seem less onerous. The rub, however, was that most women had been securing with contraceptives half of what menopause offered, and one suspects that husbands and remaining children (the nest was often far from empty) did not suddenly cook the meals and wash the clothes.

The advice literature on menopause generally urged women to think of menopause as a normal transition with few significant consequences for women who had fulfilled the demands of their biology. A few women might be bothered by hot flashes, and husbands might be bothered by their wives' irritability, but the discussion overwhelmingly assured women that menopause was nothing to worry about. Still, an easy journey through the menopausal transition should not be left to chance, or so the popular literature implied. Indeed, the popular advice had plenty of dos and don'ts for women entering her "best years." Not coincidently, the dos suggested attitudes and behaviors generally consistent with the dictates of domestic containment, even as menopause released women from its most restrictive demands.

Coping with the Change of Life

In 1952, sexologist and physician Samuel Lewin described in his book *Sex After Forty* a case of "menopause at its worst." Lewin's patient suffered from all the serious menopausal problems and "would talk about them fluently and in great detail." Although the patient gained immediate relief through hormone treatments, the remedy helped only briefly. Lewin finally diagnosed that she was "all wrapped up in herself," and he needed to find a way to direct "the patient's interest outward, away from her self." At Lewin's urging, the patient began working for a charity and discovered that she "kept so busy I haven't time to search for symptoms."[71]

This example typifies a position common among popular literature writers regarding the major problems of menopausal women and their solutions. Lewin claimed that his patient suffered because she focused too much attention on herself and talked about her problems. Lewin's treatment, by encouraging her involvement in community affairs, forced his patient's gaze outward, providing her no opportunity to brood about her shortcomings or disappointments.

To help women navigate the physical and social changes they confronted at menopause, the advice literature generally advocated strategies that reinforced gendered behaviors even as these women became less tied to social roles determined by sex. Popular health sources, written mostly by physicians, championed devotion to others and denial of self. But amid this conservative construction of womanhood, the popular discussion of menopause also suggested ways for women to chip away at gendered restrictions forced upon many white, middle-class women of child-bearing age by encouraging occupation (paid or otherwise) beyond the home. These opportunities did not allow women, however, to escape constructions of gender or to encroach upon male-gendered liberties. These expanded outlets for women were often justified as extensions of domesticity. At other times, however, they were packaged as antidotes to the dissatisfaction that domesticity sometimes engendered.

Although the popular literature argued that most women encountered few problems at menopause, the sources also acknowledged that some women might face difficult adjustments. Whether the required adjustments were physical (hot flashes), emotional (irritability), or social (what do I do now?) in origin, physicians and other medical writers generally recommended the same strategy: they urged menopausal women to seek out medical care (the medical encounter was explored in Chapter 3), and they asserted that the key to weathering the menopausal transition lay in women's own hands. Menopausal women were urged to conceal their problems, avoid introspection, exercise strict self-control, and adopt a socially useful pastime. This advice simultaneously promised a carefree menopause while reinforcing a model of middle-class womanhood that promoted service to others and denial of self.

Suffering in Silence

While physicians could offer reassurance and maybe some medications, writers of popular literature (including physicians) insisted that women themselves could do a great deal to make their menopause easier, both for themselves and for those around them. As an important first step, the advice texts entreated menopausal women to keep their troubles to themselves. Authors emphatically advised women not to talk about menopause with anyone except their physicians: not friends, nor families, nor husbands. This advice was motivated by at least two concerns; the writers felt that women's accounts of their own bodies were often false and needlessly upsetting to their listeners and that women should soothe and nurture those around them rather than demanding attention for themselves.

Physicians frequently claimed that many women learned to dread menopause from the aptly named "old-wives' tales." Edward Stieglitz, for example, maintained in 1946 that women's personal discussions posed real dangers to menopausal women. He insisted that women feared the menopause because of the "distorted descriptions" offered by their friends and relatives of what was "truly a normal phase of living."[72] Fred Trevitt and Freda White similarly commented that "if all the foolish ideas about this time of life could be gathered in a heap, it would reach higher than the

Empire State Building. This ugly pile is made up of Ignorance, Superstition, and Fear. . . . To hear some women talk, you would think that the change meant the end of everything: health, happiness and love."[73]

This condemnation of women's shared knowledge included a mean-spirited streak about the motives of older women and the value of women's networks. One particularly vitriolic comment claimed that at menopause, "the fish-wives at once begin harping upon the dangers attendant on the menopause. . . . And as soon as the menopause has been passed, a certain psychopathic element of womanhood sings the dirge which evidently she hopes will have the psychological effect of ending [her] active sex life." Another physician lambasted women who found it "personally gratifying" to excite the sympathy (and the fear) of their friends and younger women with their recitation of their miseries during the menopausal transition.[74]

In order to keep their readers from falling victim to the rants of embittered women, physicians, and other medical writers urged them to avoid stories spread by older women and to resist adding their own. Lois Mattox Miller, for example, warned, "above all don't talk about your change of life, or listen to women who are eager to tell you about theirs. For generations this has ranked with operations as a prime topic of conversation for women."[75] Despite these admonitions, the "problem" apparently continued, leading Trevitt and White to remark in 1955 that "a surprising number of women seem to think it necessary to keep their friends, or even the people they meet on a bus, informed, with ghastly details, about their symptoms—real or imaginary—during the menopause."[76]

These comments reflect both a dismissal of women's shared knowledge and a larger cultural expectation about female comportment. Throughout this period, and intensifying perhaps in the postwar era, women were widely held responsible for the affective tenor of their households. Women were expected to soothe frayed nerves, strengthen fragile egos, and calm family discord, thus providing a safe haven for their husbands and children.[77] As expressed in a 1950 *Atlantic Monthly* article, the ideal held that "it is for woman as mother, actual or vicarious, to restore security in our insecure world."[78] Consequently, women should suffer in silence, shielding their friends and family from their burdens. Physicians writing about menopause echoed these gender expectations, claiming that women "supply much of the stability that is necessary to keep mankind on an even keel in spite of atom bombs, wars and other catastrophes" and that they provided the "balance wheel of the family."[79] They argued that women who brought menopausal complaints into the family, thus calling attention to themselves, abdicated their domestic roles as peacemakers on the homefront and threatened domestic stability.

Doing for Others

The recommendation that women be stoic about their menopausal problems reflected a larger denial of the female self as a legitimate focus of consideration. The popular advice literature did not merely encourage women to keep their menopausal difficulties hidden; it insisted that they keep their minds off themselves and look outward. Assertions of this obligation were straightforward and numerous. Miller, in a 1939 issue of *Independent Woman,* urged women to "keep your mind off yourself."[80] An article in *Hygeia* similarly advised in 1940 that "when women begin to worry too much about themselves. . . . It is time to say, 'Now let's see, of what real value can I be, and how can I best serve my function as one of the mainstays of my family and a valuable member of my community?'"[81] A doctor, appealing to women's supposed vanity, claimed that a woman who occupies "herself with a job that entails doing something for someone else is the one who retains her figure, her spirit, and her good looks, menopause or no menopause." Another doctor in 1959 reminded his readers that women should derive their happiness not by indulging personal ambition but by securing the happiness of others.[82]

These comments show that despite the claim that menopause liberated women from some of the restrictions of domesticity, it did not free them from some of the restrictions of womanhood. Even after menopause and a life of sacrifice to family, women were still expected, on some level at least, to assume lives that centered on service to others and denial of self. Before and after menopause, women's most valued contributions were those made in relation to others. Before menopause, ideal women mothered children and supported husbands; after menopause, they nurtured the community. To avoid being viewed as selfish, women were urged to continue to focus their attention outside themselves.[83]

Lest women start dwelling on their own difficulties, physicians and others urged women to get busy and find outlets for their talents. Medical writers believed that menopausal women who found outside diversions would be too busy to think about themselves. Gynecologist William Danforth, for example, maintained in 1941 that "finding . . . some form of absorbing activity, either at home or elsewhere, is of itself a good form of treatment." Castallo echoed this idea in 1948. "If your mind and body are occupied, you'll have no opportunity to worry over the slight irregularities of your system, and you'll lack leisure in which to concentrate on your unpleasant symptoms."[84]

Medical writers suggested a range of appropriate possibilities. Those advocating the most traditional route recommended "grandmother" as the job most suitable for middle-aged women.[85] Others suggested hobbies.[86] Most commonly, however, the popular advice literature on menopause advocated community service as the ideal solution for the dissatisfaction of menopausal women. Gynecologist Leonard Biskind captured the essence of this advice when he noted, without irony, that after menopause "you are able to give more of yourself."[87]

While some physicians appeared to recommend community service as a diversion for women, a way to keep them distracted from their problems, others highlighted the valuable contributions older women could make. Danforth, for example, claimed that the nation's most important philanthropic work was done by middle-aged women.[88] Another physician assured women that their "social usefulness" did not end with menopause. He claimed instead that "this stage of life offers the first real opportunity for extensive social usefulness . . . [and] provides the nation with its most stable leadership."[89] Lincoln argued that "both the woman and her community are richer and happier" because of the efforts of older women. "Probably women today owe their right to vote to the fact that a sizable body of middle-aged women espoused the cause of equal rights for women . . . and spent a great deal of energy and not a little lung power in spreading their ideas."[90] These comments seem to reflect a genuine belief in the valuable contributions of middle-aged women.

These examples from the popular literature show how community service, with its commitment to others, was seen as providing a useful option for women that did not challenge gender prescriptions. After devoting a life to family, middle-aged, middle-class women could turn their domestic skills to improving their communities without challenging the primacy of domesticity in women's lives. Community work was a culturally sanctioned way for women to expand their influence, allowable because its focus on service to others simply extended the doctrine of domesticity beyond the home. Community service did not threaten men in the labor force, and it dovetailed with traditional ideas of women's work.[91] Nevertheless, the opportunities that public service provided should not be dismissed as *merely* an expansion of domesticity. Community involvement provided women with a second career (after motherhood) and gave them power and influence beyond the home. Nevertheless, this concept of community service did not demonstrate an escape from gendered expectations; rather, it confirmed the essential outline of gender constructs throughout the changes brought by aging.

Yet while much of the prescriptive literature urged community service as a way to reinforce female selflessness, some popular health writers also conveyed a second (and even contradictory) message about woman's role after her family's demands eased. A significant number of writers regarded menopause as a time for women to start living for themselves rather than for others. One gynecologist, for example, remarked that "at last she can be herself."[92] Edwin Hamblen similarly claimed that, at menopause, a woman finds before her "a good many years for herself, years in which she may find time to do many things that she has always put off." He maintained that because "the change emancipates women . . . the postmenopausal years are ones of freedom, which may be devoted to woman's own hobbies, interests and pleasure."[93] Feminist physician and sex educator Lena Levine also claimed that at menopause women need "self-realization and self-satisfaction after a life devoted almost exclusively to her family."[94]

In order to ease the transition away from a family-centered life, some medical writers urged women to begin preparing long before menopause. Physician Biskind, for example, counseled women to "develop new interests, particularly of a cooperative and communal nature" well before they need them.[95] A 1958 article in *Today's Health* similarly recommended that women "prepare for this phase of her life without waiting until her mothering job is completed." The author advised women to "keep at least one personal talent or interest alive even though she may find it difficult." In this way women could "make their influence felt in the arena of world affairs."[96] The often provocative David Cauldwell described the dangers of viewing marriage as an exchange of sexual favors and childbearing obligations for "shelter" from the pressures of public life. He insisted that women who "view the affairs of the world [as] matters for men," become "old early." With a dramatic flare, Cauldwell warned that such women "simply fade into an almost colorless form of existence."[97]

The call to prepare for life after child rearing was also voiced to help solve the "dilemma" of "modern" women in popular discussions not devoted to menopause. Women's need to fill their time "after forty" with activities beyond "numbing rounds of club meetings and card-playing" legitimated the development of interests outside the family while women were still young. Indeed, these texts insisted that by seeking activity outside the home while the nest was still full women accomplished two purposes: they became more interesting wives and mothers, and they protected society from the dangers of idleness among middle-aged women.[98]

One bold physician denounced the terms of the bargain, however, insisting that women should not have to devote their lives to homemaking throughout their fertile years. Feminist Levine complained that many women reached menopause only to find that their lives had been "wasted," that they had only used a fraction of their many talents. She related the case of Mrs. G., whose twenty-five years of marriage were filled with service to others. She worked in her husband's shop (notably, not hers), kept house, cooked all the meals, and made many of her family's clothes. She generally refused help from any of her family, believing it was her duty to care for them. At menopause, Mrs. G. began to review her life. "There was little in it but work and self-sacrifice; and when she looked ahead, she saw little else in prospect. It seemed to her that she had spent most of her life in a trap, and she blamed both herself and her family for making it."[99] According to Levine, even a hobby during the childbearing years and increased freedom after menopause could not compensate for what many women regarded as wasted years.

Many (but not all) other female writers discussing menopause did not challenge domesticity in toto, but they urged menopausal women to take paid employment rather than volunteer work. To make this point, female commentators claimed that professional women suffered less at menopause, in part because they had no time to brood about their troubles. Lois Miller, for example, claimed, "Doctors have observed that business and professional women, absorbed in a variety of interests, are least given to complaining and self-pity during the change of life. On the other hand, the overwhelming majority of housewives and unoccupied women seem to have too much idle time in which to worry about themselves. For this doctors strongly favor careers for women in middle life."[100] Maxine Davis agreed, insisting that businesswomen did not suffer at menopause. "Their plight cannot be compared with that of idle women with nothing to do but watch for symptoms and to brood over them."[101] Other women writers put a slightly different spin on professional women's reaction to menopause. Polly Allison maintained that all women experienced "identical" feelings at menopause. Professional women, however, have "made progress in educating ourselves for accepting it, and of necessity, we have hidden the symptomatic problems deeper because of the good front demanded by our work."[102]

Highlighting the various benefits of paid employment, some female commentators urged women to acquire jobs at menopause. Some writers, such as Edsall, cited financial reasons to seek wage labor. Others suggested a different reason why menopausal women should secure paychecks of their own. Madeline Gray, for example, claimed that a paying job could "make you feel you are still 'somebody.' A job to take care not only of your idle love but also of your idle hands." She admitted that "your husband may kick like a steer," but she insisted that women should "ignore him."[103]

Women, of course, did work outside the home both before and after menopause, much more than was acknowledged in the popular discussion of menopause or gender roles. A significant percentage of black women had always worked, even after marriage, and by 1960, 25 to 30 percent of middle-class white wives with children participated in the workforce, at least part-time.[104] Further, between 1950 and 1960, women over age forty-five came into the workforce at rates twice those of women under forty-five. But Americans remained ambivalent about working mothers (at least middle-class white mothers), and the popular advice on menopause reflected this ambivalence. The married career woman hardly existed in the menopause advice literature, and single women appear only at the margins, generally supplying a cautionary foil in warnings against a misspent life. Working-class women, married or single, rarely appear. Further, it seems not coincidental that female authors, career women themselves, dominated the infrequent discussion of professional women and the value of paid employment. Finally, the rare male author who admitted that women might benefit from participation in the workforce scrambled to restrict that work to the confines of domesticity. Physician and sex counselor Frank Caprio, for example, acknowledged that some wives did work outside the home, but, he insisted, a wife's primary role remained "helpmeet" to her husband, and, as a result, her career should supplement his income. "Thus her job should not be an accusation or challenge of her husband's adequacy. . . . She should think of her job . . . as a way of helping out, of sharing *some* of the burden."[105]

Menopause, then, may have made the employment of married women more palatable to society at large, but it remained a hard sell despite women's widespread presence in the workforce. By promoting employment as an alternative to middle-aged idleness, by viewing it as consistent with rather than a challenge to, domesticity, writers of popular health texts tried to persuade public opinion to accept the lived experience of many American women.

FIVE

"Casting an Evil Spell over Her Once Happy Home"

Menopause as a Family Disease, 1938–1962

In 1940, psychologist and sex educator Oliver Butterfield described a case of marital conflict:

> A New York judge tells of a case in the domestic relations court where a man and his wife had been having trouble, and in court the man complained that his wife had recently been "cold and distant" towards him. After a little inquiry the judge sent them both to a physician and in about fifteen minutes the verdict came back, "Menopause."[1]

In this example, the verdict of menopause served as the final word in understanding this couple's conflict. The blame was placed firmly on the middle-aged wife's changing physiology and, presumably, on her emotional reactions to it. The consequences of menopause, then, were seen as extending beyond the hot flashes and irritability of individual women. Indeed, menopause threatened the happiness of families and the stability of marriages.

As Chapter 4 showed, the popular discussion of menopause between 1938 and 1962 stressed the new freedoms for women that menopause made possible while simultaneously plotting a gendered course through the female life cycle. Although the popular literature acknowledged that women could begin to live for themselves after menopause, it nevertheless stressed the importance of motherhood and self-sacrifice to female fulfillment. Only after a woman had satisfied her obligations to family and "race" was she considered eligible to live for herself—and even then only

114

within specific limits. Women's behavior during the menopausal years, however, could imperil the domestic life they had spent so many years tending. Marital land mines seemed to be everywhere. According to the advice literature, a menopausal woman, by her crying jags, her incessant nagging, her careless grooming, or her sexual missteps could drive a good and reasonable husband out the front door and into the arms of a more agreeable (and presumably younger) woman. Consequently, the popular literature mapped out for women the dangerous terrain and advised them how to avoid marital discord and an appointment with a divorce lawyer.

According to popular advice literature written by physicians and other health educators, menopausal women could endanger their marriages in several ways. First, they cautioned, women's irrational behavior threatened the home as a sheltering harbor in an insecure time. Second, a woman who let herself go (or tried too hard to keep her youth) could cool a husband's ardor. Third, physicians feared that women might see menopause as the end of their sexual lives and thus limit their husband's sexual access. Finally, some women, anxious to prove they were still sexual beings, might seek sexual adventures outside of the marriage, thus challenging the model of sexual containment.

How did women react to these warnings of the potential marital woes of menopause? Did they scramble to hold their husbands' attention by donning sexy outfits or trying a new shade of lipstick? Did they blame their diminished libido for the rocks in their marital beds? The experiences related by the women surveyed in 1950 by Smith College alumna Dorothy Hamilton Brush and Hester Hoffman and by the women interviewed by Ida Davidoff in 1957 suggest that most women, at least most of these college-educated white women, did not view menopause as a threat to their marriages. Indeed, when women spoke of sexual problems, they were as likely to blame their husbands' impotence as their own aging bodies.

Disrupting Domestic Tranquility

Warnings of the familial dangers posed by menopause peppered the popular advice literature. Fred Trevitt and Freda White, for example, claimed in 1955 that at menopause a woman often "neglects her housework and children. Her attitude toward her husband is one of hatred." Rather than understanding why a woman might feel this way, Trevitt and White condemned her "self-pity" and blamed her for the "evil spell she has cast over her once happy home."[2] One physician even believed that menopausal women could disrupt their families' home lives so severely that "for the peace of their families" they should be sent to sanitoriums.[3] Another physician brought these themes together, claiming simply that menopause could "almost be called a family disease."[4]

According to the advice literature, menopausal women frequently poisoned family life by subjecting their husbands and children to a litany of complaints. Woeful tales of physical miseries, nervous anxieties, and personal slights allegedly dominated the conversations of menopausal women trying to win the attention and sympathy of their loved ones. (See also Chapter 4.) The popular advice literature frequently castigated these women for manipulating their families and wallowing in sorrows largely of their own making. Gynecologist Mario Castallo, for example, claimed in 1948 that a woman who has "so much as a grain of self-pity in her make-up will turn every day into a three handkerchief field day, all the while she's menopause-ing."[5]

Strict self-control was promoted as the best way for women to avoid burdening their families. Popular texts insisted that women could and should exercise mental discipline to keep their difficulties in check. In her 1949 book, *Change of Life: A Modern Woman's Guide,* journalist Florence Edsall, for example, insisted that menopausal women "relegate" their discomforts to "their proper place of unimportance." Indeed, Edsall continued, they must "captain the good ship self and keep a steady hand on the helm."[6] Female physician Lincoln agreed, claiming that women must "consciously cultivate emotional steadiness" during menopause. To ensure smooth sailing through these possibly turbulent seas, a menopausal woman must discipline herself, much as "she disciplines her children," firmly and consciously ironing out "the ups and downs in her feelings."[7]

If self-control failed to eliminate all menopausal difficulties, women were encouraged to keep their troubles to themselves, even if this sometimes called for outright deception.[8] Physician Miriam Lincoln, for example, urged women to make "a valiant effort to disguise" their menopause, even from their husbands.[9] Journalist Edsall in 1949 also advised a tactful lie. "When anybody—excepting, of course, the doctor—asks, 'And how are you today?' the answer should always be, very well, thank you. And you?' If, underneath, various and interesting and amazing symptoms temporarily give this answer the lie, that is a little joke the speaker has with herself."[10]

Acknowledging that some women might continue to subject their loved ones to a barrage of complaints, the popular literature also offered advice to the victimized families. Physician Marion Hilliard urged her readers to resist menopausal women's manipulations. "Don't listen to her troubles," she warned in 1957. "She'll never get stopped telling you about them. You don't console an adolescent who is crying because she can't find a yellow scarf; you tell her to pull herself together and go out and play tennis. You say it gently and you smile. This is precisely the philosophy for the menopause."[11] The comparison of menopausal women and adolescents here is telling. Both, perhaps overwhelmed by their changing hormones, should not be indulged; their personal difficulties, dare they share them, should be discounted as foolish self-indulgences.

Most popular authors insisted that menopausal women should be chastised for calling attention to their discomforts and disappointments. But not all commentators judged menopausal women's behaviors so harshly. Feminist physician and sex educator Lena Levine, whose advice to menopausal women often bucked popular trends, saw these women in a different light. She claimed that throughout their adult lives, married women generally put the needs of their family above their own, to the extent that they had no time even to be sick. At menopause, they finally had the leisure and the justification "to be sick, to pamper themselves a little." As a result, difficulties attributed to the menopause actually represented "the bursting of a dam of slight discomforts that have been piling up for years." Levine did not interpret these women's attitudes as self-pity or self-indulgence. Rather, she viewed them as an admission of and a protest against the many troubles women had suppressed all their lives, and she applauded their demands to have their own needs met at last.[12] Levine's view, by framing female stoicism as a gendered expectation, shows how the exception can prove the rule. Thus other medical writers, when they advised women to exhibit silence and stoicism in the face of menopausal symptoms, were reminding women of their obligations to soothe rather than disrupt the affective tenor of the family.

Marriage and the Menopausal Wife

While menopause allegedly disrupted the entire family, the literature depicted the relationship between husband and wife as the most endangered. Indeed, a few medical writers noted with concern that many previously happy couples divorced during the wife's menopause.[13] Reflecting on this pattern, a psychiatrist commented that "menopause . . . serves to separate women from their husbands—or, more accurately, it causes women to drive their husbands out of the home."[14] Another writer commented that "the menopause is Mary Smith's personal problem, but it may be her husband's headache."[15]

While menopausal women endangered their marriages, some of the popular literature credited men with being able to save them through sympathetic understanding or a firm hand. The literature urged husbands to "handle" their wives during these years, since menopausal women were occasionally unable to handle themselves. Physician Anna Daniels described the stakes involved, claiming that a cooperative husband "can save himself and his family from being shipwrecked in the storm of the climacteric."[16] Journalist Lawrence Galton concurred, maintaining in 1950 that it is "the husband's understanding and handling of his wife during this period that can mean the difference between hell on earth for both or a smooth passage."[17] Other physicians gave more explicit advice. One urged husbands to be "less demanding and more relenting, [so that] there will be fewer crying spells and depressions."[18] Abner Weisman reminded husbands in 1951 that menopausal women could not control their actions. "Remember, it is not she—it's her glands. Be patient, be understanding, be the sympathetic husband she married for better or for worse."[19]

If patience did not work and women did not seek medical attention on their own, doctors and others urged husbands to see that they did. Obstetrician and gynecologist Frederic Loomis, for example, maintained that a menopausal woman was an "affliction . . . to those around her." He instructed husbands to take their wives "gently by the hand to the nearest doctor for treatment." If she refused, Loomis suggested that husbands should "handle" the situation by taking her "straightway by the back hair with unmistakable firmness."[20] Nora Preddy made the same point graphically in *Minnie Pauses to Reflect,* her 1950 attempt to bring some levity to the problems of menopause. When a wife (presumably) admits to her husband that she forgot to get her hormones, he grabs her hand and rushes her to the drugstore, remarking that perhaps hormones will make her "nicer to me–for a while."[21] Drug companies likewise capitalized on family discord to promote their product. One advertisement for DES, for example, suggested that "the upset family of the menopausal woman frequently presents a greater problem than the patient's condition."[22]

As these last examples show, a hormonal fix was occasionally needed to cure domestic ferment. Although some physicians warned in the medical literature that hormones should not be used to treat domestic problems, in the popular literature their reservations were largely ignored.[23] In 1939, for example, Lois Mattox Miller recommended "female sex-hormones" to ease domestic conflicts. She claimed that "no longer need a husband fear that the happiest days of his wife's partnership with him are about to end in a baffling ordeal; no longer need sons and daughters dread the transformation of a healthy, active mother into a neurotic, complaining semi-invalid."[24] Paul de Kruif agreed. While he admitted in 1948 that estrogens were not a panacea, he maintained that "they may bring harmony to many troubled homes."[25] Another physician recounted an example from his practice. The nineteen-year-old daughter of a patient complained to him that her mother had become crabby and cross. After the doctor prescribed hormones, the mother "quickly became once more the placid person she had been."[26] These messages indicated that entire families suffered from the menopause and consequently obliged women to seek medical attention. According to one article, menopausal women owe it to themselves and their families to "take advantage of what medicine has to offer."[27] These examples highlight the obligations placed on women to adjust their behavior to prevent disrupting family harmony. If women needed a medicinal fix to restore a placid demeanor and an obliging attitude, she should submit to it.

The discussion of menopausal maelstroms and their solutions reflects larger cultural understandings of women's (at least middle-class white women's) position within the family during this period. Even as they increasingly joined the paid workforce, women were expected to foster a congenial emotional climate within the home. An ideal wife accommodated her family's needs by adjusting her behaviors and desires to match those of her husband and children. The need to secure the family peace while ignoring personal disappointments remained, throughout this period, a "peculiarly feminine task."[28] To buck up the ego of an unemployed or alcoholic husband, to welcome back a returning soldier, or to ease the tensions of the cold war, women were expected to provide a sanctuary from the pressures of public life.[29] The effects of freshly baked bread, gleaming linoleum floors, and well-scrubbed children could be ruined if the housewife complained that her efforts were unappreciated or if she nagged about another forgotten errand.

Further, the popular literature on menopause emphasized the husband's role as head of the family. Sex roles within marriage were continually negotiated and evaluated during this period, particularly as the Depression challenged a husband's breadwinner status, the Second World War necessitated his literal absence from the family, and the company demanded long days at the office. Nevertheless, throughout this period, government policies, cultural messages, and family dynamics worked to preserve male prerogatives in the workplace, in recreational spaces, and in the home. Even as popular messages and individual families approved tentative moves toward more egalitarian marital relationships, husbands remained widely acknowledged as the heads of their families, even if their role as "boss" was largely rejected. In the case of menopause, if a husband's patience and understanding wore thin, he was urged to assert his authority and "manage" his wife.

Sexual Obligations

While the nagging wife and the irritable mother could allegedly derail families during menopause, sexual problems posed the most potent threat to happy homes. Fearing that women viewed menopause as the end of their sexual lives, popular health writers between 1938 and 1962 assured women that the physiological changes of menopause need have very little effect on their sex lives. The sources assured women that their sexual desires remained robust and that their attractiveness remained intact. Indeed, because the kids may have left and birth control was unnecessary, postmenopausal sex was often heralded as the most satisfying of married life.

Although menopause posed no physical threat to sex, popular health writers nevertheless warned women that their behaviors at menopause could trouble both the marriage bed and marriage itself. Too many women, the popular literature reported, let themselves go at menopause, coming down to breakfast in a stained nightgown and curlers or putting on a few unflattering pounds in the mid-section. By contrast, other women went too far in the other direction, wearing styles meant for teenagers in a pitiable attempt to appear young. Either approach could cool a husband's ardor or encourage him to look elsewhere. Further, medical writers worried that some women might use menopause as an excuse to avoid their sexual obligations. Women were encouraged to not let distaste, either for the sexual act or for their husbands, affect their sexual accessibility. By remaining sexually receptive, women again maintained marital happiness.

In general, physicians and other medical writers scrambled to assure women that their sexual pleasures and responsibilities did not end with menopause. Married (always married) women could and should enjoy rich and rewarding sex lives well beyond their childbearing years. Popular health writers understood, however, that willing and able female flesh did not always sexual sparks make. These authors also took up the decidedly delicate task of advising aging women how to retain the sexual interest of their husbands.

To convince menopausal women that their sexual lives did not disappear with their fertility, popular texts insisted that sexual desire depended on a receptive attitude rather than on hormone levels. As a result, the popular literature maintained that most women would experience very little change in their libido. Commentators generally recognized that "the libido in women apparently has its origin in her psyche, in her state of mind" rather than in her ovaries.[30] Nevertheless, health writers acknowledged that some women dreaded the change of life because "they fear that they will no longer be 'women,' that they will no longer be interested in intercourse, or that they will be unable to satisfy their husbands."[31] Physician and sex educator Levine, incensed by this attitude, claimed that the notion that sexual functioning ceases at menopause "has done more harm to the emotional and personal lives of both men and women than any other." She was optimistic, however, because "this idea is beginning to lose its force now that women are asserting themselves as sexual beings."[32]

Some medical writers did admit that women might experience a gradual waning of desire, but they insisted that this decrease was not necessarily connected to the physiological changes of menopause.[33] These authors assured women that an increased emotional connection to their husbands would fully compensate for any physical changes. One doctor admitted, for example, that sexual desire might lose its "imperious, volcanic nature" but insisted that "it is nonetheless enjoyable and continues to play an important part in the companionship of husband and wife."[34]

Recognizing that not all women experienced satisfying sexual lives before menopause, some physicians depicted menopause as a potentially potent aphrodisiac, allowing women who had never enjoyed sex during their fertile years to finally appreciate it. Physician and sexologist David Cauldwell spoke for many when he claimed in 1957 that women "who have regarded the sex life as a form of punishment inflicted on womanhood, discover themselves as sexual creatures and, for the first time, reap the abundant health to be had through complete sex fulfillment."[35]

Popular writers explained this sexual awakening by reminding women that menopause eliminated the fear of accidental pregnancy. Endocrinologist Edwin Hamblen set the scene. "The married woman, who has suffered the coital attentions of her husband with constant fear that another pregnancy might result, really knows the freedom which the change affords."[36] Another doctor also believed that the fear of pregnancy had long "had an inhibiting effect" on many women's sexual desire. Popular health writer Maxine Davis likewise contended in 1951 that "the years after the menopause may well be the happiest ones of all your marriage." She claimed that because women will not fear pregnancy, they "will be spontaneous and relaxed. [They] will be free." Journalist Edsall agreed in 1949, noting that the freedom from unwanted pregnancy may make sex "richer and deeper than ever."[37]

Having established that women need not lose their sexual desire at menopause, physicians and other medical writers indicated that women were, therefore, obliged to maintain their libido for the sake of marital happiness. Doctors warned that women who refused their husbands' sexual demands jeopardized their marriages. Frank Caprio, for example, claimed in 1953 that many marriages break up at menopause and "a fair share of the blame can be laid to abatement of sexual love. Some wives feel that sexual activity is designed merely for procreation and the happiness of parenthood, not for gratification of the sexual urge."[38] Levine presented an example of such a woman, Charlotte F——. In her marriage, Charlotte had "not expected to find pleasure in coitus" and so was not surprised that she did not. Nevertheless, she acquiesced to her husband's demands, but she kept looking forward to menopause as a time that "would end all that." Charlotte hadn't anticipated, however, that her husband's desires would remain constant. Distressed that the relief she predicted failed to appear, she lost her ability "to acquiesce patiently. She became actively frigid." Although she tried to keep her aversion a secret from her husband, she could not. Indeed, "her incessant complaints and tears would drive him from the house."[39]

In 1957, female physician Hilliard highlighted the importance of remaining sexually available to one's husband regardless of the woman's own feelings. She acknowledged that menopause might cause a "temporary loss of sexual desire," but she downplayed the significance of this diminished passion. She assured women that after menopause they would become "renewed . . . ready to enjoy a full marriage again." She warned, however, that women's waning libido during the interim endangered their marriages. Hilliard cautioned that if women forbade intercourse during this period, men, with their sexual urges unfulfilled, had two equally undesirable options: they could remain celibate until their wives' desire returned, an "unnatural" solution at best and one that risked causing permanent impotence; or they could seek out relief with younger women, "as thousands of middle-aged men do." To avoid the potential for marital disaster, she urged women to "maintain sexual relations despite her weakened inclination. It's like keeping up the payments on her home."[40] It seemed of no consequence to Hilliard that the costs of this sexual mortgage were not distributed equally: women bore responsibility for their husbands' impotence and infidelity.

The centrality placed on a healthy sex life after menopause reflects the general importance placed on sexuality in marriage in the 1940s and 1950s. During this period, researchers into marriage and family life regarded wholesome, mutually fulfilling sexual relations as the cornerstone of a healthy marriage.[41] Medical advice literature flourished and sexual education clinics emerged, offering both technical instruction and sexual counseling.[42] According to historian Linda Gordon, "the main thrust of these efforts was not female liberation, but family stability."[43] Further, the sexual advice literature from this period marked a shift away from the importance of female pleasure, considered central to sexual success in the 1920s and 1930s, and toward protecting the male ego, weakened by the stresses of war. Many marital sex advisors worried that women's sexual demands (including the demand for orgasm) might prove too much for men. As a result, women were expected to be more thoughtful of their husbands' sexual needs. Regardless of his performance, a wife was expected to be receptive, cajoling, and grateful.[44] If women were unwilling to play along, they had only themselves to blame when their husbands started spending more time at the office (presumably with the more agreeable secretary).[45]

Despite the importance of sex to marriage, the survival of sexual desire after fertility ended posed some problems in an era when women's reproductive roles were highly esteemed. Indeed, many physicians and other social critics of the time tied women's sexuality tightly to motherhood.[46] This link did not suggest that all sex must be procreative, but it did emphasize that a woman's libido emerged from her potential fertility. In their best-selling work, *Modern Woman: The Lost Sex,* Ferdinand Lundberg and psychiatrist Marynia F. Farnham explained the connection more fully. "We are not saying that every time a woman has sexual relations she must be prepared to see them, even in fancy, result in birth. But we are saying that for the sexual act to be fully satisfactory to a woman she must, in the depths of her mind, desire, deeply and utterly, to be a mother."[47] How could popular health writers promote lifelong sexual functioning without challenging the link between female sexuality and reproduction?

Some writers maintained this link by insisting that women's past sexual transgressions (which apparently included celibacy) threatened her chances for a normal sex life after menopause. Sex educator Oliver Butterfield, for example, claimed in 1949 that a woman "who has lived a normal sexual life, who has been married and borne children" would reap the continued "dividends" from her marital "investment."[48] Endocrinologist Edward Podolsky agreed. "If her internal organs have fulfilled their true destiny by bearing children . . . she will be able to retain her sexual vigor. In the old maid, on the other hand, disuse leads to withering of the sexual organs, and this leads to the extinction of function."[49] While these doctors acknowledged female libido, they nevertheless linked sexual desire—indeed, sexual function—to reproductive goals. As a result, women who had fulfilled their reproductive obligations would be rewarded with enduring sexual fulfillment after menopause.

A woman's sexual obligations before and after menopause, however, extended beyond submitting to sex. She also had to arouse her husband's sexual interest. Deploying a strategy that was part pep-talk and part cautionary tale, popular health writers advised women on how to keep their husbands interested.

Maintaining Her Sex Appeal

The popular advice literature on menopause noted that many middle-aged women worried about losing their attractiveness. The literature portrayed these women as frantic, fearful that their allure, charm, femininity—even their womanhood—was gone. Physician Anna Daniels claimed in 1948 that these women look toward the future and see only "a dreary, dull middle age, with all the zest gone out of life." They become overwhelmed, believing that they "can do nothing to avert this catastrophic avalanche descending" upon them. They fear they have lost their femininity and their ability to charm their lovers or husbands.[50] Believing that apprehension only deepened the worry lines and darkened the countenance, popular advisors assured women that menopause did not "rob her of her feminine charm." Instead, the literature insisted that a menopausal woman maintained all the appeal she needed to "satisfy both herself and her husband."[51]

While the advice texts maintained that middle-aged women remained attractive, a few writers conceded that women's purely physical charms might wane. One physician, writing in 1953, claimed that allure was not based on woman's physical attributes but arose from her inner beauty. Consequently, he contended that women need not consider themselves less attractive at menopause because "the beauty of a woman . . . is often to be found in her personality."[52] Another physician insisted that women who were attractive before menopause because of their "pleasing personality" generally remained attractive after menopause.[53] Butterfield captured the essence of this theme when he assured women that "sexual attractiveness is not a matter of youth or physique; it is certainly just as much a matter of psychological readiness and cooperation."[54]

At the same time these writers acknowledged that the key to sex appeal was personality not physique, however, others were reinforcing women's concerns about their appearance, since careless grooming might lead husbands to more comely companions. The scenario presented by Fred Trevitt and Freda Dunlop White illustrated what they viewed as an unfortunately common problem: "For years she has come down to breakfast in a bedraggled bathrobe, her hair every which way; and her husband has had to listen to her shrill voice as she indulges in her morning tantrums."[55] Trevitt and White clearly believed that a reasonable husband could not be blamed for abandoning such a home. In 1952, physician Samuel Lewin related a similar story of a wife who had "let herself go" and a husband who consequently no longer found his wife attractive. Lewin firmly condemned the wife for this ailing marriage and demanded that she assume responsibility for the solution. He maintained of this situation that "it is a wife's first duty to make herself more attractive rather than less attractive as she grows older—that she had undoubtedly been slowly undermining her husband's ardor by her careless grooming and indifference to feminine mystery and charm."[56] Another physician commented on "the group of women who grow slack: they stuff themselves with food and add layers of fat, they grow careless in dress and grooming. . . . Suddenly they wake up to find that younger, more attractive women have stolen their husbands from them."[57] Trevitt, Lewin, and others insisted that the marital bargain required that women maintain their attractiveness, specifically to elicit an amorous response from their husbands. This position ultimately held women responsible for all sexual dysfunction.

At the same time that health writers urged women to maintain their husbands' ardor by remaining well groomed, they simultaneously condemned women for trying too hard to retain their fleeing youth. In 1947, popular health writer Bernadine Bailey declared that "there is nothing more pitiful than the woman who refuses to face the forties, the too sleek or brittle woman whose face looks as if it has suffered a long bout with struggles to look young."[58] More than twenty years later, physician and sex expert Caprio noted derisively that menopausal women still deployed the same misguided tactics, preening their feathers, donning garish clothes. "Like inmates of the harem," he noted, they desperately tried "to hold their mates."[59]

These warnings to menopausal women reflect the larger shift away from holding men responsible for the sexual success of marriage to blaming women for sexual disappointment, impotence, and infidelity. Even before menopause, a wife's neglect of her grooming or her inadequate sexual enthusiasm could be enough to send a husband into the arms of a woman who aimed to please.[60] The popular messages about menopause reminded middle-aged women that the margin of error allowed them was razor thin. They needed to abandon the vanity of their youth but nevertheless maintain their feminine charms. A skirt too tight or a dress too dowdy could sever the fragile bonds holding their marriage together.

In sum, between 1938 and 1962, the popular literature painted the postmenopausal years as a chance for sexual rebirth. If this sexual bliss eluded them, menopausal women had only themselves to blame. Perhaps they had put on too many pounds. Perhaps they wore too much rouge. Perhaps they lacked enthusiasm for their husband's amorous touch. But even if women failed to bloom sexually at middle age, the popular literature on menopause reminded them of their continued sexual obligations.

Perverse Desires

At the same time popular health writers coached aging women to remain sexually available and attractive, they also warned women of the dangers of sexual excess and adventures. Too much sexual desire, either within marriage or without, indicated pathology. Although the popular literature encouraged sexual relationships within marriage, physicians and other medical writers balked at accepting other forms of sexual expression. Indeed, some of the commentators warned that women—both single and married—might be tempted at menopause by immoral and unnatural sexual practices, such as masturbation, homosexuality, and promiscuity. Writers believed that these practices, by defying cultural expectations, challenged the primacy of marriage and family.

Medical writers expressed particular concern over some women's increased desire at menopause. Although medical writers generally agreed that couples might experience their best sexual relations after menopause, physicians and other health advisors warned that too great an increase in libido was pathological. They proposed several explanations for possible increases. One writer claimed, for example, that it was a perverse desire to take advantage of the reproductive function before it was too late, a last gasp at reproduction.[61] Others viewed it not as a reproductive urge but more as a yearning for wider experience in general. One doctor indicated in 1938 that both married and single women might experience a "strange and troublesome and sometimes disconcerting flare-up of the sexual desires." He believed that these women viewed menopause as an opportunity to "take stock of life and to ask themselves if they were ready to give up and go into old age and into their graves with only the little stock of sexual experience and happiness that they had had."[62] Other physicians claimed that an increased libido at menopause was physiological. Joseph Rety, for instance, regarded an intensification of desire at menopause as "a sort of itching in the organs, which cannot be regarded as sensuality at all."[63]

Occasionally, physicians spoke cryptically about the dangers of a pathological libido. Popular health writers worried that middle-aged women might cast aside conventional codes of behavior and embark on potentially "distressing adventures."[64] Daniels, for example, warned in 1948 that some women might adopt "a Bohemian lifestyle" at this critical period.[65] Another doctor noted that some women's sexual behaviors might "assume odd, sometimes ludicrous, forms."[66] Sociologist Laura Hutton described the situation many women allegedly faced at menopause: "It is quite characteristic at this time of life that there is a flare-up of sexual desire, and with it a longing for romance and passion which a woman may find very disturbing and feel to be very reprehensible. On the other hand, she may abandon herself to it and land herself in situations which afterwards she will regret."[67]

Other commentators painted more vivid pictures of sexuality gone awry. A few medical writers feared that older women might act on their attraction to younger men. Gynecologist Abner Weisman, for example, declared in 1951 that "the elderly widow who keeps chasing after men is definitely an ill person." He noted that newspapers chronicle the escapades of older women marrying much younger men. "Such cases are abnormal" he cautioned, "and require psychiatric treatment."[68] Rety similarly commented on some older women's propensity to chase younger men. He claimed that some women, particularly of the upper classes are "inclined to pursue men . . . and to 'make a fool'" of themselves. He believed, however, that "genuine cases of unconventional behavior due to climacteric amorousness are very rare."[69]

The popular literature also included warnings against "true perversion." Sex researcher Georgene Seward, for example, claimed in 1946 that sexual abnormalities sometimes developed at senescence because "inhibitions do not function so rigidly as at other periods." She showed particular concern about homosexuality, sadomasochistic impulses, and "pseudo-erotic advances to younger members of the opposite sex."[70] Endocrinologist Podolsky also worried that menopausal women might experience a perversion of the normal sexual impulses. Single women seemed especially prone to such troubles because of their "inability to secure the orthodox climax." This led women to masturbation and homosexual liaisons.[71]

This discussion of "perverse" sexuality reflected a national obsession with nonmarital sex during the 1940s and 1950s. Certainly, men were the most obvious targets of this obsession, as homosexual men were increasingly persecuted as threats to national security and the sexual psychopath was seen as a threat to domestic safety.[72] But women did not avoid scrutiny. Indeed, female sexuality outside marriage was seen as tempting and dangerous. According to historian Elaine May, the "sexual independence of women was feared; many believed it would weaken the family during wartime and threaten the family later."[73]

The messages in the popular culture emphasized the threatening nature of female sexuality. This was especially apparent in the movies. Film noir, for example, which evolved during and after World War II, promoted the power and danger of female sexuality. In this popular film genre, the femme fatale deployed her feminine wiles to snare her prey. While she usually died in the end (no doubt her just deserts), her duped accomplice was also generally ruined.[74] The literal and metaphorical threat of female sexuality was also symbolized during the war itself by bomber pilots' tendency to paint scantily clad women on their planes. The term *bombshell*, coined in the 1930s, gained increased use in the 1940s and 1950s, and the designer of the two-piece bathing suit named his product the *bikini*, only days after the hydrogen bomb was dropped on the Bikini Islands.[75] The popular literature on sexuality and menopause reflects this larger cultural ambivalence about women's sexuality. Within marriage, women's sexuality held marriages together; outside marriage, female sexuality could not be controlled and threatened to burst marriages apart.

Despite cultural conventions, however, some popular writers reacted fairly blandly to the sexual practices of menopausal women. In his 1958 book, *What Women Want to Know*, physician Howard Imerman, for example, noted with concern the "distressing adventures" some women launch upon to prove they were not yet old. He claimed that "aberrant behavior—promiscuity, homosexuality—occasionally appears during the climacteric among women who previously would have been appalled at the very thought." Yet while he subscribed to popular social standards of acceptable sexual behavior, Imerman begrudgingly admired women who took control of their lives. One of his case histories illustrates his ambivalence. He described in detail the case of a widow with two children who began "bar-hopping" during menopause. Imerman tried to dissuade her, noting that she had children to consider. She replied pointedly, "I gave them the best years of my life. . . . It's my turn now." Imerman, taken aback by her response, admitted that she had a point. He still hoped she'd refrain, but noted that aside from the "moral issue," "there is much to be said for this patient's behavior: it was a positive, active approach to her emotional problems."[76] He sympathetically conceded that the sexual outlets for single women were limited. Another physician exhibited similar ambivalence toward the sexual activity of older women. He noted that both single and married women "begin to act a little kittenish . . . she dresses better, she puts more rouge on her face and buys a lipstick; she learns to smoke and perhaps she develops a fondness for cocktails."[77] Although he warned against the "difficulties she must encounter and disaster that may await at the end," this physician could not quite condemn these women. Rather sheepishly he admitted that he liked "to see some of these women striking out in search of happiness and experience," and he "wish[ed] them well."[78]

These authors' ambivalence toward nonmarital sex, including lesbian relationships, seems surprising given the national mood about sex and the intense suspicion of gay men. These particular physicians regarded older women's exploits as misguided but not threatening. Although younger women's sexual transgressions challenged the integrity of the American family, older women posed much less danger. Having presumably raised their families, older women's quests for romantic adventure were undesirable and slightly ridiculous but not particularly significant.

Sexual Experiences

Although the popular literature between 1938 and 1962 worried about menopausal women's sexual accessibility and allure, menopausal women themselves did not seem to share this concern. Most of the Brush and Davidoff women indicated that their sex lives did not significantly change at menopause, a claim supported by Alfred Kinsey's late 1940s and early 1950s sex research.[79] Women with robust desires continued to enjoy vigorous sexual lives, and those with more tepid desires also remained unchanged. Caroline Torlington, for example, knew that menopause would not affect her sexual desire, and sex remained for her and her husband "a shared pleasure and close tie of affinity."[80] Another woman, who referred to herself as "frigid," also experienced no change in her yearnings.[81] The thirteen "never married" Brush respondents similarly reported no change in sexual desire. Although it is difficult to know conclusively, it does not appear that these women abstained from sexual relations altogether (although two appeared to be celibate).

But several women in the surveys did note that their sexual relationships had changed at menopause, for better or for worse. Some women enjoyed new sexual freedom because unwanted pregnancy (and messy and disruptive contraceptive methods) was no longer a concern. One survey respondent, for example, welcomed the chance "to enjoy intercourse without nuisance of contraceptives."[82] Another woman noted that with the "fear of pregnancy gone—sex life better."[83] Other women, however, reported a significant loss of libido at menopause. Mary Rathbone felt "considerably less sexual desire—almost none" since she ended menstruation. She admitted, however, that it "had been on the wane for some years" before menopause. This woman did not bemoan her loss. Instead, the "decline of the specifically reproductive urges" allowed her to value the "companionship between husband and wife."[84] Another woman admitted that sex had been "diluted" after her hysterectomy. She was unable to determine, however, whether menopause or the surgery caused the change.[85]

As the advice literature of the time predicted, some of the Brush women did look to menopause for release from sexual obligations. One woman, for example, "never cared much for the sexual act itself (although postured the usual deception of interest, etc)." She enjoyed intimate tenderness and the sense of being desired more than the physical act. "Intercourse tapered off about the same time as menstruation." Since she thought sex "should be checked off after youth," she welcomed the diminished sexual activity that accompanied menopause.[86] Another Brush respondent, Mary Clark, may also have looked to menopause as an opportunity to reduce the frequency of intercourse. Although she was "far from frigid," her desires did not keep pace with those of her "strongly sexed husband." Because of love or duty, she "never refused him, even though [she] sometimes would have preferred less gratification of his desires." Her situation did not seem to change at menopause.[87]

Other women complained about their languishing sex lives, but they generally blamed their husbands' impotence rather than their own waning libido. One woman, for example, admitted that her husband's impotence was "very hard to take" and maintained that masturbation was an inadequate "substitute."[88] Florence Manning, initially frustrated by her second husband's indifference to sex, eventually resigned herself to the situation and saw her marriage as a "nice friendship and working partnership."[89]

There is no evidence that these women held themselves responsible for their husbands' shortcomings. They did not admit to concerns about losing their sex appeal or suggest that they worried about their husbands' roving eyes. Nevertheless, the Brush survey itself suggested the pervasiveness of these stereotypes about middle-aged women. The questionnaire asked women whether they had "tried to catch hold of the tail-feathers of youth—diet, dye, youthful clothes, you know!" This question failed to resonate with the respondents; most of them simply did not answer. (One who did answer admitted to getting her first permanent wave at menopause and buying a red skirt. Racy indeed!)[90] One respondent, however, did relate to the difficult terrain that menopausal women were asked to traverse. She reminded her peers to keep up their appearance but to exercise restraint. "Don't ever pretend a youth you don't have. Be attractive at your real age level. . . . Admitting one's age doesn't mean letting yourself go. But dye, paint, uplift, and diets produce a hard veneer which fools no one and makes the woman who indulges in such . . . slightly ridiculous."[91]

Most of these highly educated, middle-class women seem to have resisted the cultural claim that it was their marital duty to preserve their sex appeal and their sexual availability. They expressed no anxiety, although perhaps some vague disappointment, about their occasionally declining sexual lives. They admitted to no frantic attempts to hold the waning interest of a middle-aged husband. They felt secure that their marriages would survive the period of diminished sexual activity, regardless of whether her lack of interest or his impotence was the source.

Perhaps these women were unaffected by the pressures to maintain their sex appeal because their sense of the role of sex in a marriage, indeed their sense of the nature of marriage itself, was forged at a different historical moment than that prevailing when they approached menopause. In the 1920s and 1930s, the wife's sexual pleasure and her sexual fulfillment were heralded as crucial to marital success.[92] Mary Clark's comment that she never denied her husband regardless of her own desires illustrates that the sexual ideal was not the sexual reality for all, probably most, women. Nevertheless, these women may have been less likely to believe that the sexual success of a marriage depended on the attributes and attitude of the wife than were women who married in the postwar years. As a result, the Brush and Davidoff women did not worry that their changing body threatened the marriage: they were just as likely to blame their aging husbands.

SIX

"Why All the Fuss?"

Middle-Class Women and the Denial of the Menopausal Body, 1938–1962

In 1950, two Smith college graduates, Dorothy Hamilton Brush and Heather Hoffman, had suffered through the worst of their unexpectedly "nerve-wracking" experiences with menopause. Blindsided by their experiences and propelled by their can-do attitude and the determination that the next generation of women should not suffer as they had, they decided to write a book about the pitfalls of menopause and how to avoid them. Putting their alumna connections to work, Hoffman and Brush turned primarily to their 1917 classmates for guidance and data. They sent out roughly three hundred questionnaires, headed by the following plea: "Two women, one married, one single, have survived the menopause—to their amazement! With your help, they propose to write a book offering every life-raft discovered for this storm-tossed whirlpool. Don't let our younger sisters drift helplessly toward The Falls. Throw them a life-line! THROW IT NOW!"[1]

The responses Brush and Hoffman received suggest the various indignant, bewildered, and delighted reactions the "Smithies" must have had to their unexpected mail. "You girls are wonderful," commented one woman. "More power to you." This seems like "a lot of bunk," remarked another woman. "Busy normal people should forget it." Yet another respondent noted her surprise that anyone would give menopause a second thought. "When menopause came, I merely skipped one month, flowed somewhat abnormally the next month, then it ceased. There was no pain, 'hot flashers,' nor nervousness." And one woman proclaimed defiantly, there is "no such thing as menopause."[2] Obviously, women experienced and interpreted menopause in vastly different ways. For some, it passed unnoticed; for others, it disturbed their bodies and disrupted their lives.

133

Women's experiences with and attitudes toward menopause between 1938 and 1962 emerge powerfully from their responses to the Brush and Hoffman survey. These responses indicated how women reacted to the transformation of their bodies, the changes in their homes, and the larger societal prescriptions for appropriate menopausal and postmenopausal behavior. Women, even women within the fairly narrow social and economic demographic represented by the Brush and Hoffman survey, did not react in any one particular way to menopause. Physiological differences among women explain why some women might be incapacitated by unrelenting hot flashes and other women might experience no symptoms at all. But physiology, as the women themselves attest, explains only some of the variation in women's reaction to menopause. Financial circumstances, marital status, employment demands, and family dynamics all influenced how women reacted to and interpreted menopause. The women did not distinguish the biological experience of menopause from its social, cultural, and familial aspects. The experience of menopause could not be separated from the lives of menopausal women.

Although women's experiences of menopause during this period certainly varied, particular themes nevertheless emerge from women's descriptions of their own experiences. Indeed, to a great extent these menopausal women insisted that menopause was a normal process that deserved very little attention. They agreed with the popular literature that menopausal women should keep quiet about their troubles, stop focusing on themselves, and occupy themselves with worthy causes. Clearly, women's reactions to menopause were guided by cultural demands for womanly behavior. But women's response to menopause—including the widespread denial of its importance—also suggests a more active, strategic reaction to the changes in their bodies. Like women physicians at the beginning of the twentieth century, many of these women were unwilling to view their bodies as a personal or professional liability. Indeed, by attending college in the early part of the century, at a time when college education for women remained relatively rare (between 1910 and 1930, the percentage of women attending college increased dramatically, but only from 3.8 to 10.5 percent), they proved that their bodies posed no handicap to their ambitions. Nevertheless, even as these women formed their own ideas about their bodies, opponents of female suffrage, education, and political participation were still using women's bodies as a reason to block their public ambitions. The women represented here, most well-educated, some professionally ambitious, understood that their bodies, or the political uses of those bodies, made them vulnerable. In response, they refused the implication that their bodies determined their destiny. Many refused to consider that their biology—their female biology—controlled their lives.

But these women had help in regarding menopause as an insignificant transition. The development of DES and conjugated estrogens at the beginning of this period bolstered women's claims that menopause should be taken in stride. A wayward body could often be brought under control with a prescription, thus making it easier to insist that menopause was no big deal.

The Menopausal Women

The data gathered by Dorothy Hamilton Brush and Heather Hoffman, as described above, provides one of the most significant windows available for examining the menopausal experience in this period. The survey they circulated asked a variety of questions intended to gauge women's emotional, physical, and sexual responses to menopause. They asked about fairly predictable symptoms: hot flashes, weeping spells, and depression. They also asked questions about sexual desire (and sexual frustrations), paranoia, and suicide. "Did you suffer from a sense of sin? Were you completely self-absorbed?" "Did you lose your sense of responsibility?" As the opening suggests, Brush and Hoffman did not merely want to know what women experienced; they wanted to know how women coped. The survey asked whether women received medical care (hormones? quieting pills? X rays?), psychiatric care (psychoanalysis? shock treatment? mental hospital?), or spiritual guidance (priest? unity? prayer?). Although many of the questions constrained women's responses, pushing them to express how menopause changed their lives, generally for the worse, the survey also invited women to describe what helped them most, whether an attentive husband, an inspirational philosophy, a steamy affair, or a prescription for "nice pink pills."[3]

Roughly 125 women responded to the survey, some merely checking a few boxes, others filling pages with their triumphs and their miseries. The respondents were typically fifty-five, the majority having been born in 1895. They certainly did not represent a cross-section of American women in 1950: 80 percent had college degrees (most from the elite Smith College), and another 24 percent had earned graduate degrees. Although their precise profiles are unknown, given the demographics of Smith College at the time, their families of origin were most likely upper and upper-middle class, white, and Protestant. They were also much more likely to be single and childless than women in general.

The research notes of Ida Davidoff provide further access to the menopausal experience of American women in the 1950s. In 1957, Davidoff interviewed fifty women to "access the impact of the women's movement . . . on women entering the postparental phase of their lifecycle."[4] The average age of these women was fifty-four at the time of their first interview, indicating most were born in 1903. Again, these responses do not capture a cross-section of American women. Although Davidoff's study included an urban and a suburban sample, the only evidence remaining is from the twenty-five suburban women (from a Connecticut suburb of New York City). All of Davidoff's subjects had graduated from college, all lived with their husbands, and all had seen their last child leave the family home. While a few of the women worked outside the home, they did not do so permanently or full-time while raising their children.

Unlike the Brush survey, the Davidoff interviews did not focus primarily on menopause; her areas of special interest were family and work. Nevertheless, Davidoff did ask a few questions explicitly about women's menopausal experiences. Using an open-ended format (with particular prompts), she asked women how menopause had affected their bodies, their relationships, and their outlook. She also asked where they gathered information about menopause, and what they had done to alleviate any physical or emotional distress.[5]

This generation of women, born near the turn of the last century, defy casy categorization. According to historian Susan Warc, they largely abandoned the fight for women's rights, instead concentrating on the rights of individual women. If Lillian Hellman, born in 1905, is at all representative of her college-educated peers, they "didn't think much about the place or problem of women." Instead, they hoped to transcend their group identity as women.[6] Even without a feminist consciousness, many of them challenged traditional notions of appropriate feminine behavior. They might have bobbed their hair and learned to smoke when it was still considered scandalous; perhaps they necked a bit in the backseat of the first Model T on their block. When they married—if they married—they perhaps insisted on the new sexual and emotional dictates of the "companionate marriage."

But despite these markers of a remade concept of a woman's role, these women lived varied yet still largely domestic lives. The Davidoff women were married with children; 10 percent of the Brush respondents were single, and 26 percent of them were childless. Many of the Brush women pursued careers, whereas none of the Davidoff women worked full-time outside the home. Nevertheless, most of the Davidoff and Brush women who offered the most detailed accounts of their experiences represented the white middle and upper class. These women (at least in the abstract) provided the models of menopausal women depicted in the popular advice literature. More significantly, these women reached menopause during World War II or in the postwar period when many women were wondering why they didn't feel fulfilled by raising their children and keeping their homes.

The women's experiences described below do not provide a portrait of a "typical" menopausal woman at mid-century. Given the importance of cultural and social factors in the experience of menopause, it seems possible, perhaps likely, that women who are underrepresented in this sample—working-class women, women of color—might have experienced and interpreted menopause in significantly different ways. Yet despite being limited to the views of women of a particular class and, presumably, race, the Brush and Davidoff studies provide a useful look into the menopausal experience. The respondents were often united in attempting to downplay the significance of the "change of life."

Although this chapter interprets women's attitudes toward menopause against the back-drop of popular advice literature, very few of the women in these studies seem to have read much about menopause. Although they often provided long lists of their reading materials, none of the Brush women, for example, noted reading anything specifically about menopause. Indeed, it was the need for more information that motivated Brush and Hoffman to create the survey in the first place. (It is useful to bear in mind that between 1938 and 1950, the date of Brush and Hoffman's survey, popular discussion of menopause was more scarce than it would be in the twelve years after 1950.) When asked where they had learned about menopause, most of the Davidoff women cited their mothers, sisters, and friends. Only a few mentioned arming themselves with published advice, either before or during menopause.[7] To the extent that their attitudes echo the popular literature, it is because the popular literature complements the broader cultural expectations of women to which the respondents were also subject.

Why All the Bother?

Many of the women who responded to the Hoffman and Brush question-naire expressed outrage at what they read. (One wonders about the reaction of the 175 women who didn't respond.) Questions about sexual affairs, suicidal thoughts, and devastating loss seemed far removed from the experiences of most women and surely outside the bounds of polite conversation. "I feel as though this were an interview of the Kinsey report," wrote one clearly indignant respondent. "Unless it is to be used for scientific purpose, I see no point in it."[8] Another woman complained that she had never noticed the "neurotic symptoms" listed on the questionnaire.[9] One shocked woman wondered why modern women would bother contemplating menopause, criticizing Brush and Hoffman for their project. Challenging the entire enterprise, she asked "whether you meant your questionnaire seriously or as a joke, rather a poor one at that. . . . Why all the fuss? Menopause is a normal period in our lives, so why dwell on it?" She found it depressing that "a Smith education and other opportunities haven't given you more interesting things to study than menopause."[10] Indeed, a few women denied that menopause existed at all.[11]

In contrast to the tone of the questionnaire, most of the Brush respondents (and the Davidoff participants) regarded menopause as a normal, perhaps even trivial, transition that caused them very little distress. Ella Davenport, for example, regarded menopause as a "normal natural process" and herself as a "normal healthy person." As a result, she anticipated no "particular trouble."[12] Another woman believed that stressing the significance of menopause encouraged an outdated view of women's functions. She maintained that "menopause should be treated as a natural, normal part of life. Just as the boog a boo [*sic*] connected with the onset of menstruation and childbirth have been, to some extent, put in their proper place so this large boog a boo about the menopause should be slain."[13] These women and others like them insisted that menopause caused them no emotional or physical distress and had very little significance in their lives.[14]

For these women, menopause was a physiological blip, a minor inconvenience perhaps, but not a significant biological or social event. Most certainly, they felt that menopause did not merit the sustained attention educated women such as Brush and Hoffman intended to give it. It is possible and perhaps likely that these women sailed easily through menopause, which would explain their disbelief that anyone would get worked up about it. But something else seems to be at play here. The tenor of the denials suggests a belief that a discussion of women's bodies, particularly the normal functioning of women's bodies, was off-limits. Although scantily-clad pinup girls displayed socially acceptable versions of the female body throughout this period, the real female body, so fleshy, so difficult to control, so prone to embarrassment, deserved to be ignored and denied.[15] In fact, even when Lucille Ball made history in 1952 by appearing on television visibly pregnant, her pregnancy could not be mentioned explicitly. In addition to the cultural denial of women's bodies, however, there seems to have been a more personal refusal to reduce female experience to *embodied* experience. Women of this generation took it for granted, perhaps, that their bodies would not hinder their aspirations, but they still defensively refuted any suggestion that their bodies represented a personal or professional liability.

Welcome Freedoms and Sobering Regret

While some women refused to give menopause more than passing notice, others embraced it enthusiastically for the physiological changes it brought and still others despaired at the loss of their fertility. Some women, for example, welcomed the relief from the monthly inconvenience and occasional pain of menstruation. These women relished the "freedom from the mess of menstruation" and the "freedom from monthly woe."[16] One avid sportswoman, for example, was delighted at menopause because she no longer needed to worry about menstrual periods while sailing.[17]

Freedom from unwanted or at least unexpected pregnancy also delighted many women. A 1962 survey (published in 1963), noted that more than three-quarters of middle-aged women welcomed the end of childbearing.[18] For most of these women, fertility had been something that required surveillance and control. After menopause, no longer did they have to cope with "messy" contraceptives or interrupted coitus. Brush respondent, Eliza Remington, noted that she "had so many children, I was glad that I no longer need wonder about possible pregnancies."[19] At least one husband was delighted too.[20]

Although most of the popular literature declared that single and childless women would suffer more than married women did at menopause, a majority of the childless women in the Brush survey expressed relief at menopause. Twenty-six percent of the Brush sample (33 women) were childless, but only five openly regretted it. Even these women seemed eager for menstruation to end. One childless single woman, for example, looked forward to menopause because she "wanted the fruitless pain over with."[21] It is difficult to know for sure what this woman felt about her declining fertility. Perhaps she was glad to be done with the physical pains of menstruation because it had neither practical nor symbolic importance in her life. On the other hand, perhaps her menstrual periods came as painful reminders of her failure to be fruitful and multiply.

But not all women were ready to give up on childbearing, and they therefore greeted the skipped periods and hot flashes of menopause with disappointment or, in the extreme, despair. A woman from Louisville, Kentucky, for example, sent a plaintive letter to the Children's Bureau in 1940. "I am wanting information," she began. "I have been told in New York some place you could get treatment to become a mother even if change of life has come. *Please.*" Another woman resented menopause and felt sad that she could not have more children. She believed that because she was no longer fertile, the "purpose of sex [was] over."[22] Another woman who had had two children admitted that the only "real grief of my life is that we *stupidly* didn't have more children."[23]

Similarly a few (but only a few) of the unmarried Brush women seemed unhappy with their circumstances. One single woman, for example, believed that menopause was harder for her because she did not have the "love and attention [married women] get." Menopause forced her to realize that she would never have a loving companion. She considered "the realization that the years have gone and that there is no more choice left— that you must accept the lonely life," the most difficult and significant aspect of the menopause. Indeed, this woman believed that her symptoms were a sort of punishment for her single life. "It seems that this lonely— (or only half-completed-state)—is the crux of the whole matter. Nature tried to make you conscious of this lack of completeness with all kinds of symptoms. There is a grand scramble by some for a new 'half' by seeking attachment, security and attention."[24]

For this woman, and perhaps others like her, menopause represented a watershed, a time of reckoning. She regarded menopause as both a biological and a social point of no return. Having no one to provide "completeness," she resigned herself to her loneliness. Moreover, she believed that her body exacted its revenge through a difficult menopause.

For most of the middle- and upper-class women responding to these surveys, however, menopause represented a largely unimportant event that brought both some minor inconveniences and some welcome benefits. By and large, it was not viewed as a time of loss. (The Brush survey specifically asked the respondents what they had lost at menopause and most had nothing to mention.) Even many of the childless women, whose menopausal experiences were described so grimly in the popular sources of the period, failed to characterize menopause as a time of intense regret or recrimination. Some of them seemed wistful, but very few seemed devastated. Rather than loss, menopause generally provided freedom from the cyclical demands of reproductive physiology, demands most of these women had been actively thwarting most of their adult lives. To the extent that menopause mattered, it loosened part of the biological hold of womanhood.

Fear and Loathing

Depending on personality or family and other experiences, some women feared menopause, anticipating it as a period of biological upheaval. For some women, the dread came from watching their mothers suffer from both the physical and mental effects of menopause.[25] Georgina Battsen, for example, feared menopause because her mother's experience had been so full of problems, both mental and physical, followed by consultations with countless doctors. She worried that she too would suffer from the "heat waves" and "possible insanity."[26] Another woman cited family history as the cause of her apprehension. All the women in her family had fallen into a "deep depression" at menopause, and at least two of them had committed suicide. In addition, her grandmother had died of a broken heart "during the change" because her husband left her. She was particularly devastated when her menopausal mother "threw herself over the 2nd story porch."[27] In explaining her fear of menopause, yet another woman remarked cryptically that menopause had been the "indirect cause" of her mother's death.[28]

Although the popular literature often dismissed the fear of menopausal insanity as an irrational superstition, at least a few menopausal women knew better. Some had heard and believed stories that you could "go crazy" at menopause; Lucy Howard, a Davidoff interviewee, knew someone who had lost her mind at menopause, and so she readily understood that it "could easily happen."[29] The women who feared menopause, who believed that it had the potential to ruin and end lives, did not harbor irrational fears. Instead, they had witnessed first-hand the turmoil menopause could bring.

Sweat, Blood, and Tears

When menopause finally arrived, some women who had feared it discovered to their relief and delight that it caused them very little trouble. Other women, however, discovered to their bewilderment that menopause was not as easy as they had anticipated. One woman who had always believed "that if one kept busy they would have no trouble" was shocked to find that a positive outlook did not prevent a miserable menopause.[30] Another woman who fully expected a carefree menopause was blind-sided when she found it dominated her life for about six months.[31]

Hot flashes were the most common symptom identified by the Brush and the Davidoff women. For the most part, however, hot flashes brought inconvenience rather than incapacity. One of the Brush respondents admitted that "it is a nuisance to throw off and on the bed clothes all night," but because she had her own room, no one else was disturbed.[32] Another woman acknowledged frequent hot flashes but denied that they were a cause for worry or embarrassment. "I remember one time, . . . I had a terrific hot flush. . . . I went to look at myself in the mirror. I didn't even look red, so I thought, 'All right . . . the next time I'll just sit there, and who will notice? And if someone notices, I won't even care.'"[33]

While a few of the Brush and Davidoff women acknowledged that hot flashes annoyed them, they were generally unwilling to admit that they were bothered by copious and unpredictable menstrual periods. One Brush woman raised the issue of "excessive flowing" only to insist that it bothered her for only one day. One Davidoff interviewee did admit that her heavy periods were her biggest problem at menopause, but she was atypical. Perhaps many women reacted like a Davidoff woman's mother, who used to say, "I'm just flooding—not the world coming to an end."[34]

The reticence about menstrual irregularities may reflect a broader cultural silence about menstrual blood. In the late nineteenth and early twentieth centuries, domestic health guides and personal products literature urged women to be as discreet and private as possible about menstruation. As a result, discussions of menstrual flooding may have been regarded as too personal and too visceral to share.

If the hot flashes and unpredictable menstrual periods troubled the Brush and Davidoff women only slightly, the nervous symptoms bothered them more. Many of the Brush and Davidoff women felt particularly unsettled by the dramatic mood swings they endured. One of the Brush women lamented that she found herself "emotionally more unstable than before."[35] Other women complained about the volatility they experienced.[36] Harriet Nottingham felt so out of sorts due to her inability to control her emotions that she quit her teaching job. In retrospect, she insisted that her frustrations with teaching and with being denied a raise were "justified," but she admitted that she "overreacted."[37] One of the Brush women described in detail the toll her instability exacted from her.

> The nervousness and entire change in my mental attitude bothered me most. . . . I was exactly like Dr. Jeckle [*sic*] and Mr. Hyde. When I had a spell of that nervousness I did not look at things in my usual way . . . I felt tired all the time, I could hardly eat. . . . I had my mother-in-law living with me and she was getting old and ill and I laid a lot of it to the fact that I had so much to do to take care of her but she died later and I still had bad feelings so I realized that it had nothing to do with her being here, although I believe everything that makes it hard for a person is magnified at that time.[38]

Depression, too, plagued a few of the Brush and Davidoff women at menopause. Georgina Battsen, for example, noted that "the symptom which still stays with me is the depression which comes suddenly and is very black and deep while it lasts."[39] Another woman noted that her menopause forced her to face her own mortality. "Death for the first time became a reality which would someday actually come to me. I never *really* thought anything *like* that could happen to me."[40] A Brush woman provided a detailed account of her depression at menopause. She spent many nights wide awake, concerned about the security of the world and paralyzed by the fear that her husband might die. In the end, she coped with menopause by steeling herself with the philosophy that "there is no security in this world today: there is only courage and faith." Despite her wrenching experiences, she advised younger women not to "worry about the menopause [because] it's really overrated."[41]

Other women who experienced depression at middle age failed to immediately connect it to menopause. One woman, for example, admitted that she felt depressed at middle age, but she did not connect it to the physiological changes of menopause. If she had made this connection, she maintained that she "would not have paid as much attention to it."[42] Caroline Torlington "felt upset for several weeks not knowing it was menopause . . . which had upset her." After she discovered her symptoms were menopausal "they disappeared."[43] These comments echo the belief that menopause itself was an unimportant concern. Once depression was linked to menopause, it too could be dismissed as unimportant and trivial.

While some women could dismiss their menopausal depression, others suffered so profoundly that they sought professional help. Mabel Stewart wrote that she had been through "several nervous experiences and finally got to the end of my rope and was in a Convalescent Home for 3 weeks. . . . I'm still fighting it but am better."[44] Myrtle Thomas "popped into Silver Hill [a Connecticut establishment dedicated to the treatment of psychoneurosis] and then out."[45] Significantly, these women did not directly blame menopause for their troubles, citing "exhausted nerves" or a nervous temperament. Nevertheless, their experiences at menopause supported the larger cultural belief that menopause caused women "to go crazy."

Curiously, although the writers of medical and popular literature noted that women became nervous and depressed at menopause, they ignored a symptom experienced by some of the Brush and Davidoff women: rage. Ethel Dasher, for example, admitted feeling an "intense anger." Because she was widely known as someone who "actually likes *everybody*," she found her anger particularly unsettling.[46] In contrast, one of the Davidoff women refused to apologize for her anger. Although she was usually a placid person, she regularly "blew my top" during menopause. Rather than guilt or remorse, she seemed almost gleeful, admitting that she was "delighted" with her outbursts.[47]

These examples suggest that many middle-class women, for most of their lives, felt compelled to be the peacekeepers in their families and were expected to placate rather than to offend. When at menopause they found themselves feeling anger, they were disconcerted by the intensity of their own rage. But as the above examples show, at least one woman welcomed this excuse for emotional release. It also seems significant that the popular literature ignored this reaction entirely or translated it into the more appropriately feminine reaction, irritability. Feminized as irritability, anger could be more easily dismissed as an irrational response to trivial annoyances.

Domestic Upheaval

Although the Brush and Davidoff women acknowledged experiences with hot flashes and mood swings, the extramenopausal aspects of middle age—financial upheavals, wandering spouses, children at war—seemed to bother them most. Although only two of the Brush women claimed that the empty nest had been hard for them, several claimed that their children's departures—to attend college, to join the war, to gain independence—required some adjustment. But the Brush women testified that the nest was not always empty at menopause.[48] Several women noted that elderly parents and in-laws moved in with them. A few women shared their homes with other women, and at least one moved in with her parents.[49] The departure of children, then, was hardly the only household shift middle-aged women confronted.

Although many women experienced middle age as a trying, difficult time, most of them were reluctant to blame menopause for their problems. Instead, they blamed personal dramas and social circumstances. Economic challenges, unhappy marriages, personal losses, and wartime anxieties were cited as the causes of, or at least contributors to, feelings of irritability, depression, and nervousness. The example of Mabel Ashton is illustrative.

> I do not think that I was quite normal for some years prior to the beginning of the menopause. My husband was called into service in 1940 and I saw him only half a dozen times until spring, 1946. The worry over keeping the home together, the loneliness (both children were at school, far away) and a feeling of insecurity as well as the extra responsibility of handling the children alone, contributed to quite an unfortunate state of mind. I felt deserted by my husband, angry that he had left me. Possibly the carryover of these feelings influenced me both mentally and emotionally during the menopause. It is also possible that the menopause actually began prior to 1946, and that the feelings here may have been caused by it, to some extent.[50]

Another woman described family changes that began the same year as her menopause. Her husband lost his business, and the couple moved in with her parents. After he admitted that he had defrauded the business, they divorced. She then nursed her sister for six months as she was dying from leukemia. After her sister's death, she had a short affair with her brother-in-law. She admitted that "I have had so many emotional strains in the past three years that I am sure that they, not the menopause, have caused any slight distress I might have had."[51] Finally, another woman remarked that her "menopause was so coincidental with my husband's changes and my children's adolescence as well as war and radical change in family fortunes, it is hard to say what was the menopause and what some bad results of a neurotic marriage during bad times."[52]

These women insisted that symptoms of menopause could not be separated from the social setting in which menopause took place. They argued that personal problems (divorce, economic missteps, death) and societal circumstance (war, unemployment) affected their bodies and their emotions. While some women admitted to feeling poorly at menopause, they refused to hold their changing bodies as more responsible for their discomforts and anxieties than their social and familial circumstances. They refused to reduce their complex reactions to mid-life to the fluctuations of their glands.

Less Discussion

While few of the Brush and Davidoff women admitted menopausal difficulties, many of them readily offered their opinion of how women should and shouldn't act at menopause. Most importantly, many of the Brush and Davidoff women insisted that women should keep mum about their sleepless nights and irregular periods. One woman noted with impatience, "If we discussed this subject less with friends and relatives, and confined ourselves to the seeking of professional advice, the majority of women . . . would weather this so-called storm more naturally and therefore more successfully."[53] Others claimed to have been "politely bored by play by play accounts of friends."[54] Agnes Bailey, for example, believed that "less discussion save at times with a doctor," would help most women.[55]

The evidence suggests that menopausal women widely believed that other menopausal women exaggerated their symptoms to elicit sympathy.[56] Olivia Fenting, for example, was "a little fed up with the way some of my friends have been carrying their menopause around on a silver platter—I have never known anyone to have a 'terrific' time that didn't have the leisure to make the most of it." Another woman refused to "put on the acts that I saw other women putting on." Similarly, Gladys Woods lamented that it had not occurred to her to "emote and enjoy all the symptoms some of my friends profess to endure. . . . For many people it is an opportunity to receive sympathy and attention."[57] Another respondent admired the behavior of an acquaintance who suffered intensely at menopause but refrained from sharing her troubles.[58]

These comments indicate that most of these women agreed with the popular advice that they should not discuss their menopausal problems.

Indeed, women who suffered stoically garnered respect from their peers. But the comments of the Brush respondents suggest that some menopausal women eagerly sought support and information from women in similar circumstances.[59] Certainly most of the women claimed to know other women who talked about their symptoms, and a few of the Brush and Davidoff respondents admitted outright that conversation with friends and relatives helped them cope with menopause. One of the women, for example, turned to her friends for help "dealing with heavy flow." Another mentioned that a friend "bolstered her up" during her dark moods.[60] This suggests that the prohibition against discussing menopause probably did cause some women to keep their problems to themselves. Nevertheless some women risked dirty looks and exasperated children by sharing their menopausal experiences as they sought relief from their fears and discomforts.

Self-Control and Busy Hands

In addition to keeping their menopausal difficulties to themselves, many women seem to have willed themselves to ignore their problems. As one woman explained, "I have always believed in the predominance of mind over matter to a reasonable extent—that is, if you brood over certain types of physical ills that can happen to you, they are more likely to happen."[61] Another woman preached: "One can control those feelings to a great extent with will power. I know I did. . . . Anyone can do anything they want if they WORK hard enough at it."[62] But achieving the state of mind over matter was no easy feat, as one Brush respondent stressed. She claimed that she was able to "sublimate" her menopausal difficulties, but she emphasized the enormity of the task. "I . . . wish to say it was not easy and I don't recommend it to anyone who is not strong minded!"[63] These women's experiences belie the position, promoted by other Davidoff and Brush women, that menopause posed no particular discomforts or problems. Indeed, these women struggled mightily against the onslaught of their symptoms. Nevertheless, by sheer force of will, they were able to act as if menopause were an inconsequential process, a trivial transformation. These women's attitudes recall the advice of women physicians at the beginning of the century. Fearing that menopausal women's "irrational" and uncontrolled behaviors might be used against all women, they urged their patients and readers to exert mind over matter. Forty some years later, menopausal women themselves encouraged the same strategy.

When asked to give her advice to younger women, one of the Brush respondents suggested firmly, "Keep busy."[64] Most of these women believed that if women had enough to do, they would not be able to "indulge" the difficulties arising from menopause. And keep busy these women did. The Brush women filled their lives with a variety of activities, ranging from birdwatching and gardening to playing the violin to working for the cause of world government. Church activities featured prominently in the lives of some women. One woman found pleasure and distraction by reading the Bible in foreign languages. Some women surveyed volunteered with the Red Cross, the SPCA, or the League of Women Voters. One woman noted that her days spent volunteering at the veteran's hospital kept her mind off her own minor aches and pains. During their busy days, these women did not neglect their physical needs. Many kept active physically with regular rounds of golf, tennis matches, and lap swimming. One woman even climbed mountains for pleasure and diversion. And, true to the stereotype, some played bridge.[65]

But while many of the Brush women's days were so filled with golf and gardening that they barely noticed their menopausal symptoms, other women's days were devoted to paid labor. Although almost all of the Davidoff and roughly 60 percent of the Brush respondents were full-time homemakers, many of those who were not saw their paid work as integral to their experiences of menopause. One part-time college professor, for example, regarded her job as one of the most important factors in her easy passage through menopause.[66] For this woman, work was an important part of her life, but she didn't need employment to support herself or her family. Other women, both single and married, needed their jobs.[67] Some women who were forced to work scolded those who had enough leisure time to indulge their symptoms. One woman described the situation that led her to full-time employment. Just before the onset of her menopause she experienced "loss of husband to another woman, loss of home, all financial support and necessity of learning to earn every cent I would spend for the rest of my life with no training." Her circumstances led her to believe that the "women who have not been able to live on the efforts of a father or a husband and have been entirely dependent financially on their own abilities, have learned to secondize uncomfortable physical feelings since they must be on the job and *alert* 50 weeks of the year."[68] Olivia Fenting agreed that nobody suffered at menopause who "didn't have the leisure to make the most of it. The gals who have had to hold a job for financial reasons and also raise a family seem to have weathered the storm."[69] As one woman recalled, "For me, the menopause came during the Second World

War. I was living on a farm, doing the housework for myself, my husband and four sons and holding down an 8 hour day shift job in the lab of a local chemical plant. I feel that I had no time to sit around worrying about myself or how I felt. I am sure that with more time on my hands I should have found it very trying."[70] These women either dismissed menopausal difficulties as the consequences of idle days or they believed that only idle women could afford to be incapacitated by their menopausal symptoms.

Don't Think about Yourself

If idle self-indulgence contributed to menopausal incapacity, several Brush women had a simple solution: stop dwelling on yourself. One woman wondered incredulously how "with the world sitting on a keg of dynamite" intelligent women could "sit around and think about menopause? Of all things!!!"[71] Another woman seemed to understand the impulse, but she too disapproved. To counter introspective tendencies, she would periodically ask herself, "Are you by any chance thinking about yourself?" This question jolted her out of her self-indulgence and led her to ignore her own problems for what she termed more noble causes.[72]

To interrupt the inward gaze, many Brush women urged menopausal women to devote themselves to the service of others. Elizabeth Archibald advised young women to "lose yourself in service for others and your own aches and pains won't seem so important." Another woman advised, "Do for others and don't think about yourself." Finally, another woman urged others to "find something more important than you are into which you can throw your full energy."[73]

While several women saw service to others as the key to a successful menopausal transition, many took an interestingly contrary approach: they believed that perhaps they had given enough to others and could now start looking after themselves. Almost 75 percent of the middle-aged women surveyed by Bernice Neugarten in 1962 agreed that "a woman feels freer to do things for herself" after menopause.[74] Brush respondent Mary Clark described her return to earlier interests: "For many years I had a great desire to write. There was no time for it because I put first my duties as wife, mother, and homemaker. Unfortunately, the habits of those many years have tended to relegate to the background the accomplishments of the writing desire. Perhaps there may still be time to try my wings after I have gotten rid of the demanding responsibilities of my home."[75]

In order to avoid this woman's situation, some women urged the next generation to develop a variety of interests and activities long before menopause arrived and the presumed empty nest of those years left them with loads of time (or at least fewer loads of laundry) but little worthwhile occupation. A woman physician, for example, recommended that women "live a regular and useful life but do have interests outside oneself in the local or national or international community."[76] Brush respondent Mary Patrick advised other women to "develop some interest outside the family to carry over the time when children leave home" while still putting "husband and home as the first call on their time and interest." Another woman warned younger women "not to get bogged down in domesticity."[77]

These comments suggest that some survey respondents, perhaps reflecting their educations, never intended to devote their lives exclusively to domesticity. While they believed that their families came first, they also intended to pursue other intellectual, artistic, political, or professional interests. But as Mary Clark indicates, that intention was sometimes impossible to fulfill while raising a family. As the popular literature in the 1940s and 1950s suggested, it may have been more realistic for many women to hold personal ambition at bay until after menopause.

For some middle-class women, menopause did provide some newly found time to fill. The Brush and Davidoff women, however, hardly viewed menopause as liberation from the constraints of domesticity. Indeed, many of them seemed obliged to find something useful and worthy to fill their time—to nurse the injured, to soothe the nation, to feed the hungry. Perhaps this suggests that they had never felt particularly boxed in by domesticity. Indeed, some of the Brush women avoided at least some of the demands of domesticity by pursuing careers or remaining single. But perhaps it also reflects domesticity's continuing hold. While there might have been fewer loads of laundry each week and fewer mouths to feed, women's household tasks did not disappear. Shirts didn't mend themselves, and shelves still needed dusting.

The Hormonal Solution

The promotion of mind over matter and the importance of undertaking worthy projects masks the contradictory beliefs these women held about menopause. While they clearly held that women could and should control their responses to menopause's physical and social changes, they also, on some level, blamed their bodies for the turmoil they experienced. The responses of the Neugarten women, in particular, suggest a conflict. While more than 70 percent of them believed that women who were troubled by menopause either expected trouble or had "nothing to do with their time," 78 percent also believed that women's troubles at menopause were caused by "something they can't control—changes inside their bodies." They seemed to believe that, on the one hand, women bring on trouble by anticipating it or by whiling away their idle days, but, on the other, that menopausal troubles are physiological and therefore beyond a woman's control. The Brush and Davidoff women also illustrate this ambivalence. Many of the same women who urged other women to get busy and ignore menopause were themselves helped through their "change" by drugs. More than 30 percent of both the Brush and Davidoff women received at least some hormone therapy. Further, most of the Brush women believed that physicians could eliminate any menopausal difficulties that self-control and determination failed to quell. One woman, for example, urged others to "go immediately to a doctor when symptoms appear."[78] Another woman got through menopause by keeping busy and "letting the doctor do the prescribing."[79]

Reading middle-class women's insistence that menopause was inconsequential against the backdrop of widespread hormone use suggests that the dismissal of menopause was a product, in part, of medicalization. Noting that one woman who urged other women to "think of it as little as possible," took hormones, suggests that willpower and voter registration drives were not always enough to guarantee regular sleep and a happy husband.[80] Surely, not all women who denied the importance of menopause were taking hormones. Without medical intervention, however, some of the others holding this opinion might have described significantly different experiences with menopause and might have been less apt to dismiss it as "a lot of bunk." Indeed, the women most disquieted by their symptoms might have been precisely those women who sought medical aid and thus could later insist that "a few pills or a shot or two can work wonders and . . . solve the problem of menopause."[81]

SEVEN

Feminine Forever

Robert A. Wilson and the Hormonal Revolution, 1963–1980

"The unpalatable truth must be faced that all postmenopausal women are castrates." So began a 1963 article by physician Robert A. Wilson and his wife Thelma, which appeared in the *Journal of the American Geriatrics Society*. In this article, the Wilsons argued that untreated menopause robbed women of their femininity and doomed them to live the remainder of their lives as mere remnants of their previous selves.[1] Detailing the dire consequences of "Nature's defeminization," the Wilsons claimed that estrogen depletion, the cause of menopausal and postmenopausal afflictions, led to hypertension, high cholesterol, osteoporosis, and arthritis. In addition, the Wilsons insisted that menopause frequently led to serious emotional disturbances; even women who escaped debilitating depression frequently acquired a "vapid cow-like feeling called a negative state." The authors maintained that these women see the world "through a grey veil, and they live as docile harmless creatures missing most of life's values." Indeed, the Wilsons believed that these women "exist rather than live." The Wilsons did not, however, abandon menopausal women to their dreary fate. Rather, they promised women a pharmaceutical escape route—estrogen replacement therapy (ERT). Robert Wilson and his wife insisted that menopause was unnecessary and could be prevented by "life-long substitution therapy," ideally from "puberty to the grave" to keep women "feminine forever."[2]

The efforts of Robert Wilson and other like-minded physicians sparked a medical movement that transformed hormone replacement therapy from a judiciously prescribed treatment for severe menopausal symptoms to a commonly prescribed therapy for the symptoms of menopause and female aging. Although most doctors did not accept Wilson's most radical claim—that all women should be treated with hormones for their entire lives—physicians during this era did prescribe hormones more freely and for longer periods than ever before.

When exploring this period in the history of menopause, many scholars have credited Wilson with fomenting the hormonal revolution by tirelessly promoting the disease model of menopause to both women and the medical community.[3] These critics have argued that sexism and misogyny infused Wilson's work and that he capitalized on women's fears of aging. According to this explanation, insecurity and anxiety planted by the popular press led women to their doctors' offices to demand hormone therapy. Although Wilson undeniably publicized the concept of menopause as a "deficiency disease," a close examination of Wilson's efforts, the medical reaction to them, and their popular dissemination suggests that critics have overstated the acceptance of this construction.

On the medical front, although most physicians who treated menopausal women did eventually add estrogen replacement therapy to their therapeutic arsenals, doctors did not overwhelmingly advise long-term estrogen use nor did they agree that all women would benefit from treatment. In addition, many physicians disputed that menopause was best seen as a deficiency disease. Many continued to regard the difficulties women encountered at menopause as the result of a natural transition and not evidence of a more significant disease. Further, Wilson and the publicity he inspired did clearly make hormone therapy attractive to menopausal women by preying on their fears of aging, but this does not fully explain Wilson's appeal. It is important to recognize that Wilson and his supporters also attracted women by placing the menopausal woman's needs at the center of medical and public discourse. Wilson portrayed himself as a friend to women, highlighting his efforts to take seriously middle-aged women and their ailments after centuries of neglect by male physicians. Acknowledging women's broadened horizons, he promised to keep women healthy and feminine and therefore better equipped to seize the opportunities newly opened to them.

Physicians' diverse opinions and practices regarding menopause were reflected in the popular literature available to women. Although many of the books and magazine articles on the subject that appeared between 1963 and 1975 did promote estrogen therapy as an attractive option for women with severe symptoms, they did not mandate ERT for all menopausal women to prevent aging or disease. Indeed, after 1975, when serious questions emerged about the safety of replacement hormones, writers in the popular media urged women to rethink their dependence on ERT, and they retreated even further from Wilson's position.

Amid the medical and popular concern about hormone replacement therapy, discussion of menopause itself and what it might mean to women both increased and decreased. Certainly, the discussion of menopause as a "deficiency disease" and a "supreme tragedy" gave new urgency and visibility to the menopausal transition and gave it a new cultural meaning as the gateway to old age and debility. Efforts to offer alternative meanings for menopause challenged its perception as a pathology, but in their scramble to establish menopause as natural, normal, and not necessarily an occasion for medical intervention, anti-Wilson physicians and popular health writers failed to articulate an understanding of menopause that did not sound defensive. Largely gone was the discussion of menopause as liberation; infrequent was the promise of golden years filled with worthy causes. Wilson and those who shared his views did not manage to furnish the only message about menopause between 1963 and 1975, but they succeeded in shifting the conversation about menopause to a discussion about treatment.

Wilson and the Estrogen Deficiency Debate

Robert A. Wilson's early medical career was unremarkable, particularly when compared to his later prominence. Born in 1895, Wilson graduated from SUNY Downstate Medical Center in Brooklyn in 1919. He then entered private practice as an obstetrician and gynecologist affiliated with Methodist Hospital of Brooklyn. Although he dedicated his practice to treating menopausal women, he began his publishing efforts only as retirement neared; his first article appeared in 1962, when he was in his late sixties.[4]

In the early 1960s, Wilson began in earnest the work that brought him national attention. In July 1963, at roughly the same time that his article on the "Fate of the Nontreated Postmenopausal Woman" appeared, Wilson launched his battle against menopause on another front by establishing the Wilson Research Foundation (WRF) in New York. The foundation hoped to "achieve the elimination of estrogen/progesterone deficiency states including the menopause."[5]

The foundation began as a family affair. The board of directors included Wilson, his wife, Thelma, and his daughter-in-law, Gretchen. His son, Robert A. Wilson, Jr., served as the executive director. The organization was not static, however, and by 1971, Leonard Brenner, a lawyer and founding board member, had taken over as the foundation's executive director.

The WRF relied on drug companies for most of its funding. In 1964, for example, the foundation received 92 percent of its funding from the combined contributions of Searle (manufacturer of Enovid, a birth control pill), Ayerst (manufacturer of the conjugated estrogen Premarin), and Upjohn (manufacturer of the progestin Provera). By its closure in 1973, the WRF had received most of its $1.3 million budget from drug companies.[6] But the foundation also turned to physicians and the general public for financial backing. Solicitation letters portrayed menopause as one of the most troubling social ills facing the country. Unlike other national problems, however, these letters proclaimed menopause as being preventable. A 1970 solicitation, for example, asked, "Do you feel helpless at times—unable to do much about such problems as inflation, pollution, the generation gap, drug traffic in our schools?" The letter admitted that solving such problems might seem beyond the reach of individuals, but the recipient could help make "menopause . . . a thing of the past."[7] Another letter presented the case even more urgently. "In view of the dreadful hemorrhaging wound this country has been suffering from, namely the Vietnam war with its dangerous drainage and depletion of our financial, cultural and especially spiritual resources, this appeal may at first seem inappropriate. . . . The problem of the estrogen deficient woman [however] is still decidedly with us."[8]

The WRF required funds to support the heart of its mission—education through information. As part of their educational campaign, representatives of the WRF presented papers at major medical society meetings and gave lectures extolling the possibilities of ERT at medical schools. In addition, the foundation sponsored an annual conference to publicize further the latest developments in replacement therapy.[9]

Although Wilson and the foundation reached out to the medical community, they seemed more intent on presenting their case directly to women. The foundation published a series of provocatively titled pamphlets for distribution to women and to doctors for display in their waiting rooms. The foundation developed a speaker's bureau that presented lectures to women's clubs, such as the National Council of Jewish Women and the local YWCAs.[10] The WRF also relied on women to carry the message to their friends and neighbors: the foundation supplied materials—including a film—for women to distribute at informal neighborhood gatherings.

Wilson and his foundation reached out to popular media outlets for further publicity. On occasion, Wilson's aggressive tactics hurt his cause. Reporter Barbara Yuncker of the *New York Times* recalled in an interview that "he and his people, especially his son, were always calling. . . . They were proselytizing like mad."[11] Gilbert Cant of *Time* claimed that "he was pestered so much by Wilson that he . . . instructed his receptionist to say he's out when Wilson calls."[12] Nevertheless, Wilson's efforts to publicize the plight of untreated menopausal women succeeded. By 1964, *Time* and *Newsweek* had published articles extolling the promise of hormone therapy to cure menopause, and women's magazines followed in 1965.[13] Writer Ann Walsh, so inspired by the coverage of Wilson's theories, wrote her own book describing her miraculous experience with estrogen therapy. In *E.R.T.: The Pills to Keep Women Young*, Walsh reported that menopause had stolen her womanhood and that ERT allowed her to "feel—and live— like a woman again."[14] Local newspapers also followed up on the story.[15] Although the popular media demonstrated a great deal of curiosity about Wilson in the early 1960s, the press coverage of Wilson, hormone replacement therapy, and estrogen deficiency disease (menopause) intensified in 1966, following the publication of Robert Wilson's best-selling book, *Feminine Forever*.

Keeping Women Feminine Forever

Feminine Forever carried a straightforward message to its readers. In prose designed to alarm, Wilson described menopause as a "deficiency disease," much like diabetes. Comparing ERT to insulin, Wilson insisted that replacement therapy could both cure and prevent estrogen deficiency disease. But unlike diabetes, menopause did not merely rob women of their health; it also stole from women their youth, femininity, and sexuality. Challenging the views in earlier popular books on menopause, Wilson dismissed as irresponsible any claims that menopause represented a positive transition. Instead, he characterized menopause and estrogen deficiency disease as a "supreme tragedy" and catalogued its horrors. But Wilson did not leave women without weapons to fight their battle against aging. Unlike his predecessors, he promised to prevent menopause entirely by tackling the problem at its source rather than superficially focusing on symptoms.[16]

By characterizing menopause as a disease, Wilson gained ammunition for his position that menopause required treatment; responsible physicians did not allow diseases to progress unimpeded. He dismissed the position that menopause should be allowed to run its natural course with two arguments. First, he claimed that doctors routinely thwarted nature. The very attempt to cure disease challenged the desirability of things "natural." Second, he claimed that estrogen therapy actually served nature's plan by maintaining the necessary hormonal balance. "The prematurely aging castrate" rather than the medically restored woman, he argued, was "unnatural."[17]

To bolster his position that menopause was a debilitating disease rather than a natural transition, Wilson focused exclusively on its negative aspects. He characterized menopause as "living decay," for example, and bemoaned the fate of women "who had shriveled into caricatures of their former selves." He claimed that estrogen deficiency led to dry skin, wrinkles, and brittle bones, adding that it also produced the dowager's hump which left women "hunchbacked." He further insisted that menopause made women more vulnerable to heart disease.[18]

Wilson did not address physical symptoms exclusively. He also recounted the emotional and mental ravages of menopause. In particular, he claimed that menopause caused once vibrant and active women to lose interest in the world around them. He maintained that middle-aged women "barely notice what goes on about them." Bemoaning the wasted potential, he described the lives of these women: "Unseeing, unfeeling, they stumble through the years that could have been filled to the brim with life's most positive values."[19]

Although Wilson acknowledged the above symptoms, he reserved most of his attention for the site of the "primary" and most devastating effects of menopause: the female genitalia. In menopause, he claimed, a "woman becomes the equivalent of a eunuch." He explained that the "entire genital system dries up. The breasts become flabby and shrink, and the vagina becomes stiff and unyielding . . . mak[ing] sexual intercourse impossible." He contrasted the plight of women with the comparatively lucky circumstances prevailing for men. "A man remains male as long as he lives," he argued. "Age does not rob him of his sexual appetite nor of the means of satisfying it." But a woman's "body ultimately betrays her. It destroys her womanhood during her prime."[20]

Even when portraying other debilitating aspects of menopause, Wilson generally traced them back to sexuality. He blamed the "menopausal negativism" that plagued middle-aged women, for example, on their unhappy marriages. He claimed that many women entered marriage filled with joyous expectations for domestic life only to discover that reality did not live up to their dreams. Until menopause, however, Wilson argued, these women continued to hope for better times; when the menopause "suddenly desexed" them, they lost all hope. At that point, realizing "dimly that the driving power of her existence has somehow failed her, [the menopausal woman] thrashes about wildly. . . . Eventually she subsides into an uneasy apathy that is indeed a form of death within life." Indeed, all too frequently, Wilson stated, "Women endure the passing years with cow-like passivity and disinterest; and a disturbingly high number take refuge in alcohol, sleeping pills, and sometimes even in suicide."[21]

After he established that menopause robbed women of their sexuality, Wilson emphasized the centrality of sexuality in women's lives. He contended that "a woman's body is the key to her fate. . . . Her physical, social and psychological fulfillment all depend on one crucial test: her ability to attract a suitable mate and hold his interest over many years." To ensure his point was understood, he continued: "a woman's physical appeal is her starting capital in the venture of life—the 'ante' which lets her into the game."[22]

Indeed, Wilson believed that estrogen therapy's "ultimate merit" was its ability to bring "enrichment and harmony to a woman's marriage at a time in her life when these qualities are especially needful to her." He assured his readers that estrogen would render women "sexually attractive and potent." Wilson did not, however, suggest that only women benefited by this boost to their attractiveness. Instead, he claimed that the promise of ERT obliged women to remain sexually receptive. In a statement that revealed a great deal about Wilson's motivations, he insisted that "every woman has the right—indeed the duty—to counteract the chemical castration that befalls her during her middle years."[23] For Wilson then, ERT was as important for maintaining a husband's sexuality at middle age as it was to maintaining a wife's.

While Wilson admitted that 15 percent of untreated women might escape debility at menopause, he insisted that no woman could consider herself safe. Even women who appeared free from menopausal torments on the surface were often plagued by debilitating fatigue, thinning bones, and philandering husbands. He argued that every woman "faces the threat of extreme suffering and incapacity" and that treatment orthodoxy should not be determined by the lucky few but by the suffering majority.[24]

To avoid the ravages of menopause, Wilson advised, every woman over twenty should visit her doctor and demand a Femininity Index to ascertain whether "her body is still feminine, or whether it is gradually turning neu-

ter." This test determined the relative incidence of three normally occurring cells in the vagina: superficial (mature), intermediate (less mature),
and parabasal (immature). In postadolescent women, the ratio of these
cells is 85:15:15. In "estrogen deficient" women, however, parabasal cells
dominate, and the percentage of superficial cells declines (10:20:70). Wilson argued that estrogen could restore the vaginal cell balance to its
premenopausal level, thereby also restoring a woman's femininity.[25]

Central to his conception of menopause prevention, Wilson urged women to remain on ERT for the remainder of their lives. Because estrogen
endowed women with their femininity, they needed a continual influx of
estrogen to prevent the otherwise inevitable decline of all their female attributes. Only by continuing to replace estrogen could women secure a
healthy and feminine future. Without the hormone, menopause and debility would promptly result.[26]

Wilson's prescription for preventing menopause and preserving femininity included a combination of estrogen and progestin, known as hormone replacement therapy (HRT). For a woman in her fifties, for example, he suggested 1.25 milligrams of estrogen taken daily for forty-two
days, with 10 milligrams of progestin added on days thirty-one through
forty-two. All drugs were then discontinued for five days, during which
endometrial shedding, or in Wilson's words "a token of your restored
femininity" occurred. On day forty-eight, the cycle would begin again.
For younger women, he suggested a much shorter cycle, one mimicking a
woman's normal menstrual cycle; for older women, he advised slowly extending the length of the cycle so that the bleeding would occur less and
less frequently.[27]

Wilson advocated this regimen to combat opponents and skeptics who
suggested that estrogen therapy increased women's risk of endometrial
cancer. He denounced the cancer concerns as "entirely false." Indeed, he
argued that HRT (with its "planned bleed") provided women with "cancer insurance." Wilson explained how the "menstrual" flow served "as a
kind of internal bath, washing out the womb" and preventing the build-
up of potentially malignant tissue. Hormone therapy did not cause cancer,
he insisted. HRT prevented cancer.[28]

At the end of *Feminine Forever,* Wilson advocated an even bolder treatment plan. Impressed that one of his patients who had taken oral contraceptives claimed to have never reached menopause, he concluded that
estrogenic contraceptives automatically prevented menopause and its consequences. He claimed, "I can now confidently assert that no woman who

uses estrogenic birth control pills . . . will ever experience menopause if she continues taking the 'pill' beyond her childbearing years."[29] By making this claim, Wilson thereby recommended estrogen from "puberty to the grave," to ensure women remained "fully sexed" throughout their lives.

Although Wilson repeatedly assured women that menopause was completely preventable, he did admit that estrogen therapy could not avoid the only universal consequence of menopause—infertility. Wilson viewed infertility, however, as an insignificant side effect of estrogen deficiency disease, barely worth noting at all. Wilson's attitude toward fertility signals an important shift in emphasis from that of past writers on menopause and reflects changing meanings of menopause and womanhood. Between 1897 and 1937, physicians considered fertility loss to be the key to understanding a woman's reaction to menopause. This framework underscored a woman's value in terms of her potential to achieve motherhood. Motherhood remained central to womanhood between 1938 and 1962, but throughout that period female sexuality also gained increased attention as an essential component of family life; women were still expected to bear children, but they were also expected to be enthusiastic and alluring sexual partners before and after menopause. In Wilson's work, however, women's value as sexual partners loomed larger than their value as mothers.

Menopause, Youth, and the Sexual Revolution

Wilson's emphasis on sexuality and youth reflects and depends upon the tenor of his time. By 1963, the United States was reassessing its attitudes toward marriage and sexuality in what some historians and contemporary observers have dubbed a sexual revolution. During this period, the popular culture increasingly acknowledged, indeed celebrated, sexual activity outside marriage. Hugh Hefner and his *Playboy* empire encouraged men to consider women as founts of sexual pleasure to be enjoyed without committing to marriage. Helen Gurley Brown, in her book *Sex and the Single Girl* and her magazine *Cosmopolitan,* encouraged women not to wait until marriage to enjoy the pleasures of the flesh.[30] Movies such as *Alfie* and *Georgy Girl* asked audiences to adjudicate the sexual revolution on the big screen.

While Hefner and Brown goaded their readers to remain single to better secure the "good life" and its materialistic trappings, another group was experiencing their own sexual revolution. The 1960s counterculture similarly eschewed traditional standards of sexual decency. In both casual and formal experiments, America's "youth" challenged traditional family structures and sexual mores. Consistent with these social trends, women's sexuality became increasingly visible and their sexual currency increasingly valued. The birth control pill, on the market since 1960, severed reproduction from sexuality and allowed women (perhaps obligated women) to indulge sexual desire and curiosity with less fear of pregnancy. Further, researchers heralded women's unique sexual abilities. Sexologists William Masters and Virginia Johnson depicted women as sexually gifted by publicizing their capacity for multiple orgasms. These changes did not mean that women were no longer valued as wives and mothers. They were. But their sexual roles and their nurturing roles no longer necessarily coincided, and they sometimes competed. As historians John D'Emilio and Estelle Freedman explained, the increased visibility of female sexuality intensified the pressure on women. "Wives could look with concern at the sexual competition they faced from women who did not have to change diapers or cook for a family."[31]

These social changes were reflected in demographic data. The marriage rate dipped sharply between 1960 and 1980, declining by more than 25 percent. Although most adults still married, they did so later in life than had the previous generation. The postponement of marriage and the widespread use of birth control (and abortion) affected birthrates. By the mid-1970s, the birthrate had slipped far below the peaks of the 1950s.[32]

At the same time that female sexuality was increasingly visible outside of marriage, older women, whose likenesses graced neither the cover of *Cosmo* nor the centerfold of *Playboy,* increasingly experienced diminished value in the sexual marketplace. As one author put it in 1969, "The furrowed brow, the wrinkled cheek, the baggy eyelid and the sagging jowl have no place in a modern America where the smooth firm flesh of youth has become a cultural totem." Susan Sontag, in her now classic 1972 essay, "The Double Standard of Aging," claimed that "for most women, aging means a humiliating process of gradual disqualification." Another woman wistfully reported, "Just as women have been given the capacity to live longer and look younger than ever before in their later years, this youth and sex-saturated society enshrines the sixteen-year-old girl as female incarnate."[33]

In response to the pressure, some women were willing to take drastic measures to retain their youth (or at least their youthful appearance). The postwar years saw the rise of the face-lift. Reconstructive surgeons, left without disfigured soldiers to fix, found in middle-aged women (and later, but always to a lesser degree, middle-aged men) a ready clientele. For a range of reasons, both economic (to keep their jobs) and personal (to keep their husbands), middle-aged women turned to surgical interventions to erase the ravages of time. By the end of the 1960s, a face-lift was not just the privilege (if it can be seen as such) of the very rich: it also became accessible to middle-class women willing to forgo new shoes and a new carpet for a newly youthful appearance.[34]

Perhaps middle-aged women were right to be anxious; the divorce rate increased by more than 90 percent between 1960 and 1980, and, most chillingly, these statistics reflected rising numbers of marriages that ended after fifteen or more years.[35] On television, the real Pat Loud and the fictional Edie Grant, both middle-aged, instigated divorce proceedings in 1973, but the sexual valorization of young women led many middle-aged women to fear divorce, or at least their husband's dalliances.[36]

Wilson's work reflected and capitalized on society's reassessment of women during this period. He connected menopause with the aged female body at a moment when an aged body accounted for women's alienation from many of the opportunities and obligations of the female and feminine body. By emphasizing an older woman's loss of femininity and sexual allure, Wilson portrayed her as an unwanted commodity in an increasingly competitive sexual marketplace. Menopausal women who wanted to hold onto their husbands (or perhaps to attract one), he argued, needed hormones to compensate for the ravages of time. Indeed, compared to a face-lift, a daily pill may have seemed like a prudent and reasonable strategy for protecting the marital investment.

Champion of Women

Central to *Feminine Forever,* then, is Wilson's unflattering, indeed disparaging, portrait of aging women. He certainly described middle-aged women as pitiable creatures. As many scholars have pointed out, his emphasis on femininity and the ability to retain a man's ardor promoted sexist notions of women and womanhood.[37] But Wilson did not merely deprecate older women and prey on their fears. In order to understand why Wilson appealed to the very women he belittled, it is critical to understand his "feminist" stance. By characterizing himself as a friend to women and a proponent of female self-determination, Wilson struck a nerve with women who felt ignored and dismissed by their doctors. Although Wilson emphasized the negative aspects of menopause and thereby intensified women's fears of aging, he also reached out to them in the guise of concerned benefactor.

A few scholars have dismissed Wilson's alleged pro-woman tactics as further evidence of his disregard for women. Katherine MacPherson, for example, claimed that by assuming "the stance of a woman's advocate" he merely "disguised his misogyny." Another critic argued that his approach merely "cloaked" his "virulent . . . misogyny." Although Wilson's depiction of older women as debilitated castrates clearly did not serve their best interests, dismissing Wilson's approach as misogynistic misses the opportunity to explore why women might have found his rhetoric reassuring.[38]

In *Feminine Forever*, Wilson cast himself as an advocate for women's needs at middle age. He blamed the current medical lack of interest in menopause and menopausal patients to "male indifference to anything exclusively female" and a dominant "anti-feminine attitude." He insisted, for example, that if male doctors experienced similar symptoms, they would not ignore them. He asked if the "man of medicine noticed his own genitalia gradually shrinking . . . [would he] be as indifferent to genital atrophy as he now appears?" Situating himself in apparent opposition to most of his male colleagues, he denounced the general medical neglect of menopause and dedicated his life to easing the suffering of menopausal women.[39] Wilson's devotion to easing women's suffering inspired Dr. Robert B. Greenblatt, professor of endocrinology at the Medical College of Georgia, to characterize Wilson as "a gallant knight" rescuing his fair lady in her "despairing years."[40]

Although he repeatedly reminded his readers of women's crucial drive to attract mates, Wilson also acknowledged that women's roles in society were expanding beyond wife and mother. This, too, gave him an opportunity to promote ERT. He argued that estrogen-deficient women missed out on the broader opportunities that were arising, making ERT necessary for women if they were to seize life's opportunities. He promoted estrogen as the "life force that motivates work, study, ambition, and that marvelous urge toward excellence that inspires the best of human beings." While he acknowledged that estrogen alone did not guarantee success, he maintained that "a woman cannot live up to her opportunities without her full quota of estrogen." The menopausal syndrome particularly handicapped women executives because it diminished the "morale of the woman's subordinates" and might "lead to serious errors of executive judgment." He underscored the problem by reminding his readers that "more and more women [were] entrusted with decision making posts in business, government, and in various institutions." The problem was exacerbated because "the syndrome develops at a time when businesswomen are at the apex of their careers and have attained their greatest range of responsibility and power."[41]

By acknowledging and affirming women's expanded social and professional roles, Wilson mirrored some of his predecessors. But his approach also explained why some women found his message so appealing. He portrayed himself as catering to modern women who were trying to make it in a modern world. In one sense, his emphasis on femininity and sexuality undercut his belief in women's professional abilities. In another, however, he provided a reassuring message: women can remain feminine as they enter middle age and middle management.

Wilson's use of women's increasing calls for power and autonomy to focus their attention back on their appearance surely had its historical precursors. The tactic became even more popular, however, in the 1970s, as advertisers co-opted feminism to sell women perfume ("I can bring home the bacon and fry it up in a pan"), cigarettes ("You've come a long way, baby"), and feminine hygiene products (New Freedom Maxi pads). Women were urged to associate increased social opportunities with the need to look (and smell) their best.

Wilson realized that not all physicians would adopt his treatment plan; indeed, he had already experienced the skepticism and indifference of his colleagues. But he consoled himself that "other medical innovators," such as Semmelweis, Jenner, and Papanicolaou, had been similarly rebuffed by their peers. Wilson believed, however, that the "general acceptance of hormone therapy . . . seem[ed] imminent." He compared those who remained skeptical to those "persons who would tear the telescope from Galileo's eyes or wrest the dissecting knife from the hand of Vesalius."[42] Wilson believed that like these illustrious scientists, he too would be vindicated.

A Medical Movement

At the beginning of Wilson's campaign, most physicians seemed unaware of his claims and the details of his treatment, and they were understandably puzzled when their patients began asking questions about Wilson and requesting hormone therapy. Some doctors wrote to the American Medical Association (AMA) seeking information about Wilson, his foundation, and his therapy. One physician, for example, sought information about the

WRF "because a patient of mine has recently been flooded with literature from them on the hormonal life." A physician from Denver, Colorado, wrote to the AMA on behalf of a family member who had received a brochure from the WRF. Like many others, he wondered about the central role of Wilson's family on the foundation's board of directors, but he retained an open mind and remarked that if "this organization is in good repute I would like to encourage this family member to continue correspondence with the foundation." Other physicians questioned the funding behind the WRF. A New York State doctor worried whether the Wilson Foundation was merely a "group of pharmaceutical manufacturers whose major premise is to sell estrogens."[43]

The letters from physicians and the public initially caught the AMA off guard. It responded to a March 1964 letter by admitting that it had never heard of the Wilson Research Foundation. Later that year, the AMA seemed better prepared, acknowledging that it was acquainted with Wilson's work. In a restrained letter, the AMA noted that Wilson's "aggressive approach" to menopause remained controversial and that the AMA believed that the therapy was "more extensive than is warranted." By 1966, the AMA issued a stronger response.

> It is our opinion that Dr. Wilson's claims of benefit exceed the available scientific evidence. Aging is a complex process. Decline in estrogen production is only one factor involved and its importance and mechanism of action is poorly defined in many aspects of human physiology. The American Medical Association does not endorse any products or regimens of treatment, but we do attempt to evaluate them in the light of available scientific evidence. Dr. Wilson's regimen is one extreme in the controversial field of estrogen therapy.[44]

Although the AMA was initially taken aback by the claims of *Feminine Forever,* Wilson was only the most visible face of a small group of doctors who were considering a broader use for hormone replacement therapy. Wilson did not originate the notion that menopause was a disease or that long-term hormone therapy could prevent its ravages. Wilson's work was indebted to the efforts of Fuller Albright and his students, who suggested that estrogen might prevent postmenopausal bone loss, and of other researchers, who suggested that the drop in estrogen might explain postmenopausal women's increased risk of heart disease. Wilson was also certainly inspired by the efforts of William H. Masters and Kost Shelton, who began promoting long-term therapy for all menopausal and postmenopausal women in the 1950s.[45] Indeed, Wilson acknowledged his debt to Shelton, referring to him as the "first beacon of enlightenment in the engulfing sea of ignorance."[46] By the 1960s, a handful of prominent (and not so prominent) physicians had begun to see hormone therapy as a judicious and compassionate response to the allegedly devastating effects of estrogen deficiency.

Inevitable Decline

Physicians who promoted long-term therapy generally regarded estrogen decline as a cause of great debility and suffering for at least some if not most menopausal and postmenopausal women. Menopause was thus considered less significant as a process in itself and more alarming as the marker of devastating and inevitable estrogen depletion. As a result, menopause was no longer a passage or even a Rubicon. Instead, it was a harbinger of loss and decay. One physician provided a long list of menopausal symptoms, including "nervousness, depression, irritability, anxiety and fear, crying spells, insomnia, dizziness, loss of memory and concentration, headaches, paraesthesia, fatigue, rapid exhaustion, state of confusion, arthralgia and myalgia, palpitations, aging appearance, dryness of the skin and mucus membranes, dysparunia, loss of libido." In addition, she claimed that declining amounts of estrogen caused osteoporosis and heart disease, with the "potential of disturbing normal function of every cell of the body."[47]

In addition to the physical consequences, some physicians claimed that women were also disabled emotionally by their diminishing estrogen. As one physician put it, at menopause, women become "a caricature of their younger selves at their emotional worst." Endocrinologist Robert Greenblatt described in 1967 the "neurotic and psychogenic" symptoms that menopause "uncloaks." He explained that "under the stress of the change of life, anxiety, apprehension, insomnia, nervousness, headaches, frigidity for some, increased sex drive for others, come to the surface." He compared menopausal women to Lady Macbeth, whom he characterized as a "bitch of the first order" and a little nuts.[48]

Some physicians who promoted long-term therapy maintained that the consequences of menopause particularly diminished a woman's "womanly" features. For example, Harvard University gynecologist Robert Kistner claimed in 1973 that the menopausal symptoms "revolve about a deterioration of feminine attributes." Menopausal women suffer from "dry or flabby skin, sagging breasts," and a "vagina which is little more than a dry, rigid tube." In sum, these physicians agreed that these physical and emotional changes "add up to a singularly unattractive future for women over 40."[49]

These texts complemented Wilson's by describing menopause as a physiological change characterized by decline. In these descriptions, menopause diminishes women, robbing them of their allure, their health, their youth. It is not merely a set of symptoms that must be weathered; it is a source of devastating loss.

Deficiency Disease

Many physicians who believed that long-term therapy served the health needs of middle-aged and older women still hesitated to call menopause a disease. Instead, they promoted the notion of "estrogen deficiency" without labeling that deficiency a disease. Endocrinologist Greenblatt, for example, referred to menopause as a physiological episode and a "hormonal deficiency state." He maintained that the "estrogen deficiency of the menopause creates an abnormal physiologic condition that endures to the end of life."[50] In 1959, endocrinologist Herbert Kupperman agreed that menopause could lead to "estrogen deficiency" but insisted that not all menopausal women were estrogen deficient; by 1967, he had adopted the more radical position that the climacteric was "a deficiency syndrome."[51]

Some physicians did promote the daring claim that "menopause is a chronic and incapacitating deficiency disease." Other than Wilson himself, perhaps the most enthusiastic promoter of this position in the 1960s was Detroit family physician Francis P. Rhoades. In a series of medical publications and conference appearances, Rhoades campaigned vigorously for the idea that menopausal women were sick. Consequently, he insisted, women did not need reassurance or a short course of estrogen therapy to help them ride out the problems of menopause: a menopausal woman needed long-term hormone therapy "to retain or regain her true femininity and sexuality."[52] Perhaps it is not coincidental that neither Wilson nor Rhoades held academic positions. Their place outside of the academy may have freed them to promote the disease model with abandon.

But caution did not prevent all academic physicians from promoting the disease model of menopause. In his often-cited 1962 article "Is Menopause a Disease?" Allan C. Barnes, chairman of obstetrics and gynecology at Johns Hopkins University, for example, declared that menopause is a "disease requiring our active treatment." Unless estrogen "deficiency" was remedied, he insisted that women would experience decades of unnecessary and rapid physical decline.[53]

Still other physicians dismissed the debate over whether menopause was normal or pathological as irrelevant to the issue of hormone use. One physician, for example, denied that because menopause might be natural or universal it was therefore "desirable for good health." Echoing the argument of Shelton nine years earlier, he insisted in 1963 that "death is universal, yet we struggle against it. Nature did not give us glasses, false teeth, anaesthesia, nor the means to fly, yet we do not hesitate to take advantage of the benefits of anything useful that we are ingenious enough to discover." M. Edward Davis, chair of obstetrics and gynecology at the University of Chicago School of Medicine, agreed in 1967 that, whether natural or not, "the sequelae of the climacteric materially threaten the well being and duration of life of our patients."[54]

Restorative and Preventive Medicine

Although physicians did sometimes address the nature of menopause, menopause itself was generally much less significant to the discussion of hormones than were the benefits the therapy could be expected to provide to women long after menopause had passed. New York City gynecologist Helen Jern, for example, believed that, once hormone therapy had begun, it should be "continued throughout a woman's lifetime." She maintained that "many female inmates of nursing homes and mental institutions could be restored to full physical and mental health through adequate hormone therapy."[55] In particular, the promise of preventing heart disease and osteoporosis converted many physicians to the cause. In a 1967 article, for example, Davis condemned as "archaic" the "current practice" of merely treating a woman's menopausal symptoms. He insisted that long-term therapy "is far more rewarding and should be continued indefinitely to retard physical atrophic changes, atherosclerosis, and osteoporosis." He promoted hormones as "preventative medicine which will help women to retain good health in their advancing years."[56]

The logic of preventive medicine thus buttressed much of the conversation about long-term therapy. As Greenblatt asked rhetorically in 1967, "would it be out of order to practice preventative medicine by anticipating the inevitable ovarian senescence to which every woman is heir by administering small doses of oestrogens in cyclic fashion?" Endocrinologist Kupperman agreed, insisting that "one should treat the estrogenic deficient female in much the same way one treats a thyroid deficiency whether or not there is a presenting symptomology." But the preventive benefits of ERT went well beyond ensuring physical health. It could also prevent family unrest. According to one endocrinologist, the relief provided by hormone therapy benefited not only the aging woman but also her "husband, children, in-laws, grandchildren and indirectly, many others."[57] Estrogen therapy was strong medicine indeed.

Gynecologists, endocrinologists, and others convinced by the evidence that hormone therapy could prevent broken hips, heart attacks, and midlife divorces considered it irresponsible, wrong-headed, and perhaps misogynistic to withhold its wide-ranging benefits. As Greenblatt put it in 1967, "to merely shrug and insinuate that the menopause is physiologic, that women must suffer through it is not [providing] the understanding nor the compassion expected of the physician."[58] Rhoades blamed "inherent male resentment of female longevity and biological superiority" for male physicians' reluctance to prescribe hormones for menopausal and postmenopausal women. He insisted that it was "logical and proper medical practice to prescribe hormone therapy for postmenopausal women."[59]

Like Wilson, several physicians argued that estrogen was especially important for women of this generation so they could enjoy the new opportunities that were opening up to them. Rhoades, for example, claimed that many women were leading active and productive lives when menopause "strikes" and "deeply resent [the] catastrophic attack on their ability to earn a living and enjoy life." He argued that only estrogen therapy could give women their lives back.[60] Davis dared to wonder what women could accomplish if they avoided estrogen deficiency. Thinking big, he maintained that "if women were universally supported with the administration of exogenous estrogens, not only through the menopause, and the postmenopausal period but throughout the rest of her life, she would take over the world."[61]

These doctors and others like them were aware that women's lives were not exclusively defined by their domestic roles. By 1968, half of all women between thirty-five and fifty-four worked outside the home, and women in the burgeoning women's rights and women's liberation movements were demanding access to lives not predestined by biology. Hormone therapy promised to keep women biologically sound so they could participate more fully in a changing society. Although they worked from sexist assumptions, these physicians cast the hormonal revolution as preparation for the fruits of women's liberation.

Before they could recruit other physicians to the cause of long-term therapy, advocates knew they had to address concerns about the carcinogenic potential of estrogen. Although researchers had suggested a link between endometrial cancer and estrogen since the 1930s, long-term estrogen advocates insisted that the alleged link was a red herring that made physicians unnecessarily cautious and women unnecessarily frightened. While they admitted that estrogen had produced cancer in lab animals, most notably rats and mice, proestrogen physicians insisted that "clinical amounts" posed no danger, at least not if prescribed with progestin.[62] Georgia gynecologist Norman Stahl, for example, conceded that estrogen-only therapy might cause endometrial cancer, but he insisted that the estrogen-progestin combination eliminated the risk. Therefore, he claimed, "there is no reason, at least on the basis of fear of inducing endometrial cancer, to withhold sex steroid therapy from anyone who clinically required such treatment." Other physicians angrily denounced physicians who cruelly withheld therapy because of the "unfounded cancer hazard." Two researchers melodramatically insisted, "If patients are to be rescued, it is essential that physicians with this negative background . . . be prepared to alter their prejudices or refer their menopause patients to a more objective colleague."[63] Indeed, many argued that estrogen therapy, coupled with the periodic shedding of the endometrium, probably prevented endometrial cancer. Family physician Rhoades, for example, suggested that a treatment regimen that included progestin and estrogen probably prevented cancer, and he insisted that women who received hormone replacement suffered fewer cases of "genital" cancers.[64]

In many ways, Robert Wilson was a medical maverick who was more interested in attracting menopausal women to hormonal replacement therapy through tales of decline and promises of rejuvenation than in making his case to the medical community. Nevertheless, Wilson's views matched those of an emerging, albeit small, medical movement. Convinced that estrogen could fix or prevent many of the infirmities attendant on female aging, a few gynecologists, endocrinologists, and general practitioners began to promote life-long hormone therapy as responsible preventive medicine. Resistance, these doctors insisted, was outdated at best and cruel at worst.

Medical Resistance

Between 1963 and 1975, the promise of long-term hormone therapy to prevent the debilitating effects of estrogen deficiency attracted some medical adherents. But these physicians represented only a small fraction of the medical profession.[65] Most physicians believed that hormone therapy might be useful to alleviate hot flashes and vaginal dryness, but they did not embrace estrogen to prevent the effects of aging. Indeed, a small number of physicians, perhaps 10 percent, refused to use hormones under any circumstances.[66] Another group prescribed hormone therapy for women with severe symptoms, but denounced long-term treatment. According to Johns Hopkins Medical School gynecologist Edmund Novak, for example, only 20 to 25 percent of his patients displayed symptoms severe enough to warrant hormonal treatment. By severe, Novak had in mind the woman who "wakes up several times a night and has completely soaked her sheets."[67]

Physicians resisted long-term hormone therapy for several reasons. Some maintained that its benefits, including the alleged protection against osteoporosis or atherosclerosis, had yet to be demonstrated. Saul Gusberg, chairman of obstetrics and gynecology at Mount Sinai School of Medicine, agreed that short-term therapy provided benefits to some women, but he rejected long-term use. "I see no evidence that those women who do not have symptoms of estrogen deficiency are benefited by being given prophylactic estrogens for the rest of their lives."[68] Other physicians who resisted long-term treatment cited safety concerns. Indeed, researchers had implicated estrogens in the increased risk of breast cancer, in addition to endometrial cancer, and in the increased risk of blood clots, strokes, and heart disease.[69] Others weighed ERT's unproven benefits against its unproven risks. In a summary statement of a 1971 conference on menopause and aging, for example, Kenneth Ryan, chairman of obstetrics and gynecology at the University of California, San Diego Medical School, wrote that while hormones should not be withheld from women for the short-term relief of menopausal symptoms, it was imprudent to "extol estrogens as a complete panacea for aging, degenerative disease, and psychic disturbances after the menopause. The concerns over thromboembolic complications and carcinogenesis cannot be dismissed." A 1974 *JAMA* editorial made a similar case. Although the author understood that the connection between cancer and estrogens remained unproven and that estrogens might yet be proved to help prevent osteoporosis and heart disease, he declared it "too risky to chase with high doses of estrogen the psychic, sexual, and degenerative changes associated with aging."[70] Perhaps two epidemiologists made the most sobering point: They claimed that between oral contraceptives and replacement hormones, the United States was moving into dangerous territory, placing millions (more than nine million by 1967) of healthy women on long-term estrogen. They concluded that the "extent of danger from widespread and long-term estrogen use remains largely unknown."[71]

This larger medical context demonstrates that the medical profession was divided over the disease model of menopause and the long-term use of hormones. Even specialists within endocrinology and gynecology did not speak unanimously. Further, it is misguided to dismiss Wilson and others like him for preying on women's insecurities just to increase drug company profits. Gynecologists, endocrinologists, and family practitioners promoted long-term therapy not solely to keep women sexually alluring and available, although this seemed a valuable benefit for many proponents. These physicians also had legitimate worries about postmenopausal women's increased risk of heart disease and hip fractures. Although the language used to promote hormone therapy clearly capitalized on and exacerbated women's fears of aging and promoted a view of women as dominated physically and emotionally by their hormones, some physicians believed that long-term therapy promised significant health benefits, in addition to perky breasts and supple skin. The evidence supports medical anthropologist Margaret Lock's claim that although "some physicians may have been self-serving, and no doubt some were misogynists, most men who devoted time and energy to the creation of menopause as a medical event were not out to benefit in any simple rapacious way from vulnerable middle-age women."[72] The medical divisions did not then reflect misogynistic physicians on the one hand and women's advocates on the other. Instead, it reflected a larger medical disagreement over the wisdom of aggressive preventive therapy that itself created possible health risks. Physicians disagreed over the acceptable risk associated with preventive care. Physicians reluctant to prescribe long-term therapy in the 1960s and 1970s call to mind the physicians of the 1940s and 1950s who avoided a systemic treatment for problems that could, they felt, be adequately handled with a less aggressive medical intervention.

Taking the Debate to the Public

Feminine Forever was a tremendous success. It sold more than 100,000 copies in the first seven months after its release. In addition, it was serialized in local newspapers and excerpted in popular magazines.[73] It had been translated into four languages by 1970. Perhaps most importantly, it generated an interest in menopause that resulted in a flood of popular articles and books between 1966 and 1975.[74]

The popular literature, particularly women's magazines, quickly carried Wilson's story to the general public, focusing particularly on middle-class, middle-aged women.[75] As in the 1940s and 1950s, this literature was often written by physicians, who discussed ERT and menopause in regular health columns in women's magazines (William Nolen's "A Doctor's World," for example), in occasional articles (for example, Kenneth Hutchin's "The Change and What Husbands Should Know About It"), and in books (such as Sherwin Kaufman's *The Ageless Woman*). In addition to these texts by physicians, popular writers typically relied on medical authorities in their descriptions of the process of menopause and the promises of hormone replacement therapy.

Although the popular discussion of menopause and estrogen therapy was often clearly inspired by ERT enthusiasts, women encountered more than one message about menopause and therapeutic hormones.[76] As historian Joanne Meyerowitz points out, popular culture is not monolithic. Instead, it is "rife with contradiction, ambivalence, and competing voices."[77] Although the popular media undoubtedly provided free publicity for estrogen therapy, it also generally emphasized the debates within the medical community, thus presenting women several competing views. Nevertheless, on a few points the popular literature did present a generally unified front: menopause was depicted as a potentially diminishing experience that responded to treatment. The overall effect was to promote estrogen therapy as a safe and perhaps miraculous cure for those women most bothered by menopausal symptoms.

Some of the articles appearing in the popular literature between 1963 and 1975 portrayed menopause as the beginning of a steep and treacherous decline into old age and ill health.[78] Physician David Reuben, for example, claimed in his 1969 best-seller, *Everything You Always Wanted to Know About Sex;* "As estrogen is shut off, a woman comes as close as she can to being a man. Increased facial hair, deepened voice, obesity, and decline of breasts and female genitalia all contribute to a masculine appearance. Not really a man but no longer a functional woman, these individuals live in a world of intersex. Having outlived their ovaries, they have outlived their usefulness as human beings."[79]

Feminist critics have appropriately latched onto this example as evidence of the misogynistic views and the negative characterizations of menopause.[80] While Reuben's depiction is extreme, other popular sources painted menopause in a similarly negative light. One article, for example, proposed that menopausal women were nature's cast-offs. The author claimed that "Nature's way just isn't all that friendly to women" after childbearing ceased; consequently, "estrogen depletion" encouraged a wide range of debilities including incontinence, vaginitis, and thinning bones.[81] Alice Lake cited a prominent woman physician who claimed that at menopause "the color of the lenses through which a woman views the world suddenly changes from rose to blue," following the assertion with a catalog of horrors attributable to menopause.[82] A first-person account in *Good Housekeeping* likewise focused on the negative aspects of menopause. This woman sought advice from her physician because she "seemed to be changing from a confident, cheerful easy-going person into a shrew."[83]

Not surprisingly, informational pamphlets published by drug companies also highlighted the negative aspects of menopause. A pamphlet published by Ayerst declared that menopause was "a difficult time, a time of general upheaval, a time when a woman needs all the help she can get."[84] A pamphlet published by a competitor described the various symptoms menopausal women faced: wrinkled skin, "flabby and sagging breasts," emotional turmoil, and "addle-headed anxiety."[85]

Significantly, however, many sources did not portray these difficulties as inevitable. After detailing the possible symptoms of menopause, one article added, "Relax. Don't worry. . . . Often these symptoms don't occur." Many authors portrayed the effects as temporary and annoying rather than debilitating. Other sources also emphasized that some women would not experience any symptoms at all. Even New York University gynecologist Sherwin Kaufman, in an article designed to reassure women that hormones were safe, admitted that "for a good many women the change of life presents no great problems."[86]

Pharmacology to the Rescue

Having established menopause as a negative experience for some women, the authors of the popular literature promoted estrogen therapy as the solution. Until 1975, virtually all the articles depicted replacement hormones positively—at least in the short-term—focusing on the "personal miracles" that ERT performed. One author, for example, recommended hormone therapy "when the ripening years act to cut off your body's supplies of much needed estrogen." In a 1965 *Vogue* article—the title of which, "How to Live Young at Any Age," belied its bias—the author painted a rosy picture of the advantages of ERT. In addition to assuring women that hormones would relieve hot flashes and vaginal dryness, the author also claimed that it was "well-established" that hormones could prevent heart disease.[87]

Occasionally, the authors goaded women into seeking out the modern solution for menopausal troubles. In a 1967 *Good Housekeeping* article, a doctor compared estrogen treatment with glasses and hair color. "If you couldn't read the fine print, you'd get glasses. . . . And you've probably tried rinses for your hair. Take female hormones in the same way—a restoration of what used to be." Another medical writer presented ERT as the modern choice for the modern woman. He claimed that "these are changing times: medical science has made such advances that change of life can be looked at in a change of light."[88]

Marital discord presented a particularly compelling justification for hormone use. The popular literature promised husbands that estrogen could deliver the bride he married. William Cooper's 1969 book, *A Husband's Guide to Menopause,* assured husbands that if a wife would "take full advantage of the medical and other options available to her today, she can look feminine, feel feminine and be feminine throughout every day of her lengthening life-span."[89] Louis Parrish maintained that for some women, menstrual periods provided critical evidence of femininity and that once women stop menstruating they considered themselves sexless. Hormones then, by providing menstrual periods, reminded women that they remained women, and, more importantly, helped them to feel womanly.[90]

A few physicians cited in the popular literature claimed that estrogen therapy could protect marriages by preserving a woman's sexual receptiveness. Harvard gynecologist Robert Kistner, for example, quoted in a 1969 *Time* magazine article, claimed that at menopause "intercourse can become painful. This leads to marital difficulties and is a factor in many cases of philandering by middle-aged husbands. If we can prevent or retard these changes . . . we can help to keep the women happier and their husbands as well."[91] Another physician spelled out the likely consequences of refusing to seek medical attention. M. Edward Davis warned wives, "The first few times intercourse becomes painful, run, don't walk, to your physician. The life of your marriage may be at stake. Certainly your sex life is at stake." He continued to muse, "When women tell me they haven't let their husbands touch them for a year, I can't help wondering what the husband has been doing to satisfy his sex drive during all that time."[92] Davis's message here was clear: If a woman makes herself sexually unavailable, her husband can't be blamed for seeking sexual release elsewhere.

Because menopause allegedly threatened marriage, some authors presented hormone treatment as a savvy preventive measure. Dr. M. Dorothea Kerr, for example, recommended that because menopausal difficulties so easily led to marital strife, women should seek out hormones to prevent divorce.[93] Another article maintained that "nearly all gynecologists recognize today that a difficult menopause can cause broken homes, broken families, lawsuits, bitter quarrels, aberrant behavior—and that many of these tragedies and semi-tragedies can sometimes be averted by estrogens."[94]

Cancer? Only in Mice!

To make hormones more attractive for the women who might be frightened off by the fear of cancer, the popular media followed Wilson's lead and assured women that estrogen therapy was not carcinogenic. In remarkably consistent language, the authors denied that estrogen had ever "caused a single case of cancer [in humans]."[95] Kerr insisted that "cancer is a needless fear in women taking estrogen."[96] One author assured his readers that estrogens were safer than "airplanes," "swimming," and "cigarettes."[97] These articles occasionally acknowledged that some doctors remained concerned about a possible link between estrogen and cancer, but the literature attempted to discredit them. The articles characterized physicians who worried about the cancer-inducing effects of estrogen as "rare," "conservative," and "diehards." A *Harper's Bazaar* article, for example, admitted that "although there is still some hesitation among very conservative practitioners, prevalent medical opinion is that the safety and benefits of estrogen therapy have been convincingly demonstrated."[98] Some of the articles called upon experts who cited misogyny rather than cancer as the true explanation for doctors' reluctance to prescribe hormones. One often-cited physician implored his colleagues not to let their "inherent male resentment of female longevity deter them from the medical responsibility of minimizing the menopause."[99]

Other articles attempted to excavate the origins of the cancer "myth" by admitting that extremely large doses of estrogen (much larger than women would ever receive) had indeed been known to cause cancer in mice genetically designed to get cancer. According to gynecologist Kaufman, "These mice were of a special strain which had been inbred over many generations, so that they were particularly susceptible to developing cancer."[100] A pamphlet issued by the Massengill company raised the question, "Does estrogen cause cancer?" In response, an illustrated image showed a woman with a bottle of estrogen in one hand, tossing a pill high into the air, her wide open mouth ready to receive it: "Only in mice," the woman glibly assured the reader.[101]

Several articles even suggested that long-term estrogen therapy might prevent cancer, echoing Wilson's assertion that combined therapy provided "cancer insurance." Relying on authorities such as Kistner, of Harvard, popular medical writers bolstered the claim that estrogen, particularly when prescribed with progestin, protected against endometrial and breast cancers.[102] These texts were carefully crafted to reassure women that estrogen therapy presented no cancer threat, even as the issue was still being debated in the medical literature. (Many women found progestin difficult to tolerate, however, so as long as the connection to endometrial cancer remained speculative, the estrogen-only therapy remained the focus of popular discussion and the more frequently prescribed hormone treatment.)

It is unlikely that these articles and books appeared solely because journalists and editors thought hormone replacement therapy was newsworthy. Indeed, some of the stories were almost assuredly prompted by representatives (understood broadly) of the drug companies. Wilson's work certainly falls into this category.[103] Even works not directly written by Wilson can occasionally be traced to parties with a commercial interest in the matter. Kerr, for example, wrote both an article for *Vogue* extolling the virtues of estrogen and a pamphlet distributed by Ayerst.[104] Similarly, Sandra Gorney, coauthor of the proestrogen book *After Forty,* was also the executive director of the Information Center on the Mature Woman, funded by Ayerst Laboratories. Further, Wilson and his foundation tirelessly pestered magazine and newspaper editors to report their views.[105] During a period when direct advertising of prescription drugs was forbidden, editorial articles provided valuable publicity for pharmaceutical manufacturers.

Medical Moderation in the Popular Media

The popular literature between 1963 and 1975 presented a generally unified position about the possible difficulties of menopause and the value and safety of estrogen treatment for some women. Nevertheless, they did not promote hormones as a necessary supplement for all aging women; this literature also reflected medical disagreement on other aspects of replacement estrogens. In particular, the popular literature did not overwhelmingly support long-term hormone therapy, the disease model of menopause, or the antiaging aspects of estrogen.

The popular literature, in other words, emphasized that most women did not need estrogen therapy or any other medical treatment to address menopause. One article reminded its readers that the "vast majority of gynecologists advise against the routine use of hormone therapy for all women."[106] Another noted that only 25 percent of postmenopausal women "have hormone deficiencies." For most women, the author insisted, "supplemental hormones are a waste of money . . . and downright silly."[107] So although these articles did "promote" estrogen therapy, they stopped short of recommending long- or even short-term treatment for all menopausal women.

The literature certainly reported that some physicians recommended long-term hormone treatments for their menopausal and postmenopausal patients. In his *McCall's* column, "A Doctor's World," William Nolen, for example, claimed that women can "take hormones for twenty or more years, avoiding menopausal discomfort indefinitely."[108] New York University gynecologist Kaufman similarly noted that, while he used to discontinue hormone treatment after a few months, by 1967 he was no longer in a "rush to stop." Nevertheless, most of the articles did not unilaterally promote long-term ERT. Indeed, many texts indicated that *most* physicians did not recommend life-long use.[109] Taken as a whole, the popular literature provided both sides of this issue, frequently in the same article. Alice Lake, in a 1965 *Good Housekeeping* article, for example, described in detail the variety of doctors' opinions on estrogen therapy, ranging from the "conservative," those who never or rarely prescribed estrogen therapy, to the "radical," represented by Wilson, who sought to preserve menstruation and prevent menopause.[110]

Magazine articles often noted that Wilson and his methods had been sharply criticized by other physicians. A 1967 *Saturday Evening Post* article, for example, mentioned that Wilson's medical colleagues had censored him for claiming that estrogen could restore a wrinkle-free face, for advocating the birth control pill as a treatment for menopause, and, most unforgivably, for using "Madison Avenue-type catchphrases" designed, as Wilson allegedly admitted, "to build sales among women readers."[111]

The popular literature also failed to characterize menopause unambiguously as a disease. Some sources promoted the idea. One article cited Kaufman, who claimed "The truth is that menopause is a deficiency state which gradually defeminizes a woman physically."[112] Another article reported with derision that "a few doctors . . . still believe that menopause is a normal condition, not a disease, and they refuse to 'tamper with nature.'" The author then acknowledged that physicians differed on the issue, but portrayed dissenting physicians as dangerously out of touch with the medical consensus of the last decade.[113]

In the popular sources, however, the disease model of menopause continued to compete with the assertion that menopause was a natural process. Obstetrician and gynecologist Sheldon Cherry attempted to dispel the myths that he believed surrounded both menopause and estrogen replacement therapy. In his 1976 book *The Menopause Myth*, he insisted that menopause was "not a disease, but . . . a natural physiological process." As a result, Cherry concluded, only about 20 percent of menopausal women required medical treatment.[114] Physician Kenneth Hutchin similarly challenged the notion that menopause was a disease. He insisted that it was not and that women should not be encouraged "to behave as if the change were a prolonged illness." He did not condemn estrogen therapy, but he maintained that it was palliative rather than curative. "You may alter the normal," he insisted, but "you cannot cure it."[115] But perhaps most significantly, many poplar discussions of menopause failed to even raise the notion that some authorities considered menopause to be a disease. Even a pamphlet written by M. Edward Davis, who claimed in the medical literature that menopause wreaked havoc on the female body, failed to promote the disease model.[116]

Finally, writers in the popular media were generally skeptical of claims that estrogens could slow the aging process, but this view did have some supporters. An anonymous physician claimed, for example, that estrogens "can retard, dazzlingly, many of the physiological signs of aging."[117] Many others took a middle position, admitting that hormone therapy could not slow aging but insisting that it could make women look and feel younger. In 1975, Dabney Rice understood that hormones could not turn old women into teenagers, but she insisted that hormones that allowed women to "feel your best, look your best, enjoying every zestful moment" were, in effect, "anti-aging."[118] A 1965 *Cosmopolitan* article conceded that estrogen could not make women "forever young," but it asserted that it would allow them to remain "forever feminine," aging "gradually without sudden loss of looks and energy."[119]

Most authors, however, challenged the idea that spent youth could ever be restored. Gynecologist Kupperman, for example, reportedly claimed that hormone therapy sometimes yielded "fantastic results," but he insisted that it was not a panacea. "Above all, you're not going to take an old woman and make her young." In the same article, Daniel G. Morton, chief of obstetrics and gynecology at UCLA, complained that the publicity surrounding ERT had created impossible expectations. He insisted that it could not deliver "the ultimate fountain of youth for all women."[120] A 1966 article similarly claimed that "no pill can make one young again, nor can a pill make one feminine—either gentle and charming in the womanly, wifely, motherly sense or 'girly' in the sex appealing, eye appealing sense."[121]

Given its internal disagreements, how can the significance of this literature to its first readers be understood? The popular media did indeed publicize and promote ERT as a wondrous cure for the negative consequences of menopause. Certainly Wilson's work and some other books and articles encouraged women to seek out long-term hormone therapy by dangling before them the negative consequences of untreated menopause and the modern miracles of hormone treatment. Although women could and probably did encounter this position while they thumbed through women's magazines, it did not represent the only view of menopause available during this period. Counterbalancing Wilson's outrageous rhetoric were articles that did not overwhelmingly assert that ERT was a necessary or desirable treatment for all women approaching middle age. Rather, ERT was presented as a valuable treatment for those women who experienced a particularly difficult menopause. Women, then, were faced with several competing characterizations of menopause and with multiple options for treatment regimens.

The popular literature between 1963 and 1975 was clearly dominated by the discussion about estrogen replacement therapy and the disease model of menopause. The more complex assessment of menopause, including discussions of its social and physical consequences, that had been the focus of publications in the 1940s and 1950s all but disappeared. The popular literature largely reduced the significance of menopause to a debate over whether it was a debilitating disease or a natural process and whether it required treatment forever or not at all.

In the midst of the publicity surrounding ERT between 1963 and 1975, the use of menopausal and postmenopausal estrogen increased dramatically. Regardless of the lingering doubts of some physicians, dollar sales of noncontraceptive estrogen more than quadrupled between 1962 and 1975.[122] As startling as these numbers are, interpreting them against the backdrop of Wilson's campaign is tricky. It is tempting, of course, to attribute much of the increase to the efforts of Wilson and like-minded physicians. Perhaps this is partially true, but the full explanation is more complex. The use of prescription drugs in most categories, for example, doubled during this period. Further, the price of estrogen itself nearly doubled between 1962 and 1975.[123] Taken together, these two facts point to a widespread medical emphasis on drug therapies and a cultural acceptance of them during this period. Estrogen advocates were therefore part of a more general trend not tied to the specific tactics of physicians such as Wilson. In addition, the generalized use of prescription drugs suggests that aging women were not uniquely targeted as consumers of pharmaceuticals. It remains noteworthy, however, that between 1965 and 1974, the number of women receiving their first prescription for estrogen replacement therapy roughly doubled.[124] In sheer numbers alone, medicine became a more prominent presence in the menopausal experience.

Estrogen Therapy and the Threat of Cancer

Between 1963 and 1975, proponents of both short- and long-term estrogen therapy acknowledged public fears that estrogen therapy could cause cancer, but many popular writers raised the cancer threat only to dismiss it. In December 1975, researchers published findings that supported women's apprehension and required a new approach to the cancer issue.

At the height of estrogen's popularity, two articles in the *New England Journal of Medicine* challenged the cavalier dismissal of the carcinogenic potential of estrogen therapy. Researchers at Washington University (Donald Smith, et al.) and Kaiser-Permanente Medical Center (Harry Ziel and William Finkle) independently discovered a link between postmenopausal estrogen therapy and endometrial cancer. The Ziel/Finkle study demonstrated an endometrial cancer rate fourteen times higher in women who had used conjugated estrogens for seven years or longer than among women who had never used them at all. Smith found that ERT posed the greatest risk to women with no other predisposing conditions, such as obesity.[125] Although researchers had proposed a link between estrogen and cancer since the 1930s, these landmark studies supplied the best evidence available at the time that ERT posed a cancer risk in humans, and they sparked further research.

Coverage of these studies did not remain buried in the medical literature. Both ABC and NBC television news ran the story, and the same day the *New England Journal of Medicine* published the studies, the *New York Times* ran a front page story under the headline "Estrogen Is Linked to Uterine Cancer." Although the article noted that the studies did "not prove that the hormones cause cancer," it also cited physicians who insisted that, while estrogen remained a useful drug, it should not be prescribed for all menopausal women and certainly not used over long periods of time.[126]

Almost immediately after the studies appeared, the Food and Drug Administration (FDA) urged physicians to proceed cautiously when prescribing estrogen. In mid-December 1975, the FDA's Obstetrics and Gynecology Advisory Committee met and concluded that the studies "provided strong evidence that post-menopausal estrogen therapy increases the risk of endometrial cancer." It recommended that the risks of hormone treatment be considered more carefully by patients and physicians alike and proposed both a warning label and a package insert to warn women more fully of the potential dangers associated with hormone treatment.[127]

The link between replacement estrogens and endometrial cancer did not go unchallenged, however. In a 1976 op-ed piece appearing in a medical journal, Robert Kistner of the obstetrics and gynecology department at Harvard Medical School, argued that the Smith and Ziel/Finkle studies, because they were retrospective, could not prove a causal link between estrogen therapy and increased cancer rates. He claimed that the research only demonstrated that "endometrial cancer is a disease of those women who have easy access to physicians."[128] Kistner maintained that estrogens did not cause cancer; physicians administering ERT were able to detect cancer in their patients. Other researchers argued that retrospective studies could never prove cause; at best, they could establish "an association between the two factors."[129] Follow-up research made the same argument. In 1978, Yale University researchers concluded that there was no difference in endometrial cancer rates between women taking replacement estrogens and those who did not. They argued that women taking replacement hormones were more likely to have their cancers detected but were not more likely to develop the cancer itself.[130]

Because medical doubts remained about the causal connection between endometrial cancer and estrogen therapy, some physicians continued to promote its use. A 1976 American College of Obstetricians and Gynecologists technical bulletin, for example, cited "considerable doubt" about the cancer connection and continued to recommend short-term use of estrogen for the treatment of menopausal symptoms and long-term use for the prevention of osteoporosis in women with no contraindications. Kistner agreed. In 1977, he claimed that while the "precise duration of therapy in the postmenopausal woman is controversial, most 'authorities' on menopause suggest ad infinitum." He threw his own hat in with the "authorities," claiming that "when estrogen therapy is initiated in the postmenopausal woman, I believe it should be continued indefinitely."[131]

Eventually, however, the preponderance of evidence supported the claim that long-term unopposed estrogen therapy increased a woman's risk of contracting endometrial cancer.[132] By 1979, several more studies indicated that the prolonged use of replacement estrogen increased the likelihood of endometrial cancer.[133] A few other studies associated estrogen with an increased risk of breast cancer. On the basis of these studies, the National Institute of Aging concluded in 1979 that ERT substantially increased the risk of cancer.[134]

Even with this new evidence, some physicians refused to abandon long-term ERT and the women who "needed" it; the promise of preventing hip fractures and heart attacks remained seductive. Gilbert S. Gordan (a student of Fuller Albright) and C. Vaughn, for example, argued in 1979 that because estrogens were effective in preventing postmenopausal bone loss, "the benefits outweigh the risks." They highlighted the disability caused by osteoporotic hip fractures, noting that "many are completely bedridden for the remainder of their lives." As a result, Gordan and Vaughn promoted prevention through hormones as "the only ethical solution to this major public health problem."[135] Duke University endocrinologist Charles Hammond made a similar plea for the role of estrogen therapy in preventing cardiac disease and hypertension.[136]

To secure the alleged benefits of estrogen while reducing or eliminating its hazards, including the risk of endometrial cancer, researchers and clinicians increasingly promoted the benefits of combined progestin and estrogen. Although some physicians had long favored HRT (at least in writing), it became therapeutic orthodoxy for women with uteri only after the cancer revelations.[137]

Drug companies scrambled to find ways to minimize the effects of the negative publicity. Soon after the 1975 *New England Journal of Medicine* publication, Ayerst sent physicians a letter acknowledging "a controversy" involving estrogen replacement therapy and its role in endometrial cancer. The letter did not cite the studies or describe the findings. Instead, Ayerst concluded that "it is fair to state that, amid the welter of complexities surrounding this condition . . . it would be simplistic indeed to attribute an apparent increase in the diagnosis of endometrial carcinoma solely to estrogen therapy."[138] Ayerst also turned to a prominent New York public relations firm, Hill and Knowlton, to help battle the impact. In a December

1976 letter to William Davis, the president of Ayerst, Stanley Sauerhaft of Hill and Knowlton outlined his proposal. He advised a media blitz "to restore perspective" and to counteract "unfavorable publicity incidents as they occur." He recommended that Ayerst saturate the media at every level: TV, newspapers, women's magazines, general magazines, and film. He also proposed recruiting a "television spokeswoman," who, if "properly prepared and rehearsed," could come across as providing a "public service." Sauerhaft warned, however, that these efforts required a focus on menopause rather than estrogen replacement therapy. He claimed that this approach "multiplies the numbers of outlets that will accept and publish materials and the message can be effectively conveyed by discreet references to 'products that your doctor may prescribe.'" Sauerhaft also insisted that Ayerst anticipate all "potentially dangerous developments," such as the publication of a negative medical article, by gathering favorable information that could be quickly distributed. Finally, he called upon Ayerst to prepare at least two executives who could respond to "critical situations . . . confidently and convincingly."[139]

The Hill and Knowlton strategy was originally publicized and decried in a feminist newspaper *Majority Report,* but other media outlets quickly carried the story to a wider audience. The *Washington Post* ran the story and condemned Hill and Knowlton for treating the "cancer risk as a PR problem." Although critical of the public relations firm, the *Washington Post* piece allowed Ayerst to take the moral high road. An Ayerst spokeswoman (did the company take the advice of Hill and Knowlton?) claimed that the company "flatly rejected" the Hill and Knowlton proposal, claiming that it "seemed insensitive to the concern about cancer and estrogen therapy."[140] In contrast, Morton Mintz and Victor Cohn, writing for the *Progressive,* did not absolve Ayerst of responsibility so easily. While Mintz and Cohn acknowledged that Ayerst ignored Sauerhaft's advice, they pointed out that "an attempted rape is not stripped of criminality because it did not succeed," and they condemned Ayerst for claiming that estrogen treatments could prevent genital cancer.[141]

In general, the enthusiasm of writers in the popular media for long-term estrogen therapy cooled significantly in the aftermath of the cancer studies, but most articles in women's magazines assured women that short-term estrogen therapy remained both safe and beneficial. A 1976 *Vogue* article, for example, maintained that "20 percent of women undergoing menopause do need estrogen, for a limited period, and are tremendously helped by it. But they don't need it for the rest of their lives." A *McCall's* article published the same year voiced a similar position. Citing Saul Gusberg, the article maintained that "no woman should take estrogen unless she really needs it" but went on to say that short-term hormone treatments could provide a great deal of benefit while providing very little risk.[142]

Other articles focused on the continuing medical controversies. In a 1977 article, for example, Paula Weideger reported on the 1975 studies linking cancer to replacement hormones, but she emphasized the continuing doubt about these studies. She insisted that conclusive evidence had not yet been found to prove a causal link between estrogen therapy and uterine cancer, and she cited physicians who challenged the accuracy of the conclusions. She highlighted the position of the American College of Obstetrics and Gynecology, which concluded its statement on the issue with these words: "There is no evidence to indicate an increased risk of breast cancer or other malignancies in women using estrogen therapy."[143] An article in *Today's Health* similarly presented the range of medical opinion on hormone therapies for menopause. Marion Steinmann quoted Robert Greenblatt (who wrote the introduction to *Feminine Forever*) in his claim that estrogen "can help a woman grow old with dignity"; he concluded that it was "close to criminal" to withhold estrogen treatments from menopausal women. Steinmann contrasted Greenblatt's enthusiasm with the reservations of Dr. Robert Morris. Morris, associate director of obstetrics and gynecology at New York University Hospital, admitted that he had never embraced estrogen therapy; he now believed it was "potentially very dangerous" and prescribed it very rarely for women who still had their uterus.[144]

The coverage of ERT in *Vogue* appeared especially dismissive of the cancer risk. Two articles by health editor Melva Weber appeared intent on discrediting the cancer studies. A 1976 article called on three experts who asserted that the misgivings about estrogen therapy were overblown. These physicians reminded *Vogue* readers that "solid evidence" did not exist to prove that "estrogens do cause cancer of the endometrium." Kistner of Harvard admitted in numerous interviews that an "overdose" of estrogens might lead to endometrial cancer, but he insisted that regular screening could eliminate the danger. Finally, another physician suggested that "*untreated* menopause" rather than estrogen therapy "is itself a cause of cancer." Despite their claims that women need not fear estrogen therapy, these physicians conceded that replacement therapy should be used cautiously and supervised carefully by a physician.[145] In a 1978 article, Weber reported continuing doubts that estrogen alone caused endometrial cancer and cited new evidence that suggested that natural estrogens might prevent both breast and uterine cancers. She concluded by quoting a physician who emphatically supported estrogen replacement, declaring it "a necessity if women want to remain physically active after the menopause."[146]

Other sources were more critical. Some consumer groups and publications aligned with the political left characterized ERT as an unnecessary medication most effective in raising profits for drug manufacturers. *Consumer Reports,* under the headline "The Dangerous Road to Shangrila," described estrogens as a $80,000,000 a year bonanza for the drug industry. The article insisted that hormones were "potentially dangerous drugs" and warned women to avoid physicians who enthusiastically recommended ERT. Sidney Wolfe, director of the Washington-based Health Research Group, insisted in a 1978 *Mother Jones* article that physicians and drug companies had long known that estrogens were "one of the most potent cancer-causing agents known." He believed that women would eventually reject ERT as they learned more about its risks.[147]

Cancer and ERT Prescriptions

The immediate impact of the earliest studies on the prescription of estrogen appears to have been minimal. Twelve private-practice physicians surveyed the day the Ziel/Finkle and Smith reports were published indicated that most physicians remained unconvinced that estrogens "directly cause cancer." They argued that "in the absence of such proof . . . no drastic change in practice [was] warranted." A San Francisco gynecologist Rubin Clay continued to promote menopause as a "deficiency disease" and planned to continue prescribing estrogens "for virtually all menopausal women for an indefinite period." He admitted, however, that he would lower the dosage for some women who had "requested it."[148]

As drug manufacturers feared, however, the cancer research eventually slowed the prescription rates of ERT. In 1975, physicians wrote more than twenty-eight million prescriptions for replacement hormones; in 1980, they wrote only fifteen million.[149] A survey of thirteen New York state physicians indicated that many who had readily prescribed long-term estrogen treatments in 1974 would no longer do so in 1981. Although 65 percent of the physicians would still prescribe estrogen in 1981, they lowered the dosage and shortened the duration of treatment. Furthermore, these physicians would also more likely combine estrogen with progestin to counteract the cancer risk. On the other hand, the percentage of women taking hormones dropped 18 percent between 1975 and 1976 and another 10 percent between 1976 and 1982. The physicians surveyed had reconsidered their practices in response to the medical literature, the FDA warnings, and patient reservations.[150]

Of crucial importance for women in this period, however, the discussion of ERT had largely displaced the conversation about the social and cultural significance of menopause. While the popular literature generally denied that menopause was a debilitating disease, meaningful discussion of what menopause might mean for women and what it represented to the culture did not emerge.

But thus far the menopausal women themselves have been absent from this examination of menopause between 1938 and 1962. It is to them I now turn to explore women's role in the increased use of hormone replacement therapy and to learn whether they viewed their menopausal bodies as diseased and aged, annoying and perplexing, or strong and liberated.

EIGHT

"At the Will and Whim of My Hormones"

Women, Menopause, and the Hormonal Dilemma, 1963–1980

In the early 1970s, a fifty-three-year-old woman responded to a survey about her experiences at menopause. Before menopause, she had always thought of herself as "a calm person," someone who was able to "cope with the responsibilities and pressures" of being a minister's wife and raising a large family. Although her mother and two of her sisters had sailed easily through menopause, it hit her "like a ton of bricks." Suddenly, "the ordinary chores of the home seemed like mountains" and she was repelled by anything that required responsibility. She began to withdraw from everything and everyone. She couldn't even stand to be near her husband. She spent more and more time crying and less and less time sleeping, always believing that everyone was against her. Her family suffered in confusion and disbelief, wondering "what had happened to their tower of strength."

Desperate to recover her old self, she visited her family physician, who seemed unconcerned that she "was crawling the walls and crying" all the time. He chocked it up to menopause and prescribed butesin, which she believed was a mild sedative, assuring her that she would be fine. She wasn't. Instead, she lived in misery for the next fifteen years! Finally, she went to the doctor who had delivered her children, and he prescribed hormones. Her relief was immense. "I am so much better, thank God! After 15 years of nightmares, I feel like a human being again."

This woman blamed the medical profession for her years of misery. "It seems a disgrace that the medical profession does not have the knowledge and ability to do anything in the difficult (almost disastrous) years. . . . I would have flown almost anywhere for help but had no idea where there was a physician who would take my case seriously enough to try to help me. I very nearly lost my mind . . . because I couldn't find a doctor that really cared." She asked on behalf of all menopausal women, "Must we go on suffering forever?!!"[1]

This woman was clearly caught within the confusion over medical controversies about the best way to treat menopause and menopausal symptoms, but she eventually found relief by taking hormone treatments. Her story illustrates several themes that dominated the discussion and experience of menopause in the 1960s and 1970s. First, this woman's story suggests an experience of profound transformation caused by menopause: she did not merely suffer menopausal symptoms; menopause changed who she was. Second, she condemned the medical profession for not understanding the needs of menopausal women and for not caring about them; she felt dismissed and angered by this inattention. Third, even in an era of increased publicity for hormone replacement therapy, many women, even those who called upon the medical profession, found they needed to fight to receive estrogens. Apparently, not all physicians, despite Robert Wilson's activity in the cause, willingly offered hormones from puberty to the grave.

It is also instructive to note what this woman did not say about menopause. She did not describe menopause as a disease or even a process that inevitably required treatment. Indeed, her mother and sisters had done fine without. Further, she did not seem to seek medical care to prevent the consequences of aging. Her reasons for taking hormones did not include the desire to preserve her sexual allure or to prevent osteoporosis. Instead, she wanted something to alleviate her despair and confusion. This woman's testimony suggests that many women who sought hormones were not looking for a fountain of youth or a cure for their deficiency disease. Read against the backdrop of Wilson's campaign to keep women feminine forever, this woman's story asks us to consider carefully the impact of Wilson's work on the experiences of menopausal women between 1963 and 1980. How did menopausal women react to Wilson's characterization of their changing bodies? Did Wilson convince menopausal women they were diseased? Did women seek hormones to ensure their femininity?

Perhaps inspired by the depictions of menopause in the popular literature, women in the 1960s and 1970s were more willing to believe that menopause was a significant physiological upheaval that would leave them always altered and, often, diminished. As a result, they were more willing than their mothers had been to call upon medicine to ameliorate their symptoms, restore their personalities, and conserve their health. They did not, however, widely embrace the notion that menopause left them diseased. Further, at the same time that menopausal women were becoming more likely to believe that menopause was a significant event that warranted medical intervention, they were less likely to trust medical judgments and defer to medical authority. Perhaps Wilson's campaign to "prevent estrogen deficiency disease" should be regarded as a resounding success, as most menopausal women never acquired the disease in the first place.

Three sets of documents provide first-hand insights into the thoughts and feelings of menopausal women in this period. Most important are the records of Women in Midstream (WIM),[2] a support group and informational clearinghouse for menopausal women sponsored by the Seattle YWCA. The WIM records include the results of a nationally circulated survey as well as a collection of letters from menopausal women seeking advice and consolation. The women who responded to the WIM survey constituted a much more diverse group than those in the Brush and Davidoff samples examined in Chapter 6. They included wealthy and poor women, urban and rural residents. Most of these women were married, and three-quarters of them had at least one child; one-half had three or more children. Although the evidence is incomplete, most of them seem to have been between forty-eight and fifty-eight at the time of the survey, although some were in their early forties and several were in their seventies and eighties. The WIM records span the years 1973 to 1978.[3]

A second set of useful records are from the American Medical Association. After Wilson and his supporters championed estrogen therapy as a cure for menopause, menopausal women and concerned physicians flooded the AMA with requests for information on Wilson and his methods. The AMA collected these documents along with literature about Wilson's activities in files kept by their department of investigation. These records, dating from 1964 through 1970, do not indicate the age, marital, or economic status of the female correspondents.[4] Finally, the sociological research of Marjorie Lowenthal Fiske provides a further window into the experiences of menopausal women. In 1968 Fiske and two research assistants began a longitudinal study of adults facing life-course "transitions." This study included twenty-seven women who were facing the "post-parental" stage of family life. The women were urban, white, and middle-class.[5]

These archival materials, taken together with evidence gleaned from published sources—including physicians' case studies, informal interviews appearing in the popular literature, and other published survey data, most notably a survey circulated in 1974 by the Boston Women's Health Book Collective—allow a look into experiences of menopausal women during a period of tremendous social change.

Still a Natural and Normal Phase

Although many popular sources dating from after 1963 painted menopause (at least for some women) as the beginning of decline and debility, most women apparently rejected these dire characterizations. Most women, for example, did not seek medical attention at menopause.[6] The groundbreaking feminist health guide *Our Bodies, Ourselves,* originally published in 1971, reported that roughly two-thirds of the menopausal or postmenopausal women who responded to their survey about menopause "felt neutral or positive about the change they experienced."[7] Among the respondents to the Women in Midstream survey, 41.4 percent reported an easy or a relatively easy menopause.[8] Norma Neuman represents the experience of many women in the survey when she claimed that menopause did not "affect [her] at all": "I took no medications and I didn't have any nervous problems or anything like that."[9] Although another woman had "a few hot flashes," she found menopause "extremely uneventful" overall.[10]

Many of the WIM survey respondents agreed that menopause posed no special challenges but, they insisted, much like their predecessors in the 1950s, that a positive attitude had protected them. One woman, for example, "never had any trouble with menopause," claiming that she failed to notice any symptoms. She believed she had created her own good luck because she "didn't expect anything untoward." Another respondent maintained that the right attitude was crucial in creating a positive menopausal experience. She hoped to convince other women that "menopause . . . is a natural process and can be accepted and handled if one understands what to expect" and works with "the various functional changes instead of fighting them," as she thought most women did.[11]

Some menopausal women during this period relied on a strategy promoted by the women of the Brush sample twenty-five years earlier—stay busy and you won't have time to suffer at menopause. A WIM survey respondent espoused the familiar argument. Because she worked full-time, she did not "have either the time or inclination to analyze all my twinges . . . during menopause." Another woman's life was so filled with Girl Scouts, bike riding, playing bridge, and working forty hours a week that she had "no time to have menopausal symptoms." Yet another woman rather testily insisted that her "very busy life" had afforded her very "little time to dwell on any minor complaints."[12]

For some women, their busy schedules included a return to college. One woman began working toward a teaching certificate as she approached middle age. As a result, she felt "so happy and interested in my work that I never realized I had gone through menopause." Another woman, after dispatching her domestic obligations, "simply decided it was my turn. I got so absorbed in school and the university . . . that I don't think I really had time to sit down and think about it."[13]

This last comment suggests a shift in women's thinking about how they should spend their menopausal and postmenopausal years. While many of the Brush women urged others to seek worthy causes as a strategy to avoid introspection and self-pity, at least some of these women embraced the menopausal years as a chance to put themselves first. A college education allowed women to meet their own needs, to satisfy their own ambitions. These women did not seek to continue lives of sacrifice and service but devoted some well-deserved attention to themselves. Surely this would have been widely condemned as selfish in the 1950s, but it seemed more permissible by the 1970s.

Although some women believed that a busy schedule and a positive attitude were the most important elements of an uneventful menopause, they did not necessarily shun pharmaceutical assistance. One woman believed "that a woman can go through menopause beautifully with the right mental attitude." She conceded, however, that she "happen[ed] to need a little boost to help control [her] mental process."[14] Another woman noted that no one need suffer at menopause as long as they keep a "positive attitude" and "seek medical help early."[15]

In many ways, these women expressed views of and experiences with menopause that coincided with the experiences of their mothers' generation. They saw it as trivial or at least amenable to a positive attitude, a packed calendar, or a prescription for hormones. But most women, at least most women whose experiences are recorded here, did not vehemently insist that menopause was normal and thus inconsequential. For the most part, these women felt disturbed and diminished by menopause, moody and miserable, hot and bothered.

Menopausal Distress

As members of their mothers' generation had learned, keeping busy did not always stave off menopausal problems. Julie Schaffer voiced her frustration with the claim that a full life prevented problems at menopause. "Yes," she said, "I do keep busy, involved in several organizations, as well as carrying 12 credits at college, plus 3 children. However, the symptoms are nonetheless real and severe, and I begin to feel I am at the whim and will of my hormones, to say nothing of a misunderstanding medical profession." Beth Cauldwell, another WIM correspondent, had believed that maintaining a busy schedule would protect her from menopausal symptoms. She discovered, however, that although she worked full-time as a secretary and had to "rush home to do the cooking, cleaning, laundry, etc.," she still experienced hot flashes and insomnia.[16] Another woman related her surprising discovery that a full life did not prevent physical symptoms. "As a modern liberated woman, the major myth I had to overcome was the one which maintained that menopause was only a problem for neurotic women. I was taught that if a woman was physically active, busy, enjoying life, career-oriented and fulfilled, she would not experience any special discomfort during menopause, as these symptoms are all neurotic and psychosomatic. I am healthy, very busy and active and was amazed to discover that certain physical menopausal symptoms did indeed occur." These women, and others like them, discovered that, despite their best intentions, menopause often caused discomfort; it sometimes caused misery.

Night sweats and hot flashes topped the list of the troublesome physical symptoms of menopause, experienced by roughly 25 percent of the WIM survey respondents. Although hot flashes were not necessarily seen as debilitating, they could be inconvenient and annoying. A woman vividly described her experience in *Our Bodies, Ourselves:* "Suddenly, without warning, my temperature seemed to skyrocket about a hundred degrees. It wasn't the sensation of standing in front of an open oven . . . but the breathless feeling of having stayed too long in a hot shower. . . . I was hot, I was wet, and I was breathless. Charging across the room I slammed up the window and began to gulp down the cool, comforting fresh air."[17] Another woman admitted that her embarrassment over her copious sweating was her biggest problem with menopause.[18]

Some women did not mind the hot flashes at first, but when they continued for several years, these same women expressed their impatience with them. One woman began experiencing hot flashes at forty and was "thrilled" that menopause was at hand. Seventeen years later she still had regular menstrual periods and wondered despondently, "Will this menopause never end?" Hester Newman, at sixty-three, noted grimly that the average healthy woman might have to deal with her symptoms for "the rest of her life."[19]

Menopause and Mental Instability

While hot flashes were disruptive, embarrassing, and tiresome, the mental and emotional effects of menopause plagued more women and seemed to bother them more severely. These effects varied widely. More than a third of the respondents to the WIM survey felt burdened by irritability, nervousness, depression, and fatigue, and nervous symptoms also led the list of complaints from the Fiske women.[20] One woman became afraid to drive alone and often panicked in crowds. Another had trouble expressing what she felt beyond describing "peculiar feelings" in her head. One woman began to crave liquor at menopause; another became anxious and irritable. Yet another wondered "when will I come back to me? My ambition, my energy, my feeling of belonging again." These women complained that menopause changed who they were, how they navigated through their lives, and how they responded to others.[21] Most of these women admitted feeling annoyed rather than debilitated by their unstable nerves and uncontrollable emotions, but some women required intense medical and psychiatric intervention.

Many women struggled with bouts of menopause-induced depression. One woman pleaded for information on how to overcome it. She kept up a very active social life but she despaired that activities "only help during the time I'm actually participating in them. The moment I'm alone the depression and sense of futility overwhelm me."[22] Alice Stone became similarly depressed when at forty-five she endured a "very bad series of family problems." When the depression did not disappear, she visited her gynecologist who attributed her condition to menopause. She accepted the physician's explanation for the depression but insisted that without her other problems she would not have suffered so at menopause.[23]

Some of these women found relief through sedatives and tranquilizers, much as their mothers had. One woman, for example, declared menopause "hell" and despaired that "most women just keep their mouths shut and try to tough it out." She claimed that "Librium is the only medication that has ever helped." Another woman only felt better after her dentist gave her Valium. Indeed, 42 percent of the respondents to the WIM survey reported that they were taking some kind of tranquilizer or sedative. Other women found relief from a combination of hormone and sedative therapy.[24] Clearly, the rhetoric of "feminine forever" did not displace these older forms of menopausal treatment.

But many women found tranquilizers and sedatives useless against their menopausal difficulties and discovered relief from their sometimes quite serious mental problems only through hormones. One woman, for example, who feared she was losing her mind because she "imagined [she] heard voices," experienced no relief when her physicians prescribed sedatives and sleeping pills for her "nervous tension." Only massive doses and injections of hormones relieved her suffering.[25] Another woman received tranquilizers from three different doctors and began to think that she was "getting neurotic." After a year, she still felt "extremely nervous and I felt I was about to flip," so she went to yet another doctor, a gynecologist, who put her on Premarin. As a result, she "became a changed happy person," feeling better both "mentally and physically."[26]

Hormones seemed to cure even the most severe mental illness. One woman who became psychotic at menopause published an account of her ordeal in a 1969 *Reader's Digest* article. In "My Dark Journey through Insanity," Kathleen Seegers described her experience with "involutional psychosis"—an experience that included electric shock treatment and six weeks in a state mental hospital. After her reason returned, her doctor explained that her troubles were "caused largely by endocrine imbalance that was likely triggered by menopause." Consistent with this diagnosis, he treated her successfully with Premarin and tranquilizers.[27]

A few of the WIM participants recalled similar experiences. One woman related her struggles with her emotions and with the psychiatric profession. She had started to feel ill when she was about forty, and, after visiting several doctors, she finally sought out a psychiatrist. She described her harrowing experience. "He couldn't help me either, and said I was 'emotionally ill.' He stuck me in the psycho ward in the University of Washington Hospital. That was a terrible experience and didn't help me either." Finally she found a doctor who treated her successfully with hormones.[28] Another woman recounted her similarly troubling experiences. She underwent a drastic shift in her personality when she reached menopause, changing in one year from a "happy, outgoing" person into a "recluse." Ultimately, she spent six weeks in Crown Hill "undergoing 18 electric shock treatments which I abhorred and regret to this day." She insisted that hormone treatments and sensitive physicians would have solved her problems better and without the "long-lasting" and "unpleasant" effects of her hospitalization.[29] Because these women and their doctors looked to hormones to cure these episodes of mental illness, their expectation and belief clearly was that menopause could cause mental disturbance.

What explains the grim experiences and descriptions of menopause in the 1970s? In part, the sources of these reports account for their bleak tone. In general, women impelled to write the AMA and Women in Midstream for advice and guidance probably were experiencing a menopause more troubling than the average. Their stories became a matter of record because menopause was a significant enough event for them that they sought help or volunteered to share their experiences to help others. But menopause does not occur in a vacuum, and larger social and cultural developments also influence women's experiences and how they react to them. Most obviously, Robert Wilson and others recruited women to the hormone cure by focusing on the negative aspects of menopause and, simultaneously, by conflating aging with menopause. This certainly heightened some women's anxieties about menopause and enlarged the scope of symptoms considered menopausal. During an era of intense valorization of youth, the characterization of menopause as the beginning of old age and the cause of diminishing physical appeal surely encouraged some women to regard hot flashes and irregular periods as harbingers of old age and loss. Further, the proliferation of popular literature on menopause and its treatment heightened public awareness and discussion, engendering a culture in which women felt free to admit their menopausal troubles, unlike the earlier generations' embrace of stoicism. The women's movement, particularly the women's health movement, in its infancy at the beginning of this period but gaining momentum throughout, insisted that women had a right to know about their bodies and encouraged the trend toward more open communication.[30] So in different ways, the misogyny of Wilson and the empowerment of the women's movement simultaneously encouraged women to admit their menopausal troubles and to interpret their troubles at middle age as menopausal.

But some middle-aged women in the 1960s and 1970s, like some in the 1950s, remained unconvinced that menopause was responsible for their depression and other mental upsets. One woman, for example, suffered from insomnia during menopause, but she and her doctor agreed her sleeplessness was caused by "the difficult circumstances of these years." She had nursed her husband through a fatal illness and then nursed her daughter "through a similar illness ending in her death." She declared that "it would give a saint insomnia." (I must agree.) Another woman blamed the arrival of her semisenile mother-in-law for her fear that she was losing her mind. One woman wondered whether her depression was caused by menopause or by her children's departure, leaving her feeling "totally useless" and fearing that her "productive life" was over.[31] Judy Bartlett frequently worried that she was losing her mind at menopause, but she was unsure what was to blame. "I've had a pretty tragic time—widowed twice in four years, teenage troubles, broken romance, so I wonder what is causing my problems. My time of life or my past?"[32]

Other women expressed frustration that people around them attributed all angry outbursts or episodes of depression to menopause. One woman fumed, "Most people seem to think if you get mad or upset it's because of menopause. Just as if you should never be upset at this age."[33] Another woman complained that her son and husband dismissed all her anger as menopausal. They claimed she yelled and screamed because she was "going through menopause." She countered that she was always "screaming and yelling" ever since she was a young woman, and she resented the implication that she had somehow changed during menopause. In the most drastic example, when Eleanor Lang's next-door neighbor committed suicide at middle age, the victim's husband blamed menopause. Lang objected to this conclusion, insisting that the husband's behavior, his "stepping out, looking for younger women," contributed more misery than the menopause.[34] These women bemoaned the impulse to blame women's bodies for their behaviors, perhaps harkening back to women's efforts to ignore or conceal any menopausal complaints for fear that menopausal symptoms would be used to discredit women and women's professional and personal ambitions.

Menopause and the Marital Bed

Compounding their emotional problems, many women reported that marital difficulties emerged at the same time they entered menopause. Jennifer Stang, for example, noticed that about when she reached menopause her husband "suddenly went berserk over women." He eventually moved out to live with a woman who dressed like a "hippy" ("no offense intended to any hippy," she insisted). She complained that he was no longer anyone she knew. He became a "wild, woman chasing, alcoholic," and she wondered how she would cope.[35] Another woman asked her husband for a divorce about one year after her menopausal symptoms began. She admitted that "at the time of the divorce I was inadequate in marriage," but she insisted that "he was not at all adequate in providing emotional support." She believed that the "menopausal symptoms" were "the last straw," although she believed that the "divorce would have been inevitable . . . with or without menopause."[36] Another survey respondent complained that her "husband was absolutely rotten when I was going thru this," and she felt that his attitude probably contributed to their divorce. She also blamed her physician for withholding estrogen: "Lack of estrogen caused my divorce," she maintained.[37]

Several women noted that menopause produced sexual problems, and many others had anticipated that it would. Although one-half of the women responding to a 1974 *Our Bodies, Ourselves* survey felt no change in their sexual desire at menopause, some women did notice disagreeable consequences.[38] A forty-seven-year-old woman, for example, feared that she was losing her sexual desire. Until she hit menopause, she had had "regular orgasms," but she experienced them only infrequently after menopause. She regarded her inability to focus sexually as even more disturbing. She railed against her situation. "I feel inadequate and cheated that sex desire should end so early in life."[39] Another woman similarly bemoaned the erosion of her sex life. Although a combination of estrogen-androgen restored her flagging desire, she still missed the intense sexual drive she had once felt at ovulation. She complained that male doctors (not knowing what they missed) dismissed her disappointment by claiming that desire was in her head. She insisted that it was biological, like "estrus," and she mused that her present situation was "like settling for a dish of jello when you know what strawberry shortcake was like."[40] Susan Price complained that her inability to "respond normally during intercourse . . . took on enormous proportions." She began to lose heart about "getting [her] marital relations in order." After estrogens failed to cure the problem, her doctor prescribed a book on sex to her husband "which he read and manfully tried to follow."[41]

Sometimes husbands and wives differed in their view of menopausal sexual dysfunction. One husband, for example, blamed his wife's "frigidity" on menopause, but he concluded that her attitude might be connected to his viewing sex as a "physical process." His wife understood that her sexual rejections made him "unhappy," but she was just no longer interested in "anything like that." She didn't know whether it was the "change of life or what it is, but I'd just as soon not have any relationships. I won't always cooperate in that."[42]

Robert Wilson had asserted that menopause caused marital strife by making women physically unappealing, emotionally off-putting, and sexually unavailable. Were these women fulfilling Wilson's model? Some of these women may have internalized Wilson's message, leading them to blame their declining estrogens for their marital problems, but most did not. Even when women complained a bit about changes in their sexual lives, they did not usually report that these changes had caused marital problems. The woman who was begrudgingly settling for Jell-O, for example, reported only her own sexual disappointment; she did not indicate any effect on her partner's sexual pleasure. When sexual problems did threaten the happiness of marriages, "inadequate" husbands shared the blame with unresponsive wives.

Women and Their Physicians

While some women complained of frustrations in their marriages, many more described frustrations with their doctors. The Women in Midstream respondents, in particular, complained that their physicians failed to meet their needs. This stands in stark contrast to the experience of the Brush women in 1950 who reported a great deal of faith in and satisfaction with their physicians.

Many women believed that physicians were ill equipped, both educationally and emotionally, to care for menopausal women. Heidi Hauser protested that "medical school gives only a couple of periods to menopause so doctors seem [to] go along hit and miss in dealing with women who suffer the depths of their little hell."[43] Another woman blamed women's suffering at menopause on the medical profession's reluctance to learn about women's needs; she believed that a gynecologist would "rather work with any other type of patient, but a menopause patient." She concluded that physicians "do not know enough about menopause. They are afraid of it." Because of their indifference and ignorance "they cannot give you a straight answer."[44] Iris Pushkin likewise maintained that "most doctors seem to know very little about [menopause] and seem to care less. When I ask questions, I get answers of 'don't worry about it.' Unfortunately, that does not alleviate my ignorance."[45] Indeed, one woman claimed that her physician intentionally kept her in the dark. She noted impatiently that he "refuses to discuss pros and cons of what's going on for fear, I'm sure, of putting ideas into my head of new symptoms to have."[46]

Noting what they considered their physicians' disregard for their needs at menopause, many women felt their doctors belittled them and their symptoms. One woman protested that "I've about had it with this 'it's all in your head, honey' attitude."[47] Diane Bates listed her grievances: "After 10 months of no treatment, maltreatment and mis-treatment, I realized these doctors had the attitude, a) she's neurotic, b) she's to be patronized. Change of life, you know, c) It's all in her head."[48] Another woman complained that doctors "either joke about it, belittle it, or frankly admit they haven't the slightest idea why I should feel as I do." She was encouraged by the efforts of WIM, because, she insisted, "Something needs to be done and I sincerely hope your organization will find the answer. It would be a Godsend to millions of women."[49]

Many women documented their struggles to have their menopausal symptoms taken seriously. Dee Sutter, for example, hoped that WIM would "not just chalk up menopausal ailments to sheer neurosis; for the sufferer, ailments are real and sometimes quite frightening and devastating."[50] This dissatisfaction reflected a larger cultural dissatisfaction with the medical profession. While in 1942, 83 percent of Americans reported that they were satisfied with their medical care, in 1966 satisfaction levels had dropped to 73 percent, and by 1976 it had declined even further, to 42 percent.[51]

The significance of Robert Wilson's campaign on behalf of all women and especially menopausal women becomes more apparent against this backdrop. Wilson acknowledged that physicians had for generations belittled and ignored the concerns of menopausal women, but his work demonstrated that the medical profession could be responsive to aging women's needs. He explicitly positioned himself—and the estrogen replacement therapy he advocated—as taking menopausal women and their complaints seriously, and he decried the tendency of other physicians to dismiss suffering women as neurotic. His message of hope to women was that compassionate physicians who understood the gravity of menopause did exist, and this encouraged some women to continue to seek adequate, responsive medical care.

Did Wilson and his followers create the problem they proposed to cure? Without Wilson's input, would women have continued to view menopause as a trivial event that excited little concern? Surely, some women had always suffered at menopause. Wilson did not invent night sweats, vaginal dryness, nervous tension, or marital discord. Further, women have long sought medical solutions to their gender-specific needs, shopping around for particular treatments for menopause, contraception, and infertility.[52]

Further, Wilson did not create the cultural milieu that made aging in the United States particularly difficult in the 1960s and 1970s. Wilson did, however, tie menopause to the most negative aspects of aging. Further, he broadened the number of complaints and consequences associated with menopause, thus increasing the reasons for women to seek medical care and intervention.

HRT: A Great Boon to Women

Despite their dismay with their physicians, many menopausal women sought medical intervention. Some of them may have headed to the doctor because they had heard of the wonders of hormone replacement therapy and they wanted in on it. Others probably first heard of estrogen therapy when they received a prescription. Either way, hormone replacement therapy became an increasingly common accompaniment to menopause in the 1960s and early 1970s. Estimates of the number of women who used hormonal replacement therapy vary widely. A 1975 survey undertaken in the Seattle, Washington, area claimed that 51 percent of all postmenopausal women had used estrogen for at least three months, and the median length of treatment was more than ten years.[53] More in line with other estimates, one epidemiological study claimed that the percentage of women between the ages of forty-five and sixty-four using estrogen rose from 5.8 in 1962 to 12.9 in 1967. Not surprisingly, women who used hormones were overwhelmingly white and middle class.[54] Roughly 75 percent of the WIM survey respondents received hormone replacement therapy as did 61 percent of the women responding to the Boston Women's Health Book Collective questionnaire. At least 33 percent of the Fiske women, who, given the nature of the survey, were possibly less affected by their menopause, received hormones; this number may have been even higher, since some of the Fiske sample women received medication but were unsure what it was. (At 33 percent, hormone use in the Fiske sample roughly matches that in the Brush and Davidoff samples from the 1950s.) The numbers for all these groups are skewed high because they include women who had had hysterectomies, and physicians routinely provided long-term hormone treatment after "artificial menopause."

We should not assume that doctors foisted these hormone treatments on their patients. Indeed, many women sought out physicians who would prescribe hormones for them. One woman noted that she changed doctors at menopause because both her gynecologist and her general practitioner resisted treating menopause as "a deficiency disease."[55] Another woman ignored her "male doctor's" advice that she "grit [her] teeth and bear it" and "insisted that [she] be given estrogen."[56] One survey respondent advised other women to follow her lead and secure a physician who would provide hormones, saying she "finally found a Dr. that took an interest in my problem and gave hormones." She admitted that it "takes a lot of patience to find the right help . . . but after you find the right Dr., it is well worth all your effort, time and money spent."[57]

This occasional reluctance to prescribe hormones should not be interpreted as evidence of widespread resistance to the judicious use of hormone therapy. By the end of this period, most physicians willingly prescribed hormones for some of their menopausal patients. Physicians, however, did not believe that all menopausal women needed estrogen. Further, physicians insisted that medical judgment rather than patient desire or demand should dictate therapeutic decisions.[58]

Some of the women who demanded hormone treatment did so after reading about menopause and ERT in the popular literature. Writer Ann Walsh, for example, felt so inspired by *Newsweek's* 1964 article, "No More Menopause?" that she immediately wrote to Wilson to find out where she could find a doctor sympathetic to estrogen therapy.[59] Walsh's account, in turn, inspired another woman to ask her doctor for ERT.[60] Complaining about her patients' unrealistic expectations, a woman physician reported that "she had been besieged by women patients who [brought] Dr. Wilson's book in to her with paper clips attached to various pages."[61]

Some physicians were concerned and frustrated by women's demands. Sherwin Kaufman, although an important promoter of limited estrogen use, believed that women's requests were often unreasonable. "The situation has gotten ridiculous," he complained. "Women come in asking for 'the youth pill' and they say 'check my estrogen level.' From what they've read, they think it's as easy as driving into a gasoline station and having their oil checked."[62] Another physician complained about excessive demands from his women patients: "They've read Dr. Wilson's book . . . and they insist that I give them the pills. When I don't, they accuse me of being a 'medical reactionary.' . . . One perfectly normal young woman . . . wanted to take estrogen 'preventatively' . . . [W]hen I told her to come back in twenty years, she walked out in a huff."[63] These examples indicate that physicians, even physicians who supported long-term estrogen use, attempted to dissuade their patients from believing the most radical claims of Wilson and other hormone advocates cited in the popular literature.

When they did secure hormones, women often testified that their battles had been well worth the effort. One woman wrote excitedly, "I couldn't live without them and my doctor agrees! Great boon to mankind."[64] Another woman reported, with evident relief, "After 15 years of nightmares, I feel like a human being again."[65] Still another woman noted that hormones lived up to their reputation, and the Premarin that she fought for "made all the difference in the world" to her; she only wished she "had rec'd help sooner."[66]

Although women were obviously encouraged and perhaps inspired by the depictions of estrogen therapy in the media, it would be a mistake to assume that all women rushed directly to their physicians after reading about hormone therapy and demanded preventive treatment. Perhaps some did. But others proceeded more cautiously, researching both the treatment and the doctors supporting it. One woman, for example, when she discovered that her physicians disagreed about the appropriate use of estrogen, headed to the UCLA medical school library to do her own research. Other women turned to the AMA for advice. A woman from San Leandro, California, for example, wrote to the AMA after receiving literature from the Wilson Research Foundation. The literature claimed that menopause was unnecessary and could be avoided. She thought this sounded "marvelous, fantastic, and scary all in one." She was already receiving hormone shots but she believed they were "inadequate." She wondered whether the Foundation's research was sound and whether she should seek out "planned bleeding."[67]

Cancer concerns encouraged other women (and their physicians) to proceed cautiously, even before 1975. A sixty-year-old woman, for example, although still experiencing hot flashes, stopped taking hormones "in fear they are dangerous." She was concerned, however, that the experience of menopause itself might endanger her health, "since my pap test proved my hormone level is atrophic." Another woman had to be "taken off" hormones because of spotting and uterine irregularities. Her physician informed her that after a hysterectomy "hormones could be used with less side effects." She wondered whether a hysterectomy was "ever advised" to allow the continuation of estrogen therapy.[68]

Although some women actively sought out hormone therapy, others showed little concern about what sort of medication their physicians prescribed. Indeed, many women did not know what they were taking.[69] Fay Price explained her situation. Her doctor gave her "this pill, which keeps me from getting nervous." When she didn't take the pill, she became irritable. She admitted that she didn't know the name of her medication. "I don't know what the name of it is, I really don't. I just—you know, the doctor gave me them five years ago and I just keep calling my druggist and saying 'send me some more.' And I really don't know what it is."[70] Della Swanson took "the big yellow pumpkin pill" that she hoped would "slow the aging process."[71] Claudia Thomas knew only that when she forgot to take her "tablets," she became "a little confused."[72] Obviously not all women challenged medical authority. These women seem to have believed that their physicians knew what was best for them, and they readily accepted their advice and treatment.

Several factors contributed to women's eagerness to secure prescriptions for hormone therapy. Some scholars have claimed that popular depictions of menopause and menopausal women fed women's insecurities about aging and thus seduced women into seeking treatment.[73] In her 1994 book, *The Menopause Industry,* Sandra Coney claimed that because women were bombarded with negative portrayals of their aging bodies, they felt they had no choice but to seek out hormones.[74] But this position cedes too much power to the popular media. As Dorothy Nelkin has shown, deliberate attempts by the popular media to influence behavior have often failed. People did not quit smoking just because the press urged them to, nor did they line up for the Salk vaccine. At times, of course, the popular media did affect consumer behavior. In the aftermath of the toxic shock publicity, for example, the sales of certain brands of tampons plummeted. According to Nelkin, however, the media does not by itself change the public's actions. Rather, consumers act on information in the media "mainly when it corresponds to their prior inclinations."[75]

Nevertheless, some women, frightened by Wilson's gloomy depictions and florid prose, did seek hormones to protect against aging. The popular literature provides several examples of women searching for "anti-aging pills,"[76] and the archival sources provide further examples of this trend. One woman who reported "no trouble" at menopause, nevertheless took a "post-menopausal pill . . . to slow the aging process."[77] A WIM survey respondent admitted that "I'd like to see menstrual periods continue through medicine. . . . I guess I like feeling young, looking young and energetic."[78] Another woman sought hormones after her hysterectomy in order to feel like "a woman again."[79] A few women also acknowledged taking hormones to prevent menopause altogether. Doris Lauer, having taken hormones for four to five years, had heard that "as long as you take hormones, you never experience [menopause], so I'm hoping that's right."[80]

But we should not dismiss these women's desire for a youthful body as a desire to remain appropriately feminine or as a concession to a culture that revered unlined faces and firm buttocks. Surely some women did hope to retain "their looks" as they aged. But aging does sometimes lead to a body that betrays through infirmity. Women who used estrogens, thinking they would prevent heart disease and osteoporosis, may have felt as responsible as those taking multivitamins and getting plenty of exercise. One woman described her complex motivations: "I feel so good with monthly hormone shots and vitamins that I plan to continue until my last days so as to have a healthy body, clear mind, and avoid osteoarthritis, osteoporosis and the shrinking that seems to occur as one gets older."[81] Although this woman was influenced by the medicalization of preventive health measures, she does not appear more victimized than those women who take calcium supplements and head to the gym three times a week.[82]

The surveys provide no evidence that women, even women with menopausal difficulties, regarded menopause as a disease or their symptoms as signs of illness. Indeed, the evidence points away from acceptance of menopause as a deficiency disease. A survey of women aged forty to sixty, for example, demonstrated that they overwhelmingly rejected the illness model of menopause.[83] Other women's comments support this. Alice Rand, although she took "b.c. pills" for menopause, nevertheless believed that it was "stupid" to make too much of a "natural process."[84] Another woman took hormones for her menopausal nerves but she regarded menopause as "just a phase to adjust to." She later amended that opinion, deciding, ultimately, that menopause required "no special adjustment." Sarah Keenan endorsed hormone treatments but insisted that "too much stress has been put on a problem that is a natural process of nature."[85] These women accepted hormone therapy without embracing the disease model.

Despite widespread hormone use, Wilson's rhetoric had not won the day. Many other threads in the popular literature encouraged women to embrace hormone therapy. First, the enormous publicity surrounding ERT brought menopause and its treatment to the attention of middle-aged women. Unlike earlier periods, when women were urged to ignore menopause, this publicity dared women to assess their own reactions to menopause and to decide for themselves whether they should "grit their teeth" or find means to ease their suffering. Bolstered by reassurances that their misery was unnecessary, many women did seek pharmaceutical help. Second, menopausal women experienced real symptoms—some annoying, some debilitating. Virtually all of the popular literature unambiguously recommended ERT for severe cases of hot flashes and genital atrophy and suggested that hormones might prevent brittle bones, heart disease, and marital discord. For women who suffered from severe symptoms or who feared future debility, the popular literature validated replacement hormones as a legitimate choice.[86] Third, the popular literature encouraged women to shop around for a physician who would provide hormonal relief. Lila Nachtigall, for example, advised her readers to find a doctor who "is willing to go along with the kind of treatment you want."[87] Another writer, himself a doctor, urged women to "insist" on hormone treatment and if "he refuses, find another doctor."[88] This empowered women by encouraging them to be active participants in their own health care. Taken together, these incentives provided women with the permission and the impetus to secure the modern treatment.

With a few exceptions, women did not seek hormones to prevent aging, to cure a disease, or to reclaim their lost femininity. They turned to hormones at menopause for the same reasons their predecessors had, to relieve the more mundane, but potentially debilitating, consequences of menopause: hot flashes, insomnia, headaches, genital atrophy, and nervousness. Clearly, while women increasingly accepted ERT as a beneficial—occasionally fantastic—therapy for menopausal symptoms, they did not necessarily view ERT as a miraculous cure for their diseased bodies.

Cancer Concerns and Hormonal Comforts

After 1975, the mounting evidence that estrogen therapy increased the risk of endometrial cancer led many women to reconsider their reliance on replacement hormones. Frightened, or at least sobered, by the publicity in the popular literature, women increasingly tried to weather menopause without hormones.[89] According to a *Vogue* article, "women in droves quit estrogen" in response to the publicity.[90] The letters received by Women in Midstream after 1975 reflected women's fear of cancer along with their enduring desire for relief from menopausal symptoms. Many women wanted to stop taking estrogens but could not. One woman wrote that she had been "taking Premarin for 17 years and would like to stop" but admitted that she needed the help.[91] Another woman who had taken stilbestrol for twenty-one years "tried to wean herself off" after she learned of the cancer risk. Without the drug, however, her "hot flashes were almost unbearable and seemed to gain momentum as time passed. . . . After suffering through three weeks of this," she fell back on the medication.[92] Another woman remained on estrogen although her physician urged her to stop because of her past diagnosis of breast cancer. (He did continue to provide the prescription, however.) She tried to stop, but her experience with hot flashes, four to six each night, forced her to resume them.[93]

Some women were reluctant to use hormones regardless of their doctors' advice. One woman explained that her physician, who normally discouraged hormone treatments, nevertheless thought she would be a "good candidate" for a short course of low-dose estrogens. Although she was "exhausted all the time," and had to fortify herself with Valium before leaving the house "to help with the pressure," she remained determined to avoid hormones "as long as I have the strength."[94] Another woman claimed that physicians were "too quick" to advise hormones. Two of her friends had died of cancer within a year of starting hormone treatment for menopause, and another had been diagnosed with cancer. As a result, she refused estrogen therapy, relying instead on Librium to relieve her menopausal headaches.[95]

These women were clearly affected by the publicity surrounding the link between estrogen and cancer, and they hoped to secure a safer path to easing their menopausal difficulties. Nevertheless, they believed that they needed some form of assistance to fortify their bodies and their spirits. Further, they did not necessarily regard their physicians as the only legitimate source of medical information. Instead, they relied on their own research and experiences to guide them through their decision-making process.

Women did receive less estrogen therapy in the years right after 1975. Physicians wrote fewer prescriptions (twenty-eight million in 1975; fifteen million in 1980) and fewer women took the drugs. According to one survey, the number of women taking replacement hormones dropped by 18 percent between 1975 and 1976 and by another 10 percent between 1976 and 1977. Estimates for the percentage of women aged forty-five to sixty-four using replacement hormones in 1977 ranged from 7 to 14 percent.[96]

Thus, although many women did respond to the popular literature by asking for—perhaps demanding—hormone therapy, some did so only after arming themselves with information that allowed them to accept ERT to treat their symptoms while simultaneously rejecting the most egregious characterizations of menopause and menopausal women.

At the same time Wilson was referring to aging women as castrates, a burgeoning feminist movement was urging women to revise their relationships with their bodies. Feminists, particularly those dedicated to wo-

men's health, encouraged women to accept their bodies as a site of pleasure and a repository of strength, and they emphasized the importance to
women's emancipation of controlling one's body. Feminism's influence
on the understanding and experience of menopause is the subject of the
next chapter.

NINE

"What Do These Women Want?"

Feminists Respond to Feminine Forever, 1963–1980

In 1963, the same year that Robert Wilson declared postmenopausal women castrates, a part-time housewife, part-time journalist identified "the problem that has no name." In *The Feminine Mystique*, Betty Friedan documented the growing unrest among college-educated, middle-class, white women with the demands and limits of domesticity. While it clearly did not foment the feminist revolution, *The Feminine Mystique* testified to the smoldering dissatisfaction among women that led, within a few years, to the women's movement. Both *The Feminine Mystique* and Wilson's 1966 *Feminine Forever* invited women to reconsider the meanings of womanhood and their roles within American society.

The convergence of Wilson's campaign and the emergence of the women's movement raised many issues. The disease model of menopause and its proposed hormonal cure presented several dilemmas for the fledgling women's movement. Should feminists shun the "medicalization" of their normal physiological processes or should they demand even more medical attention? What were the social costs of regarding menopause as a "deficiency disease" requiring pharmaceutical intervention? Were menopausal symptoms caused by defective physiology or a sexist society? Did medical technology help or hinder the cause of women's liberation?

Between 1963 and 1980, some feminists wrestled with these questions as they confronted the popular characterizations of menopause and the increased popularity of estrogen replacement therapy. In the beginning of this period, some feminists embraced Wilson as a benefactor to aging women, while others highlighted the dangerous implications of regarding

209

female aging as pathological. In 1975, studies linking ERT and endometrial cancer challenged the wisdom of the routine prescription of
hormone therapy. Although this concern shifted the tenor of the feminist
discussion, feminist consensus about the meaning of menopause or its
treatment remained elusive. Despite these divisions, the feminist discussion of menopause revealed a larger women's health agenda. Whatever
their views of ERT, feminist health activists demonstrated an unyielding
belief that women should retain control of their bodies and participate
fully in making decisions about their health. By controlling their bodies,
they believed, women could ultimately seize greater control of their lives.

This larger philosophy, rather than any one particular recommendation
regarding hormones, represents the most important feminist contribution
to the discussion of menopause. Significantly, while the feminist discussion
of menopause was limited to a fairly small number of participants, the
broader agenda reached well beyond this narrow circle. The women's
movement affected the experience of many menopausal women not otherwise aligned with feminism. As they demanded that their doctors provide
ERT or sought out other women to talk with, many menopausal women
between 1963 and 1980 were influenced by the feminist approach to
women's health. The varied feminist responses to menopause and its treatment and the effect of feminism on the experience of menopausal women
outside the women's movement are the subjects of this chapter.[1]

Feminism and Women's Health

The women's movement of the 1960s and 1970s can be divided roughly
into two strands: the women's rights movement and the women's liberation movement. The women's rights movement drew its constituents primarily from among middle-class, professional women. Their campaign attempted to secure for women the same opportunities for professional and
political advancement traditionally enjoyed by men. The women's liberation movement generally attracted younger women whose dissatisfaction
with women's roles in the civil rights and New Left movements engendered a more radical, more militant approach to attacking social problems.
The campaign for women's liberation, however, was not itself a unified
movement. Indeed, it was characterized by internal dissension over goals,
tactics, and the roots of women's oppression.[2]

By the end of the 1960s, concern for women's health in both the
women's rights and women's liberation movements had coalesced into a

women's health movement. In 1969, for example, participants in a women's conference in Boston raised the issue of "women and their bodies" as an appropriate focus for feminist consideration. This gathering led to the formation of the Boston Women's Health Course Collective.[3] This pathbreaking group published their first collection of articles in 1971. Inspired by the example of the Boston organization, women in New York sponsored the first Women's Health Conference in March 1971. A nationwide survey, circulated in 1974, testifies to the willingness of the women's movement to embrace health issues as an important plank in its platform. The survey found that more than twelve hundred women's groups offered some sort of health service, and "tens of thousands" of individual women considered themselves participants in the women's health movement.[4] As part of their health education efforts, feminists published books and articles, gathered and analyzed information, sponsored workshops, designed and taught courses, and supported "consciousness raising" (CR) groups.

Initial feminist health efforts focused primarily on reproductive issues, including childbirth, birth control, and abortion rights. The first edition of *Our Bodies, Our Selves* only mentioned menopause in passing, as part of a larger discussion of the ovarian cycle.[5] This reflected, perhaps, the youth and interests of early feminist health activists.[6] But even within these discussions, feminists challenged the traditional doctor-patient relationship in which patients relinquished control of their bodies to the more "knowledgeable" professional. As a strategy to loosen the medical profession's hold on female patients, feminist health activists urged women to be wary of the intentions of male physicians. Barbara Ehrenreich and Deirdre English, for example, claimed that misogyny was built into the medical profession and argued that medicine had been used as an agent of social control to preserve patriarchy and to oppress women.[7]

Despite general agreement about the need for medical reform, feminists did not share a common vision of women's health care. Some activists sought to avoid entirely the male dominated medical profession and promoted female self-help and lay-controlled health facilities. Other feminists acknowledged that the medical profession had much to offer women but sought to establish health facilities that embraced feminist principles. One prominent activist even proposed that only women should be allowed to become obstetricians and gynecologists and that all research on women should be carried out exclusively by women.[8] Feminists also disagreed about the nature of their bodies. According to Ehrenreich and English, feminists "seem to alternate between accusing the medical system of treating us as if we were sick and accusing them of not appreciating how sick we are."[9]

The feminist discussion of menopause between 1963 and 1980 reflects the larger divisions within the women's health movement. Nonetheless, two aspects of the larger movement provided the scaffolding for later feminist responses. Activists agreed that women must retain control of their bodies by refusing to see all bodily occurrences as medical events and by participating actively in the doctor-patient relationship. The self-help gynecology movement, for example, encouraged women to demystify their bodies and to use self-exams to diagnose gynecological disorders. The natural childbirth movement, while not exclusively feminist, urged women to see childbirth as a natural event rather than a medical emergency. Both movements acknowledged that medical intervention was sometimes required, but they insisted that women remain the ultimate decision makers in matters that concerned their bodies. These themes became central to the feminist discussion of menopause and estrogen therapy.

ERT: Welcome Treatment or Risky Medicine?

Many scholars of menopause have rightly credited feminism with challenging both the disease model of menopause and the use of estrogen therapy to treat menopause.[10] It would be a mistake to assume, however, that feminists immediately rejected the message of *Feminine Forever* and the widespread use of ERT.[11] The evidence indicates that feminists did not overwhelmingly dispute either the disease model of menopause or the use of ERT, at least in print.[12] Indeed, before 1975, very few feminists discussed menopause at all, at least in print.[13] Those who did engage the issues surrounding menopause displayed a great deal of ambivalence about how to regard menopausal bodies and how best to cope with menopause's changes.

Far from rejecting Wilson and his ideas, some feminist health activists maintained that Wilson's model of menopause as a disease with estrogen therapy as its cure provided powerful weapons in women's fight for liberation. Research scientist turned writer Belle Canon, for example, railed against the medical profession's general neglect of menopause and the women who suffered from it. During a trip to the public library, she tried to find helpful information about menopause but only discovered an endless stream of medical platitudes that menopause was normal and that its symptoms would eventually pass. She interpreted this to mean that it was woman's fate to feel ill at certain periods of her life. To Canon's relief, she discovered *Feminine Forever* and Wilson's assurance that women need not feel ill at menopause. She enthusiastically accepted Wilson's claim that menopause was a deficiency disease, a disease that could be easily cured.[14]

Canon credited Wilson with providing the "first and only stimulus to public and medical discussion of menopause." She noted that his revolutionary treatment had engendered a great deal of controversy and acknowledged that many physicians retained an "old-fashioned" view of menopause by insisting that women weather the storm, but she urged women to take charge of their relationships with their bodies and their physicians. After promoting estrogen therapy as the cure for menopausal difficulties, she complained, "You may or may not get it, depending upon how your doctor feels about it and depending no less on how actively involved you, yourself become to get relevant information and to demand help to be given to you."[15] Canon's own fight to receive estrogen therapy lasted two years, but she believed that "the results turned out to have been worth every minute of the battle."[16]

British journalist Wendy Cooper embraced estrogen therapy even more enthusiastically, seeing it as an important tool in securing women's liberation.[17] Because estrogen allowed women "to control the biology that had for so long controlled them," Cooper believed replacement therapy could lead to a biological revolution. She argued that until women could control their bodies, they could not "compete . . . on something like equal terms with men." She challenged the assertion that because something was natural it must be allowed to progress unimpeded. She claimed that this argument had been used to prevent access to contraception and thereby kept women constrained by the demands of biology.[18]

Cooper lauded Wilson for taking menopausal women and their unique problems seriously, and she celebrated the choice that estrogen represented. "No longer need any woman, unless she chooses, be fobbed off during the menopause with palliatives such as aspirin, Librium or Valium, or worse still, be dismissed with the words, 'It's just your age. There is nothing I can do. You must put up with it.'"[19] Indeed, Cooper believed that estrogen allowed women to "age in a way that parallels that of a man."[20]

Cooper blamed misogyny for physicians' general neglect of menopausal women and cited the words of Dr. Francis Rhoades, who urged doctors to reconsider their relationships with their menopausal patients: "The physician should not let inherent male resentment of female longevity and biological superiority deter him from his medical responsibility. Because men do not experience the dramatic and often devastating changes represented by the menopause, they have come to regard it as normal for women to suffer the consequences of cessation of ovarian secretion." Cooper described Rhoades' contention as "splendid ammunition for Women's Liberation."[21]

Cooper drew inspiration from Robert Wilson and *Feminine Forever*, but she adjusted Wilson's message to fit her needs. Uncomfortable with Wilson's obsession with keeping women young and feminine, she amended his interpretation to place "less emphasis on femininity and more on feminism and on the right of women to have more say in decisions, medical or social, which affect their own bodies and their own lives."[22]

Medical anthropologist Paula Weideger did not embrace the disease model as enthusiastically as did Canon and Cooper, but she similarly encouraged estrogen therapy as the best treatment for menopause. Although Weideger admitted that some problems of menopause represented "responses to society's evaluation of the older woman's status," she embraced estrogen deficiency as a more satisfying and comprehensive explanation for women's physical and emotional symptoms.[23]

Weideger's widely cited 1976 book, *Menstruation and Menopause: The Physiology and Psychology, the Myth and the Reality,* did not explicitly recommend long-term ERT, but it tacitly communicated her leanings in several ways. First, Weideger implied that women's bodies were not designed to live without the benefits of estrogen. She allied herself with Dr. Herbert Kupperman (and others), claiming that because medical science extended a woman's life span "much beyond her reproductive potential," medicine had an obligation to keep a woman healthy during her "extra" years. Weideger conceded that nature acted wisely by ending fertility at middle age, but she suggested that nature goofed by simultaneously decreasing the supply of ovarian hormones. Noting that natural selection could not shape women's postreproductive years, she complained that "women had to live with the results of nature's error." As a consequence, she claimed, menopausal women needed science and medicine to step in and fix the flawed design.[24] Weideger refuted the idea that because menopause was natural, it should not be treated medically. Rather than rely on the ability of women's bodies to adapt, she put her faith in medicine as a way of improving women's lot.

Weideger simultaneously scolded physicians who withheld estrogen treatment until menopausal symptoms occurred and condemned a medical system that neglected preventive medicine. She suggested that a doctor "is a participant in the culture that views 'female complaints' as women's fate," and she denounced the too common practice of ignoring the problems of menopause until women experienced a "menopausal crisis." She blamed this attitude on the sexism inherent in both medicine and society.[25]

Finally, Weideger believed that women who chose ERT challenged society's perceptions of their bodies by insisting that menopause "need not be an infirmity." Weideger claimed that ERT allowed women simultaneously to affirm the physiological roots of menopausal symptoms and to diminish the significance of those symptoms in their lives. By taking ERT, women relieved their unpleasant symptoms but also challenged the long-held belief that women's suffering was all in their heads. Weideger saw both of these situations as empowering to menopausal women in the face of a sexist medical establishment.[26]

Despite her generally positive characterization of replacement estrogens, Weideger admitted that "any woman who now chooses ERT, is a guinea pig and a gambler." She insisted, however, that the risks associated with estrogen therapy were less than those younger women faced with oral contraceptives. She argued that ERT, unlike oral contraceptives, merely brought "estrogen levels back up to the hormonal levels of the fertile years."[27] In the end, Weideger conceded that the safety of ERT was not guaranteed and that it could not cure all menopausal difficulties. Therefore, women must make their own choices—guided perhaps by friends and physicians.[28]

The views of Canon, Cooper, and Weideger reflect a feminist tradition of belief in biomedical technology as a complement to the goals of women's liberation. These feminists denied that the natural order of things— whether the functioning of women's bodies or entrenched gender relations—inherently benefited women. As Shulamith Firestone argued in her feminist classic, *The Dialectic of Sex* (1970), "humanity has begun to outgrow nature: we can no longer justify the maintenance of a discriminatory sex class system on grounds of its origin in Nature."[29] She insisted that technology promised to help women escape from the tyranny of their biology. She believed that before the technological development of birth control women "were at the continual mercy of their biology—menstruation, menopause, and 'female ills,' constant painful childbirth, wetnursing and care of infants, all of which made them dependent on males . . . for physical survival," and she demanded more technological developments to weaken further the biological demands of womanhood.[30] Feminists who enthusiastically embraced hormone treatment similarly denounced the conflation of "natural" and "desirable" and insisted that technology could and should sever women's dependence on the demands and difficulties presented by their bodies.

Other feminists before 1976 were more ambivalent about estrogen and *Feminine Forever* than were Canon, Cooper, and Weideger. While they rejected Wilson's negative portrayals of menopause, they nevertheless thanked him for focusing much-needed medical attention on menopause and for publicizing a treatment that could alleviate the real suffering of many women. They tried to describe menopause in more positive ways while they simultaneously embraced hormone therapy as a valuable tool for menopausal women.

The position of the Boston Women's Health Book Collective reflects this attitude. As noted earlier, the first edition of *Our Bodies, Ourselves* (1971) only mentioned menopause in one sentence: "At the time of menopause, when a woman runs out of follicles, she gets an estrogen deficiency."[31] The 1973 edition downplayed menopause's negative aspects, condemning popular images that portrayed menopausal women as "haggard, irritable, bitchy, unsexy and impossible to live with."[32] The collective extolled the value of adequate information about menopause in order to demystify (and thereby ease) the experience. Further, the authors emphasized a woman's right to demand "good medical care and advice."[33] At one point, they chided physicians who did not offer treatment (or at least an explanation) to women who were feeling tired during menopause. They repeatedly admonished the medical profession for not devoting more research to menopause and for failing to discover more "cures," insisting that if "every male doctor went through menopause," a more thorough research program would be in place.[34] They noted that "some doctors have gone so far as to declare menopause 'an estrogen deficiency disease,' which they claim can be 'cured.'" While the authors noted that most physicians supported a more conservative position, the collective did not dismiss or even challenge the disease model.[35]

The collective accepted estrogen replacement therapy, regarding it as a valuable tool for alleviating menopausal symptoms such as hot flashes and vaginal dryness. Moreover, they suggested that estrogen was "necessary" for other areas of women's health. They described its ability to maintain "general skin tone" and to prevent osteoporosis and heart disease. Although they also mentioned the benefits of diet, rest, and exercise in preventing the negative effects of menopause, the membership of the collective nevertheless presented estrogen therapy as an effective treatment for a wide range of physical and emotional symptoms. Nevertheless, they also suggested that ERT posed potential risks that women should discuss with their physicians.[36]

Despite the widespread acceptance of hormones and a grudging respect for Wilson and his work, a few feminists spoke out against Wilson's portrayal of menopause and menopausal women. Joan Solomon, writing for *Ms.* magazine in 1972, provided an early feminist voice of concern and caution.[37] Unlike most of her feminist contemporaries, Solomon challenged the idea that menopause was a disease, asserting instead that it was "as inevitable and natural as menstruation." She did not, however, reject hormone treatments. She noted that estrogens were neither a "sexual godsend" nor a fountain of youth, and she reminded her readers that drug companies "are tremendously excited by the notion of 'estrogens forever.'" She also warned that many of the claims for ERT, that it prevented osteoporosis and heart disease, for example, remained unproven; the risks, she argued, were clear. While her portrayal of estrogen therapy clearly indicated her bias against it, she in no way condemned its judicious use, declaring unambiguously that a woman must make her own decisions. "It's a decision you alone must make, keeping in mind your medical history, psychological needs, and physicians' advice."[38]

Barbara Seaman, who had already led the fight against the widespread use of contraceptive estrogens, similarly challenged the marketing of replacement hormones in a 1972 *Prime Time* article. Seaman attacked the characterizations of menopause promoted by Robert Wilson and others that encouraged women to believe that their bodies and minds needed estrogen to avoid debility.[39] Although Seaman clearly believed that physicians and drug companies had the most to gain and menopausal women had the most to lose from hormone therapy, she did not explicitly recommend that women avoid it. In her 1972 book, *Free and Female,* Seaman was harsher on drug manufacturers and more leery of estrogen, particularly because of its possible connection to cancer. Nevertheless, she concluded that "this whole area is so 'iffy' that one cannot take a blanket stand against estrogen replacement therapy." As a result, Seaman, like Solomon, recommended caution and urged women to seek out physicians who treated their patients as "fully functioning autonomous adults."[40]

Between 1963 and 1975 feminists did not promote one particular position on the disease model of menopause or the use of estrogen therapy.

Feminists did, however, agree on a larger issue that affected menopausal women. Seaman voiced the opinion supported by all feminist health activists: "We cannot gain autonomy over our minds unless we gain autonomy over our bodies as well. We must reject the majority of doctors who push us around or patronize us, and take our business to the few who are willing to treat us as full partners in our own health."[41]

Increased Concern

As described in Chapter 7, new evidence emerged at the end of 1975 that linked unopposed estrogen therapy with an increased risk of endometrial cancer. Researchers at Washington University (Donald Smith, et al.) and Kaiser-Permanente Medical Center (Harry Ziel and William Finkle) independently concluded that long-term estrogen therapy posed a health threat to women with a uterus.[42] Although a few researchers had suspected a link between estrogen therapies and cancer since the 1930s, the claims of these landmark studies gave the alleged dangers new legitimacy. The news quickly spread beyond medical circles and into the national press, suggesting that what had once been seen as a medical miracle cure might well have made at least some women gravely ill.[43] Consequently, these studies encouraged menopausal women and their physicians to carefully weigh the alleged benefits of long-term estrogen therapy against its sobering dangers.

These studies also awakened an increased feminist interest in menopause and a more critical examination of hormonal therapy. Alerted to the ideological and physical price of considering menopause a disease by the cancer disclosures, more feminists condemned the widespread use of long-term hormone treatment. Feminists remained divided, however, over the benefits of short-term treatments. Although feminists on both sides of the estrogen divide continued to affirm a woman's right to decide her own coping strategy, they urged women to think more broadly about the consequences of treatment.

Despite this continued ambivalence about the prudence of ERT, after the 1975 studies feminists emerged newly united on the need to consider carefully the meaning and significance of menopause. Feminists realized that menopause marked a social as well as a physical transition; as a result, they insisted that the real solution for menopausal difficulties required changes in women's relationships with their aging bodies and in their roles within society. In particular, feminists united around three alternative approaches to menopause and the problems faced by menopausal women.

First, they denied that menopause was a disease, portraying it instead as a natural transition. Feminists believed that characterizing menopause as a normal life event eased women's symptoms by dispelling apprehension. Second, they urged women to break free of their socially sanctioned roles and to establish lives beyond home and family. Third, feminists insisted that individual choices would not eliminate the larger problems faced by menopausal women. They claimed that only women's liberation would solve the ultimate problems of menopausal women. In short, many health activists interpreted the difficulties women faced at menopause as symptoms not of physical illness but of social pathology.

The feminist reconsideration of ERT emerged after a series of medical episodes that disproportionately affected women. In the early 1970s, for example, researchers began publishing startling findings about the increased incidence of an extremely rare vaginal cancer. Boston physician Arthur Herbst, for example, reported eight cases among adolescent girls in his practice. Eight cases of this cancer among women would have gained attention, but the cancer had previously been unknown in girls; the evidence shocked the profession. Cancer experts quickly connected vaginal cancer in girls to the use by the girls' mothers of diethylstilbestrol (DES) to prevent miscarriage.

DES had first been prescribed as a treatment for menopause in the 1940s,[44] but it gained popularity in the late 1940s and early 1950s as a preventive for miscarriage. Although the exact number is unknown, experts estimate that physicians prescribed DES to more than three million pregnant women, making the potential scope of the problem huge by epidemiological standards. Further research linked the use of DES in pregnancy to other abnormalities in daughters and, more recently, in sons. In 1975, enraged that the FDA still allowed the administration of DES as a postcoital contraceptive, feminists urged the FDA (unsuccessfully) to withdraw approval of DES for all women.[45]

At roughly the same time, the dangers of the Dalkon Shield caught the attention of the women's health movement. In the 1960s and 1970s, the IUD (intrauterine device) emerged as a popular form of contraception among American women. Unfortunately, since the FDA did not consider "medical devices" part of its jurisdiction, manufacturers of IUDs were not required to test their products for safety or effectiveness. Although complications appeared with several models of IUD, the Dalkon Shield proved particularly dangerous. By 1974, thirty-six American women had died and thirty-five hundred had been hospitalized as a result of complications from the Dalkon Shield. Feminists, angered that women were being fitted with such potentially dangerous devices, lobbied the federal government to intervene. Partly in response to feminist efforts, in 1976 the FDA added medical devices to the list of products that must be proven safe and effective before being put on the market.[46]

These events prompted feminists to reconsider their relationship with medical technology, and while most health activists did not reject all medical developments, they learned to keep a watchful eye on the industry. As a result, some feminists were primed to condemn ERT at the earliest sign of danger.

In her 1977 book, *Menopause: A Positive Approach,* feminist health activist Rosetta Reitz presented several of the feminist positions that emerged after the cancer studies. First, Reitz denied that menopause was a disease, insisting instead that it was a normal and natural process. "I accept that I'm a healthy woman whose body is changing. No matter how many articles and books I read that tell me I'm suffering from a 'deficiency disease,' I say I don't believe it. I have never felt more in control of my life than I do now and I feel neither deficient nor diseased."[47] Consistently, she downplayed the significance of both the physical and the emotional effects of menopause. Reitz claimed that only 50 percent of menopausal women experienced hot flashes at all, and she insisted that, even at their worst, hot flashes were "harmless." She maintained that "the worst thing about them is that they may be uncomfortable, but they are unaccompanied by pain."[48] Reitz urged women to accept "yourself and your hot flashes"[49] rather than looking for a drug to treat them. Reitz approached depression at menopause the same way she viewed hot flashes: she urged women to accept it. "You don't have to run for help from a pill. Go along with the feelings; do not try to deny them. . . . By allowing 'uncomfortable' feelings their full range, you are experiencing a fuller range of yourself. That is a way to get in touch with yourself."[50]

Because Rosetta Reitz denied the severity of menopausal symptoms, she easily condemned all but "natural" approaches to their relief. She began her chapter on ERT with the bold statement, "Estrogen replacement therapy is dangerous. It will raise your cancer risk. It may lead to vascular disease. It may even kill you." Just as Weideger saw choosing ERT as a revolutionary statement, Reitz viewed rejecting ERT as a political one. "If our refusal to tolerate carcinogens could become universal, we would shake the very fabric of this culture."[51]

Feminist publications widely promoted Reitz's position,[52] and many health activists adopted her views. Nevertheless, other feminists acknowledged that some women suffered greatly at menopause and insisted that medical intervention was an appropriate decision in those cases.

Although they refused to condone the routine use of estrogen therapy, feminists nevertheless wanted tools to relieve menopausal symptoms. The 1976 edition of *Our Bodies, Ourselves* reflects the continuing ambivalence some feminists felt toward estrogen. While the 1973 edition had accepted ERT, the 1976 version was more circumspect. The authors in both editions hoped to "reduce the anxiety that results from a lack of knowledge," but whereas the 1973 edition indicted physicians for not taking their menopausal patients seriously, the 1976 edition denounced "doctors who put every woman on medication and, equally, . . . those who tell us that our symptoms are 'only in the mind.' There are situations when severe symptoms *may* require treatment, and we have a right to medical help that will provide such treatment."[53] The 1976 edition shared with the 1973 edition a belief that women should exploit what medicine had to offer, but it also acknowledged the risks of ERT and advised women to proceed with caution.[54]

Other feminists took an even bolder position, condemning Reitz and others who dismissed as trivial the real suffering of some menopausal women. Irma Levine, a founding member of a menopause support group, for example, agreed that menopause was natural, but she argued that many women suffered severe symptoms nonetheless. She insisted that for these women, it is no more helpful "to say they should just take calcium and vitamin E than it is helpful to say if they just keep busy it will all go away." Levine asserted that women should not feel guilty for feeling bad at menopause or for turning to the medical profession for relief, and she resisted the notion that right living guaranteed an easy menopause.[55]

Although after the cancer revelations about estrogens feminist health activists did not promote any one position on ERT, they did agree that social factors contributed to women's experiences at menopause. The 1976 edition of *Our Bodies, Ourselves,* for example, contended that the "most unpleasant aspects of menopause" might be social rather than physical because menopause arrives "at a time in a woman's life when her relationships may be changing."[56] Maintaining that social problems demanded social rather than pharmaceutical solutions, some feminists proposed women's liberation as the ultimate solution to women's menopausal difficulties.

Marriage and family counselor and part-time college instructor Vidal S. Clay agreed that women's troubles at menopause were not primarily medical but social. "A woman does not go through the climacteric . . . in a vacuum. How she deals with this continuing development of her life is determined by her feelings about herself as a woman at this time in her life. These feelings will reflect society's notions about women, about women who do not reproduce, about women who are middle-aged and growing older."[57] In order to address the dilemmas of middle age, Clay called for a feminist revolution that would improve life for middle-aged women by improving life for all women. She insisted that "women must work together to continue to exert pressure for social change," and she considered the women's liberation movement the "most significant social force working for women today."[58]

Other feminist health activists agreed with Clay. Sociologist Pauline Bart and her part-time collaborator Marlyn Grossman, for example, denied that "individual solutions" could ultimately improve conditions for menopausal women. They insisted that the real remedy for menopausal depression depended on the "organized efforts of many women working together to structure alternatives for themselves and others." Only women's liberation, they argued, could improve the lot of menopausal women by supporting alternative lifestyles and deviations from prescribed roles. Women's liberation would help all women discover and develop their own potential.[59] The authors of the *Ms. Guide to a Woman's Health* similarly recommended that menopausal women turn to the feminist movement, claiming that "it is preventative medicine for the awful feeling that you are suddenly in the denouement before the end of the play."[60]

After the 1975 cancer revelations, more feminists turned their attention to menopause, and they increasingly discouraged women from seeking a pharmaceutical solution for a natural process. Nevertheless, health activists did not unanimously adopt this position. For the most part, feminists continued to support short-term estrogen use for women whose other efforts to find relief from severe menopausal symptoms had failed. But the feminist discussion of menopause did not focus exclusively on treatment options. Rather, they examined the difficulties many women experienced at menopause against the social backdrop. These women claimed that women's social roles as wives and mothers led to emotional depression and physical ailments when women felt forced into "retirement" by menopause. As a result, feminists believed that changing women's role in society was a critical strategy for improving the lives of menopausal and postmenopausal women.

The Women's Movement and Menopausal Women

The feminist discussion of menopause between 1963 and 1980 was limited to a small group of women writing primarily in feminist publications such as *Our Bodies, Ourselves, Prime Time,* and *Ms.* The influence of the women's movement on the understanding of and response to menopause was not limited, however, to the women who read these periodicals or who participated directly in feminist organizing. Indeed, feminism empowered a wide spectrum of American women to reexamine their relationships with the medical profession and with their individual doctors. It also affected many women's views of themselves as consumers of medical knowledge, and it allowed women to regard the doctor-patient relationship as negotiable.

The women's movement affected many women's experiences at menopause in at least four ways. First, feminism encouraged women to take control of their bodies and their health care decisions. As a result, some menopausal women demanded both respectful treatment and specific therapies from their physicians. If their demands were not met, they took their business elsewhere. Second, prompted by the feminist critique of patriarchy, women began to articulate their dissatisfaction with their medical providers in terms of misogyny and male chauvinism. Third, women rejected the "suffer in silence" approach to menopause advocated by their mothers and grandmothers and turned to one another for support. And finally, realizing that their reaction to menopause was influenced by their limited social options, some women saw women's liberation itself as the cure for menopausal difficulties.

By 1973, doctors, particularly obstetricians and gynecologists, began noticing a change in their patients and responded variously with hostility, perplexity, and acceptance, wondering what had come over their once pliable patients. "What is behind these demands that threaten the staid orderliness of the doctors' office? What is it that has caused many patients— even the more docile, soft-spoken ones—to suddenly start questioning every procedure, every prescription; to come out with shocking statements on pre-marital sex, lesbianism, and childless marriage. . . . What do these women want?"[61]

Physicians realized the far-reaching influence of the women's movement on women as medical consumers. "The philosophy has permeated far beyond the activist movement. Women who don't regard themselves as liberationists are embracing the new health care goals much as they have the right to equal pay."[62] Many physicians came to understand that "today's woman wants considerate respectful treatment from her physician, wants complete information about her bodily condition, and wants a voice in medical decisions that affect her."[63] Indeed, the actions of many menopausal women reflected these very demands.

After 1963, women experiencing menopause had a great deal of information at their disposal. Books and popular magazines publicized the issues surrounding menopause, Robert Wilson, and hormone replacement therapy. As a result, many women apparently felt empowered as "informed" consumers to demand from their doctors hormone prescriptions. If a physician refused, some women took their demands and their money elsewhere, insisting that finding the right doctor was worth any effort.

As Chapter 8 demonstrated, however, even though women were obviously encouraged and perhaps inspired by the publicity surrounding hormone therapy to seek it for themselves, not all women, immediately rushed to their physicians demanding the femininity pill. Perhaps some did, but others proceeded more cautiously, seeking further information to better weigh the benefits of ERT against its risks.

It may seem peculiar to argue that feminism led women to demand a treatment promoted in part for its potential to keep women "feminine forever." Close reading of the evidence, however, suggests that menopausal women rarely sought hormones solely to maintain their femininity. Rather, as the previous chapter showed, women generally turned to hormones at menopause to relieve its more mundane but potentially debilitating symptoms: hot flashes, insomnia, headaches, genital atrophy, and nervousness. Feminism, and particularly the women's health movement, encouraged women to trust their perceptions of their own bodies and to refuse to be dismissed by patronizing physicians who regarded hot flashes and other menopausal symptoms as temporary inconveniences. Further, the women's health movement urged women to view their physicians as hired consultants possessing valuable skills but not mystical powers. As one health activist advised, "view him as you view your accountant or TV repairman, or the seller of any other service."[64] Many women seemed to take this message to heart as they negotiated for the treatment they thought would best meet their needs.

This is not to say that before the women's liberation movement women eagerly turned over complete control of their medical care to their physicians. Indeed, as Judith Walzer Leavitt and Elizabeth Watkins have demonstrated for twilight sleep in childbirth and oral contraceptives, respectively, women have frequently demanded particular treatments.[65] Further, the feminist critique of the medical profession coincided with a larger consumer movement that similarly recommended a healthy distrust of all so-called experts.[66] In the case of ERT, however, at least in the late 1960s and 1970s, feminism provided the theoretical foundation and social momentum that encouraged women to challenge the authority of their physicians to control all medical decisions.

The women's liberation movement also influenced women's experiences at menopause by providing a political framework within which women could understand their relationships with medical practitioners. Feminism invited women to form expectations for their treatment and to express dissatisfaction when those expectations were not met. Unlike women of previous generations, menopausal women during this period expressed a great deal of dissatisfaction with their physicians. Even more significantly, these women at times accused their physicians of misogyny.

A few women claimed that male indifference to women's needs or men's inability to empathize with female patients led to unsatisfactory care at menopause. One of the Women in Midstream survey respondents blamed her perceived mistreatment on male physicians' lack of interest in things female. She believed that "if more doctors were of the female sex, they would have been more interested in solving these problems."[67] Another menopausal woman complained that her "male doctors simply felt I should grit my teeth and bear it."[68] Another survey respondent reported that two weeks before she attempted suicide, "a male chauvinist doctor" belittled her distress by insisting that she was "psychoneurotic and narcissistic."[69] Although their specific complaints varied, women during this period clearly began to believe that their physicians' "maleness" compromised their ability to treat female patients with sensitivity and respect.

Lynn Laredo, writing in the feminist publication *Prime Time*, articulated the grievances of many menopausal women. She admitted experiencing some physical and emotional difficulties at menopause, but she nevertheless sensed a misogynistic agenda behind much of the popular literature on menopause. Consequently, she claimed that menopausal women were set up by the medical profession: women were expected to fall apart at menopause because they are unable to adjust, and they were simultaneously expected to "bear up and keep smilin'." "I begin to smell a (m.c.) pig," she said, one who punished women for "daring to outlive" their fertility.[70] Another woman discovered misogyny where she expected it least.

Annette Henkin Landau's menopause rap group had invited a woman gynecologist to provide a medical point of view. Landau soon realized that "the doctor believed we were entitled to know only those things about our bodies that she thought we should know." The gynecologist refused, for example, to list common symptoms of menopause, claiming that menopausal women were "so suggestible that they might produce symptoms simply by knowing them." The experience with this gynecologist led Landau to conclude that "male chauvinism is a point of view, an entrenched attitude not always related to the sex of the chauvinist."[71] Clearly, then, the women's liberation movement gave women both the conceptual framework and the language to articulate their dissatisfaction with their medical experiences.

Having challenged the absolute authority of physicians, many women in this era rejected another medical position: that menopausal women should keep their difficulties to themselves. Whereas earlier in the twentieth century menopausal women believed (or said they believed) that menopausal distress was best borne in silence, women in the 1960s and 1970s eagerly sought out other women with whom to share their experiences. The variety of topics these women hoped to discuss testifies to the range of social and physical changes they encountered at menopause.

Not surprisingly, some women wanted to know how other women coped with menopause's physical and emotional symptoms. One woman, for example, wrote to Women in Midstream hoping to learn how other women "weathered menopause and were able to work and be with people without becoming very nervous." She hoped to discover how other women kept their "self confidence" and avoided "panic." Cathy Smith, suffering from "the worst part of my life so far," sought other women for "any information" that would ease her suffering.[72]

But many women who sought information and emotional support from other women understood that their experiences with menopause were not exclusively biological: they also sought guidance for their changing social role. Several women wanted to discuss the feelings of uselessness that had emerged after their children left home. One woman, for example, wanted help "adjusting to life when home and children [were] no longer [her] main interest."[73] Another wanted to "talk to other ladies about the empty nest syndrome."[74] Yet another woman wanted to learn how "to remain sane through the process of aging and changing your values as life itself forces you to adjust to a new you and a lack of purpose when your children no longer need you."[75]

Women also sought advice for coping with the dissolution of marriage at mid-life, either through divorce or death. One despondent woman wrote to Women in Midstream seeking guidance. Her husband had recently "decided to live elsewhere." She had never lived alone in her life and "would like to know about going back to work . . . how to master my emotions, how to begin establishing a social life."[76] Another woman had recently lost her husband and wanted information on "finances, home care, car care, job training, making new friends, etc."[77]

One woman experienced mounting anxiety at menopause and regarded "contact with other women" as the best way to understand her feelings and their origins. She called self-help centers in her area looking for a menopause "rap" group. When she found none, she started her own. Although the group initially focused exclusively on menopause, the discussions quickly moved on to the "middle-age syndrome and problems of the older woman in our society."[78]

The influence of feminism can be seen here on at least two fronts. The rap or consciousness raising groups that some women sought at menopause were an integral tactic of the women's liberation movement. Consciousness raising taught women to recognize their oppression and thus constituted the first step to overcoming it. Further, the women's health movement held that women themselves were a legitimate and valuable source of information about their bodies. Classic texts such as *Our Bodies, Ourselves* shared women's experiences in print and urged women to do the same in person.

Finally, the influence of the women's movement can be seen in women's understanding of the roots of their menopausal problems. While some women sought a hormonal fix for their deficiency disease, others blamed their difficulties on broader social ills. In particular, some women blamed their constricted roles in American society. One woman explained the context for her menopausal depression: "I worked until I was 37 in outside employment—mostly offices—then stayed home with two small children. This seemed like a forced confinement to me—like being a shut in. However, this was considered being a good mother and my kids have 'turned out well.' Yet I feel I've missed the whole boat. . . . If our whole life is bent toward procreation without satisfaction—then we should change our thinking toward enjoying what we can while we can."[79] Another woman wrapped up the situation more succinctly, claiming that menopausal problems were "caused by the role of women in our culture— over-emphasis on youth—fear of aging—lack of meaningful occupation."[80]

Taking this understanding one step further, another woman claimed that the women's movement cured her menopausal symptoms. She had read about menopause before she reached it and had come to fear the "desperation and foolishness" she had heard was inevitable. She believed what she read and found herself at menopause severely depressed. She called upon a psychiatrist who told her that she should be happy because "you still have a husband, a lovely home, three beautiful children and soon you can look forward to being a grandmother." Unfortunately, none of husband, home, or children relieved her depression, and she didn't look forward to becoming a grandmother.

On the eve of her fiftieth birthday, her daughter told her about the women's movement. "I got so excited that I called my friend Sylvia (also menopausal and not looking forward to being a grandmother)," and they visited a Women's Center in New York City. Although they needed a couple of stiff drinks for courage, they made it to the center and "have been in the Women's Movement ever since." Now "I never think about my lack of estrogen, tragedy of declining breasts, loss of youth and beauty. . . . But best of all since that day Sylvia and I made it to the Women's Center, I have never again been depressed."[81]

Epilogue

Menopause at the Turn of the Twenty-First Century

In September 2002, Phyllis Bogen of Cresskill, New Jersey, shared her dismay and confusion with readers of the *New York Times:* "As a result of the flurry of negative data recently in the news media, I have discontinued [estrogen replacement therapy], but I am not sure I have done the right thing. It's more confusing than amusing. How's a women [*sic*] to know?"[1] Although so reminiscent of the confusion women felt in the late 1970s over the possible connection between estrogen replacement therapy and endometrial cancer, Bogen and millions of other women in her position were reacting to the latest blow against menopausal hormone treatments. On July 10, 2002, the *New York Times* reported that a large study of women taking estrogen and progestin had been halted prematurely because researchers concluded that the regimen "was doing more harm than good when taken for several years."[2]

The study in question was a section of the Women's Health Initiative, the largest experimental study to date on the effects of hormone replacement therapy on postmenopausal women. Begun in 1993, the trial followed 16,600 postmenopausal women to assess the benefits and risks of long-term combined (estrogen and progestin) hormone therapy. While researchers agreed that the combined regimen lowered the risk of colorectal cancer and hip fractures, it also increased, albeit slightly, the risk of stroke, breast cancer, and coronary heart disease.[3] Many women and their doctors reported shock and disbelief at the results (after all, ERT had been prescribed as part of a "healthy heart" program), but the conclusions were not unprecedented; indeed, they underscored and vindicated the efforts of many biomedical researchers and feminist health advocates who had long

229

claimed that the benefits of hormone therapy (particularly combined therapy) were unproven and the risks unknown.

In the aftermath of the 1975 cancer studies, how did millions of women find themselves taking replacement hormones? How does the ongoing controversy over hormone treatments inform the history of menopause? The late twentieth century saw a resurrection of menopausal and postmenopausal hormone therapies, despite feminist resistance to their widespread use and the reexamination of the meaning of menopause.

Heart Attacks and Broken Bones

Although the link between estrogen therapy and endometrial cancer temporarily disrupted the widespread use of hormone replacement therapy in the mid 1970s, it began to rebound in the early 1980s. The number of prescriptions for replacement estrogens rose from 13.6 million in 1982 to 31.7 million in 1992.[4] Estimates of the number of women actually taking HRT vary a great deal, but a 1998 survey found that 34 percent of women aged fifty or older used HRT (up from 23 percent in 1993).[5]

Several factors, both medical and social, help explain the recovery. First, the aging baby-boomer cohort swelled the ranks of women facing menopause. Between 1970 and 2000, the number of women between forty-five and fifty-four increased by roughly 56 percent (or more than 6.5 million women). Second, these women continued to want relief from hot flashes, vaginal dryness, and other menopausal discomforts. Hormones effectively relieved at least some of these symptoms. Third, physicians routinely added progestin to the estrogen treatment, creating a regimen that significantly reduced the risk of endometrial cancer. While this combination had been prescribed for years, it became the standard hormonal therapy for women with a uterus only in the 1980s. Fourth, the prevention of osteoporosis and heart disease emerged as the primary indications for sustained hormone use. Although some medical researchers had championed estrogens to prevent these diseases for decades, only in the late 1970s (for osteoporosis) and the 1990s (for heart disease) did they figure prominently in the marketing of hormone replacement therapy.[6]

By the 1990s, the use of replacement hormones as preventive medicine helped create something like a medical consensus around the claim that long-term estrogen therapy was good medicine.[7] With heart disease the number one killer of women and hip fractures a significant cause of death and debility, why not prescribe an allegedly safe regimen to help secure the health of aging women? Many physicians were convinced. A 1997 survey of American gynecologists, family physicians, and general internists showed that nearly all favored long-term hormone therapy for these patients.[8]

The profile of hormone replacement therapy was boosted by savvy marketing. Soul star Patti Labelle touted the benefits of Prempro in national television and print ads, appealing to black women (who used hormone replacement therapy in much lower numbers than did their white counterparts) and other women who wondered where their groove had gone. Lauren Hutton, a former "super model," made the rounds of the talk shows and appeared in *Parade* magazine promoting the wonders of estrogen therapy. While touting the preventive value of estrogen for heart disease and bone loss (she turned to hormone therapy after losing an inch in height), she spoke with especial authority when she noted that "if I had to choose between all my creams and make-up for looking good and feeling good, I'd take estrogen." For all her personal disclosures, she never mentioned that her appearances were paid for by Wyeth-Ayerst, makers of Premarin.[9]

Guinea Pigs and Cash Cows

But HRT had its detractors. Feminists, while not alone, led the challenge against the widespread use of hormone therapy with three interlocking critiques. While generally claiming they weren't "antihormone," feminists criticized the claim that aging women were diseased and required treatment to keep them well; they characterized the widespread use of hormone therapy as a medical experiment with unproven benefits and identifiable risks; and they highlighted the huge profits for drug companies if healthy postmenopausal women used hormones for the rest of their lives.

Many feminists maintained that menopause, even though it might cause unpleasant and disruptive symptoms (or "signs" as some critics insisted), was not a disease nor were postmenopausal women "estrogen deficient."[10] While these critics of medicalization did not rule out hormones to ease severe hot flashes, they insisted that nonmedical alternatives—soy rich food, herbal preparations, and an electric fan—helped many women. Further, they noted that woman-controlled efforts, in particular diet and exercise, could lower women's risk of heart disease and osteoporosis. Finally, they suggested that the medicalization of women's bodies depoliticized women's (and the public's) health. In 1989, for example, the National Women's Health Network claimed that proposing a pill as the fix for osteoporosis deflected attention from the political and cultural forces that leave women (and men) vulnerable to falls. Individual solutions for osteoporosis, they argued, precluded efforts toward social changes that would potentially benefit everyone.[11]

In her characteristically bold manner, long-time women's health activist Barbara Seaman recently dubbed the widespread use of HRT "the greatest experiment ever performed on women."[12] Other feminists agreed, highlighting the possible risks of hormone therapy (increased risk of breast cancer, blood clots, endometrial cancer, iatrogenic diseases) and insisting that the benefits had yet to be demonstrated (including reduced rates of heart disease). While they didn't generally deny that estrogen therapy could slow the rate of bone loss, feminists did challenge the construction of osteoporosis as a result of menopause. Further, they disputed the conflation of thin bones (as diagnosed with a bone scan) with fractures.[13] In short, feminists insisted that too much remained unknown about the long-term effects and benefits of hormone therapy to support the "knee jerk tendency of most doctors to hand you a prescription for hormones as soon as you seem to be menopausal."[14]

Feminist and other critics insisted that the "great experiment" could not be understood without examining the financial stakes involved. Skeptics of hormone therapy emphasized that the long-term treatment of potentially all women over fifty was clearly "a glittering prize" for the pharmaceutical manufacturers.[15] The tactics used to lure women into hormone therapy, thus increasing drug company profits, were also attacked. Feminists particularly denounced the scare tactics that constructed and exacerbated women's fear of disease, of aging, and of dependency. They also attacked drug companies for co-opting a tenet of the women's health movement—preventive care—to further their own bottom lines. Critics alleged that physicians, drug companies, and a culture worried about the potential social burden of the aging baby-boomer generation were conspiring to construct health as "the new virtue for women as they age." As a result, women were held responsible for what happened to their bodies.[16]

However, feminists were not the only ones skeptical about the long-term benefits of HRT. Many menopausal and postmenopausal women also remained largely unconvinced that the alleged benefits of HRT were worth the costs (or the bother). Admittedly, in the 1990s, more American women received prescriptions for replacement hormones at menopause than ever before. Further, women increasingly used this therapy to prevent illness, in addition to relieving menopausal symptoms. Nevertheless, in 1999, at least 66 percent of American women over fifty, despite the hard sell by the drug companies and the efforts of well-intentioned physicians, failed to embrace medical intervention.[17] Further, most women who began hormone therapy discontinued the treatment after the first or second year, causing a flurry of concern about the "problem" of the "noncompliant" patient.[18] Certainly, some women may have wanted hormones, but limited access to medical care thwarted their desires. Other women, perhaps influenced by the feminist critique of medicalization or encouraged by a willingness to seek alternative healing paths, intentionally looked elsewhere for ways to cope. Some found relief by using soy products and black cohosh. Others renamed hot flashes "power surges" and embraced them as a source of feminine inspiration. Still others gritted their teeth or bought a fan. And finally, some women barely noticed their menopausal symptoms. At the apex of hormone replacement use, many menopausal women continued to seek out and employ alternatives to medical treatments.

Declining Fortunes Once Again

At the same time that the medical consensus was indicating that hormone therapy was good medicine, the results of several clinical trials, often regarded as the "gold standard" of medical research, began to expose its weaknesses, indeed, its dangers. The results of the 1998 HERS study (Heart and Estrogen/Progestin Replacement Study), for example, legitimized skeptics' fears. Not only did the estrogen-progestin combination not reduce the number of coronary events (a heart-related death or a nonfatal heart attack), it led to a higher incidence of thromboembolism (blood clots) and gall bladder disease.[19] Then the July 2002 report from the Women's Health Initiative study confirmed what other researchers had already suggested.

After the July 2002 WHI report, the news only got worse for HRT and the women who depended on it. The estrogen-only regimen was implicated in an increased incidence of ovarian cancer, and the research on combined therapy suggested that it might increase the risk of Alzheimer's disease and other forms of dementia. As the risks mounted, the benefits faded. In March 2003, researchers from the WHI reported that hormones did not improve postmenopausal women's quality of life. The therapy had "no significant effects on general health, vitality, mental health, depressive symptoms, or sexual satisfaction." In March 2004, researchers stopped the estrogen-only arm of the study, citing an increased risk of stroke and no reduction of coronary heart disease.[20]

But not everyone saw in this research a reason to change course. Some physicians warned against an impulsive backlash against hormone therapy. The chairman of obstetrics and gynecology at the University of Southern California Medical School insisted, "I don't think we should throw out the baby with the bath water just because of this one study." Even small-town local newspapers introduced the WHI conclusions with headlines such as "Much Ado About Nothing."[21] Women, too, were conflicted about the findings. Some women taking preventive hormones—perhaps as many as half—stopped taking them within six months of the initial WHI report.[22] Others insisted that hormones made menopausal and post-menopausal life bearable. Perhaps most women who were taking hormones as the damning evidence mounted were somewhere in the middle: dismayed, confused, and angry.[23]

By May 2005, a consensus among clinicians and researchers in the United States against the use of preventive hormones had reemerged. But although most physicians abandoned the *routine* use of preventive hormones, some awaited the results of further research before stopping their patients' long-term hormone use altogether. Short-term therapy for menopausal symptoms continued to be considered safe.[24]

Reclaiming Our Menopause

How does this story of the second rise and fall of hormones inform our understanding of menopause? It certainly complicates understanding of the medicalization of menopause at the close of the twentieth century. The treatment that once helped gauge the level of medical involvement in menopause had become a generalized therapy for the consequences of female aging. The medicalization of menopause may not have intensified at the end of the twentieth century; menopause may have merely provided the gateway for the medicalization of female middle age. As others have noted, the wider use of hormones increased the medical surveillance of middle-aged women and their chances of developing iatrogenic diseases.[25]

Although the medical world after 1980 largely abandoned the study of menopause in favor of investigations into the value of hormones for post-menopausal life,[26] the cultural conversation about menopause continued.

As we have already seen, the hormone debates shaped some of this discourse. Some physicians highlighted menopause as the beginning of estrogen deprivation and regarded it as a trigger for beginning hormone therapy. Some feminists, in contrast, argued that menopause was normal and that the body provided all the estrogen it needed at various stages in life.

Two best-selling books of the 1990s, however, took the conversation about menopause beyond the debate over whether it was natural or pathological. Although both books engaged the estrogen debate, their primary purposes were to give meaning to the menopausal transition itself. Quite different in many respects, these books reached similar conclusions about the significance of menopause in the 1990s.

In her 1991 book, *The Change: Women, Aging and the Menopause*, Germaine Greer regarded menopause as a time when women would be less driven by their sexual needs and less concerned about their ability to attract a man, eerily echoing the 1900 claim that menopause represented a time when women were beyond the reach of sexual storms. Rather than resisting the "change" through hormone treatments and other efforts to retain youth and beauty, Greer urged women to see menopause as the beginning of a new phase of life. She encouraged women to accept their sexual decline, to embrace themselves as witches and crones, and to seize the "accumulated spiritual power" earned by aging women.[27] A startling assessment indeed for a woman who made her national reputation in 1971 by promoting the sexual liberation of women.[28]

Although it never occurred to Gail Sheehy to embrace her inner crone (though she does embrace hormone therapy), she made a remarkably similar argument about the meaning of menopause in her 1992 book, *The Silent Passage: Menopause*. Sheehy, known for her examination of other life passages, chatted with celebrities and various less well-heeled women and concluded that, after menopause, a woman can't "be the person she was before." Sheehy urged women to let go of "the aspects of femininity that define" women and to begin a path of "meditation and spiritual exploration." Able to unite their "masculine and feminine sides," postmenopausal women, Sheehy claimed, could thrive in their "Second Adulthood," freer to speak their minds and contemplate the eternal.[29]

Both Greer and Sheehy emphasized menopause's potential as a gateway to personal transformation and an opportunity for spiritual growth.[30] Like many authors of the past, they also saw menopause as a chance to escape from some of the constraints of womanhood, of femininity, and of sexuality. But for both of them, the means of escape was biological; the woman's changed body altered who she was, what she cared about, and how she was viewed. Note the difference from the discussion of liberation in the 1940s and 1950s, when menopause allowed women to take up new challenges without changing their identities. Unlike the menopause described by Sheehy and Greer, menopause in the 1940s and 1950s changed a woman's social obligations but not the woman herself.

Looking for Meaning in Menopause

This history of menopause in the United States has shown that menopausal women's bodies have been used to discuss and debate larger social concerns: the nature of womanhood, the role of women, the practice of medicine. Physicians, popular health writers, and menopausal women themselves have all constructed meanings for menopause against a changing social and medical backdrop. As the expectations of women changed and the connection of womanhood to the female body shifted, menopausal bodies have been used by various parties to further a wide range of social, medical, and economic agendas. Opponents of female political rights have used menopause to demonstrate women's unsuitability for public life. Popular health writers have used menopause as a symbol of the necessary compromise between a life devoted to others and a life of one's own making. Physicians have used menopause to discuss the nature of medical practice and the parameters of preventive medicine. Feminists have used menopause to demonstrate the need for "woman suffrage" and "women's liberation." Drug companies have used menopause to improve their bottom line. Menopausal women's choices have also been inspired by larger agendas. By demanding medical attention for menopausal symptoms, some women have refused to be derailed by the whims of their bodies. By refusing medical care or by denying the need for it, some women have challenged others' construction of their bodies as pathological. By embracing the physical and psychological changes of their "second adulthood," some women have surrendered to the "power" and "wisdom" of the aging female body.

The history of menopause reveals two points about the relationship of menopause and its historical and cultural context. First, menopause only gains meaning when read against the changing cultural understandings of womanhood. The social landscape did not forge medical and personal reactions to menopause in any purely deterministic way. The messages about womanhood have always been too diverse, and the personal life courses of women and the professional stances of physicians too varied, for any deterministic model to apply. The social context, however, supplied the blocks with which women and physicians constructed and interpreted the menopausal transition. Second, the bodies of menopausal women have been used to create new roles for women and new understandings of womanhood. Their changing menopausal bodies have been used by women and others to demand social change.

Menopausal women in this history, particularly middle- and upper-class white women, have struggled to cope with the often unsettling, sometimes disruptive, and occasionally devastating changes in their bodies. Some women resolved to give it no thought at all, while others battled mightily to control with their intellect the upheaval of their bodies. Others filled their lives with activity, allowing themselves no time to "indulge" any menopausal discomforts they might experience. Some returned to the unfulfilled ambitions of their youth—a college education, paid employment, artistic aspirations—while others took up social causes, taking their domestic talents into the broader community.

For some women, however, an active life and willpower did not quell the disruption of night sweats or alleviate the discomfort of a dry vagina. When something more was needed, women had a variety of options. Some women relied on patent medicines like Lydia Pinkham's Vegetable Compound; more recently, women have turned to "natural" therapies such as soy-rich foods and herbal remedies. Others headed to the doctor, eagerly accepting his (or perhaps her) prescription for a long vacation, a sedative, or hormone therapy. And still others have demanded estrogen treatment from their sometimes reluctant physicians.

Significantly, some women throughout this period have maintained that individual coping strategies, whether volunteer work or hormone replacement therapies, did not sufficiently address the problems they faced. These women called for a more political treatment of menopause. In 1918, Stanford physician Clelia Duel Mosher suggested that "votes for women" might solve the problems menopause posed for middle-aged women and the threat middle-aged women posed to society. In 1979, another physician, Susan W. Cooke, maintained that only women's liberation would relieve the suffering of menopausal women by treating the larger social ill of women's oppression. Although separated by sixty years, these commentators shared a common perspective. They believed that women's experiences at menopause were not influenced merely by their "raging" hormones, but also by their place in society.

What can this history of female agency, social construction, and medicalization teach us as we ponder the future of menopause, women's bodies, and women in twenty-first century America? Perhaps most vividly, it illuminates women's efforts to gain control of their bodies. Whatever means they used to control their flushing, sweating, shrinking, bleeding bodies, many women gained personal relief. But because "raging" menopausal hormones have been used to disqualify women from certain aspects of public life (a menopausal president, it has been said, could not have handled the Bay of Pigs), we should also see the desire of some women to control their menopausal bodies as a larger struggle for women's rights. By keeping a stiff upper lip, by embracing a charitable cause, by demanding hormone therapy, some women have refused to allow their menopausal difficulties to be used to undermine the political, professional, and social aspirations of all women.

But what happens when some measure of bodily control becomes possible? History has suggested how the *ability* to control one's body frequently shades into the *obligation* to control one's body. While making it easier for women to say yes to sex, has the birth control pill also made it harder to say no? Has the right of some women to control their fertility created the obligation in others? The history of menopause and its relationship with estrogen therapies has demonstrated how slippery the slope can be. Where is the line between allowing women to remain sexually active after menopause and obligating women to remain sexually alluring and accessible? Where is the line between allowing women to feel less anxious and expecting women to be agreeable and placating? Where is the line between helping women to avoid osteoporosis and expecting women to medicalize their aging bodies in the name of preventive health?

Further, individual, medicalized responses to illness prevention and female aging can ultimately depoliticize women's bodies. Popping a pill to prevent hip fractures and heart disease deflects public attention from the larger need for safer homes and nutritious diets. Relying on hormones to escape the effects of aging reinforces the cultural expectation that women should always look good by looking young. Without movements that denounce the denigration of aging women and demand universal health care, individual women will be left to fend for themselves. Rather than helping women look and feel young, we need a movement that values aging women as they are or choose to be and that secures the health of everyone to the extent possible.

Finally, this history highlights the limits of the "empowered patient."

As the risks and benefits of hormone replacement therapy continue to be debated, physicians have increasingly insisted that the HRT decision belongs to the female patient. At a moment when many clinicians are themselves "bewildered" about what the evidence really means for women,[31] it does not empower women to guess what might be best for them. (Although perhaps it protects physicians in the event of a malpractice suit.) In the face of inadequate research, "women's choice" places the burden of the hormone decision on individual women, who have little or no ability to command the direction of biomedical research. Only collective insistence on safe medical treatments will lead to a truly empowered patient.

Menopause is both a cultural construct and a physiological transition. Although rewarding work and hormone replacement therapy have helped countless women to cope with their changing bodies, the larger issues faced by middle-aged women cannot be addressed by using prescription drugs. As so many women in this story have insisted, the significance of menopause extends well beyond the boundaries of middle-aged women's bodies. The construction of menopause has political, medical, and social consequences for women of all ages and for society at large. Consequently, the battle to control the effects of menopause must target both women's bodies and the body politic.

Notes

Introduction

1. Marilyn Bender, "Doctors Deny Woman's Hormones Affect Her as an Executive," *New York Times,* July 31, 1970, 33.
2. Ibid.
3. David Brinkley, NBC News, July 31, 1970; Sam Donaldson, ABC News, July 31, 1970; Bender, "Doctor's Deny," 33.
4. There are also hundreds of self-help books, some written by "activists" of one kind or another, offering women advice and truisms. See, for example, Susan M. Love with Karen Linsey, *Dr. Love's Hormone Book: Making Informed Choices about Menopause* (New York: Random House, 1997); National Women's Health Network, *The Truth about Hormone Replacement Therapy* (Roseville, CA: Prima Publishing, 2002); Marcia Jones and Theresa Eichenwald, *Menopause for Dummies* (New York: For Dummies, 2002); Carolyn Scott Brown, *The Black Woman's Guide to Menopause: Doing Menopause with Heart and Soul* (Naperville, IL: Source Books, 2003); and Linda Ojeda and Jeffrey Bland, *Menopause without Medicine* (Alameda, CA: Hunter House, 2003). There are also various collections of first-person accounts. See, for example, Joanna Goldsworty, ed., *A Certain Age: Reflecting on Menopause* (New York: Columbia University Press, 1994); and Dena Taylor and Amber Coverdale Sumrall, *Women of the 14th Moon: Writings on Menopause* (Freedom, CA: Crossing Press, 1991).
5. Margaret Lock, *Encounters with Aging: Mythologies of Menopause in Japan and North America* (Berkeley: University of California Press, 1993), xliii. See also Emily Martin, *The Woman in the Body: A Cultural Analysis of Reproduction* (Boston: Beacon Press, 1987); and Yewoubdar Beyene, *From Menarche to Menopause: Reproductive Lives of Peasant Women in Two Cultures* (Albany: State University of New York Press, 1989).
6. This literature is vast. For a small sampling see Susan E. Bell, "Changing Ideas: The Medicalization of Menopause," *Social Science and Medicine* 24 (1987): 535–542; Susan E. Bell, "Gendered Medical Science: Producing a Drug for Women," *Feminist Studies* 21 (1995): 469–500; Patricia A. Kaufert and Sonja M. McKinlay, "Estrogen Replacement Therapy: The Production

of Medical Knowledge and the Emergence of Policy," in *Women, Health, and Healing: Toward a New Perspective*, ed. Ellen Lewin and Virginia Olesen (New York: Tavistock, 1985), 113–138; Kathleen I. MacPherson, "Menopause as Disease: The Social Construction of a Metaphor," *Advances in Nursing History* 3 (1981): 96; Sharon Scales Rostosky and Cheryl Brown Travis, "Menopause Research and the Dominance of the Biomedical Model, 1984–1994," *Psychology of Women Quarterly* 20 (1996): 301; Renate Klein and Lynette J. Dumble, "Disempowering Midlife Women: The Science and Politics of Hormone Replacement Therapy (HRT)," *Women's Studies International Forum* 17 (1994): 327–343.

7. Although some of this work has been historically informed, few historians have yet entered this discussion. Notable exceptions include Carroll Smith-Rosenberg, "Puberty to Menopause: The Cycle of Femininity in Nineteenth-Century America," in *Disorderly Conduct: Visions of Gender in Victorian America* (New York: Oxford University Press, 1985), 182–196; Alison Li, "Marketing Menopause: Science and the Public Relations of Premarin," in *Women, Health and Nation: Canada and the United States since 1945,* ed. Georgina Feldberg, Molly-Ladd Taylor, Alison Li, and Kathryn McPherson (Montreal: McGill-Queen's College University Press, 2003), 101–120; Elizabeth Siegel Watkins, "Dispensing with Aging: Changing Rationales for Long-Term Hormone Replacement Therapy, 1960–2000," *Pharmacy in History* 43 (2001): 23–37; and Joy Webster Barbre, "Meno-Boomers and Moral Guardians: An Exploration of the Cultural Construction of Menopause," in *Menopause: A Midlife Passage*, ed. Joan C. Callahan (Bloomington: Indiana University Press, 1993), 23–35. See also Barbre's 1994 dissertation, "From 'Goodwives' to Menoboomers: Reinventing Menopause in American History" (Ph.D. diss., Univ. of Minnesota, 1994).

8. Carol Groneman, *Nymphomania: A History* (New York: W. W. Norton and Company, 2000); Londa Schiebinger, *The Mind Has No Sex? Women in the Origins of Modern Science* (Cambridge: Harvard University Press, 1989); Thomas Laqueur, *Making Sex: Body and Gender from the Greeks to Freud* (Cambridge: Harvard University Press, 1990); Ornella Moscucci, *The Science of Woman: Gynaecology and Gender in England, 1800–1929* (Cambridge, UK: Cambridge University Press, 1990); Carroll Smith-Rosenberg and Charles Rosenberg, "The Female Animal: Medical and Biological Views of Woman and Her Role in Nineteenth-Century America," *Journal of American History* 60 (1973): 332–356.

9. Andrew Fay Currier, *The Menopause: A Consideration of the Phenomena Which Occur to Women at the Close of the Child-Bearing Period* (New York: Appleton, 1897), 35.

10. In many cases, the socioeconomic status of the women remains unknown to me. When I have clues about class, however, the evidence suggests that these women were overwhelmingly middle class. Race is an even bigger mystery. While I do not assume that all these women were white, I know of only one

individual who was definitely not. But again, circumstantial evidence indicates that most of these women were probably white.

11. Charles E. Rosenberg, "Framing Disease: Illness, Society, and History," in *Framing Disease: Studies in Cultural History,* ed. Charles E. Rosenberg and Janet Golden (New Brunswick, NJ: Rutgers University Press, 1992): xvii–xxvi.

12. Currier, *The Menopause.*

13. Robert A. Wilson and Thelma A. Wilson, "The Fate of the Nontreated Postmenopausal Woman: A Plea for the Maintenance of Adequate Estrogen from Puberty to the Grave," *Journal of the American Geriatrics Society* 11 (1963): 347–362; and Robert A. Wilson, *Feminine Forever* (New York: M. Evans and Company, 1966). For the rise and fall of estrogen prescriptions, see Peter Greenwald, et al., "Endometrial Cancer after Menopausal Use of Estrogens," *Obstetrics and Gynecology* 50 (1977): 239; and Nancy Worcester and Mariamne Whatley, "The Selling of HRT: Playing on the Fear Factor," *Feminist Review* (Summer 1992), 4.

14. See, for example, Wendy Mitchinson, *The Nature of Their Bodies: Women and Their Doctors in Victorian Canada* (Toronto: University of Toronto Press, 1991); Elizabeth Lunbeck, *The Psychiatric Persuasion: Knowledge, Gender, and Power in Modern America* (Princeton, NJ: Princeton University Press, 1994); Mary E. Odem, *Delinquent Daughters: Protecting and Policing Adolescent Female Sexuality in the United States, 1885–1920* (Chapel Hill: University of North Carolina Press, 1995); Ann-Louise Shapiro, *Breaking the Codes: Female Criminality in Fin-de-siecle Paris* (Stanford: Stanford University Press, 1996); and Rickie Solinger, *Wake Up Little Susie: Single Pregnancy and Race Before Roe v. Wade* (New York: Routledge, 1992).

15. Shapiro, *Breaking the Codes,* 129.

16. For the classic articulation of this view, see Ann Douglas Wood, "'The Fashionable Diseases': Women's Complaints and Their Treatment in Nineteenth-Century America," *Journal of Interdisciplinary History* 4 (1973): 25–52. Regina Markell Morantz adroitly challenged Wood in "The Perils of Feminist History," *Journal of Interdisciplinary History* 4 (1973): 649–660.

17. Roy Porter, "The Patient's View: Doing Medical History from Below," *Theory and Society* 14 (1985): 192.

18. Barbara Duden, *The Woman beneath the Skin: A Doctor's Patients in Eighteenth-Century Germany,* trans. Thomas Dunlap (Cambridge: Harvard University Press, 1991). See also Lunbeck, *Psychiatric Persuasion.*

19. Sheila M. Rothman, *Living in the Shadow of Death: Tuberculosis and the Social Experience of Illness in American History* (Baltimore: Johns Hopkins University Press, 1994). For other patient-centered histories, see Judith Walzer Leavitt, *Brought to Bed: Childbearing in America, 1750–1950* (New York: Oxford University Press, 1986); Roy Porter, ed., *Patients and Practitioners* (Cambridge, UK: Cambridge University Press, 1985); Mary E. Fissell, *Patients, Power, and the Poor in Eighteenth-Century Bristol* (Cambridge, UK:

Cambridge University Press, 1991). Other historians who incorporate patients' (or subjects') perspectives include Regina Morantz-Sanchez, *Conduct Unbecoming a Woman: Medicine on Trial in Turn-of-the-Century Brooklyn* (New York: Oxford University Press, 1999); Joanne Meyerowitz, *How Sex Changed: A History of Transsexuality in the United States* (Cambridge: Harvard University Press, 2002); Baron H. Lerner, *The Breast Cancer Wars: Hope, Fear, and the Pursuit of a Cure in Twentieth-Century America* (New York: Oxford University Press, 2001).

20. Paul Starr, *The Social Transformation of American Medicine: The Rise of a Sovereign Profession and the Making of a Vast Industry* (New York: Basic Books, 1982), 14.

21. Leslie Reagan has demonstrated that medicine was a "negotiated terrain between physicians and patients." Leslie J. Reagan, *When Abortion Was a Crime: Women, Medicine, and Law in the United States, 1867–1973* (Berkeley: University of California Press, 1997), 7.

22. See, for example, Susan Bordo, *Unbearable Weight: Feminism, Western Culture, and the Body* (Berkeley: University of California Press, 1993); Linda Gordon, *Heroes of Their Own Lives: The Politics and History of Family Violence, Boston, 1880–1960* (New York: Viking, 1988); Elizabeth Haiken, *Venus Envy: A History of Cosmetic Surgery* (Baltimore: Johns Hopkins University Press, 1997).

23. Kaufert and McKinlay, "Estrogen Replacement Theory," 130–132.

24. See, for example, Kathy Peiss, *Cheap Amusements: Working Women and Leisure in Turn-of-the-Century New York* (Philadelphia: Temple University Press, 1986); and Nan Enstad, *Ladies of Labor, Girls of Adventure: Working Women, Popular Culture, and Labor Politics at the Turn of the Twentieth Century* (New York: Columbia University Press, 1999).

25. Judith Leavitt, *Typhoid Mary: Captive to the Public's Health* (Boston: Beacon Press, 1996); and Emily Martin, *The Woman in the Body: A Cultural Analysis of Reproduction* (Boston: Beacon Press, 1987).

26. Nancy Tomes, "Merchants of Health: Medicine and Consumer Culture in the United States, 1900–1940," *Journal of American History* 88 (2001): 523.

27. Irving Kenneth Zola, *Socio-Medical Inquiries: Recollections, Reflections, and Reconsiderations* (Philadelphia: Temple University Press, 1983), 295. See also Ivan Illich, *Medical Nemesis: The Expropriation of Health* (New York: Random House, 1976), 39–124.

28. See, for example, George Chauncey, "From Sexual Inversion to Homosexuality: Medicine and the Changing Conceptualization of Female Deviance," *Salmagundi* 58–59 (1982): 114–146; Peter Conrad, *Identifying Hyperactive Children: The Medicalization of Deviant Behavior* (Lexington, MA: Lexington Books, 1976); Peter Conrad and Joseph W. Schneider, *Deviance and Medicalization: From Badness to Sickness* (St. Louis: Mosby, 1980).

29. Frances B. McCrea, "Politics of Menopause: The 'Discovery' of a Deficiency Disease," *Social Problems* 31 (1983): 113.

30. Rostosky and Travis, "Menopause Research," 301. See also Klein and Dumble, "Disempowering Midlife Women."

31. Leavitt, *Brought to Bed,* 128–141, in particular.

32. Ibid., 137. See also Catherine Kohler Riessman, "Women and Medicalization: A New Perspective," *Social Policy* 14 (1983): 3–18.

33. Margaret Marsh and Wanda Ronner, *The Empty Cradle: Infertility in America from Colonial Times to the Present* (Baltimore: Johns Hopkins University Press, 1999); Elizabeth Siegel Watkins, *On the Pill: A Social History of Oral Contraceptives, 1950–1970* (Baltimore: Johns Hopkins University Press, 1998); Morantz-Sanchez, *Conduct Unbecoming,* 138–155.

34. Margaret Morganroth Gullette, *Aged by Culture* (Chicago: University of Chicago Press, 2004); Lois Banner, *In Full Flower: Aging Women, Power, and Sexuality* (New York: Knopf, 1992); Christine T. Field, "'Are Women . . . All Minors?' Women's Rights and the Politics of Aging in the Antebellum United States," *Journal of Women's History* 12 (2001): 113–137; Pat Thane, "Social Histories of Old Age and Aging," *Journal of Social History* 37 (2003): 93–111.

1. "Menopause Is Not a Dangerous Time"

1. Andrew Fay Currier, *The Menopause: A Consideration of the Phenomena Which Occur to Women at the Close of the Child-Bearing Period* (New York: D. Appleton, 1897), v, vii–viii.

2. See, for example, Anna M. Galbraith, "Are the Dangers of Menopause Natural or Acquired? A Physiological Study," *American Gynaecological and Obstetrical Journal* 15 (1899): 291–314; G. H. Mallett, "Notes on Some of the Symptoms of the Menopause," *American Gynaecological and Obstetrical Journal* 11 (1897): 193–197; Philander A. Harris, "On the Dangers of Certain Faulty Impressions Regarding the Menopause," *Transactions of the Medical Society of New Jersey* (1898): 317–325.

3. Paul Starr, *The Social Transformation of American Medicine* (New York: Basic Books, 1982); Ellen Garvey, "Reframing the Bicycle: Advertising Supported Magazines and Scorching Women," *American Quarterly* 47 (1995): 66–101; Leslie Reagan, *When Abortion Was a Crime: Women, Medicine, and Law in the United States, 1867–1973* (Berkeley: University of California Press, 1997); and Carroll Smith-Rosenberg and Charles Rosenberg, "The Female Animal: Medical and Biological Views of Woman and Her Role in Nineteenth-Century America," *Journal of American History* 60 (1973): 332–356.

4. Ornella Moscucci, *The Science of Woman: Gynaecology and Gender in England, 1800–1929* (Cambridge, UK: Cambridge University Press, 1990); and Regina Morantz-Sanchez, *Conduct Unbecoming a Woman: Medicine on Trial in Turn-of-the-Century Brooklyn* (New York: Oxford University Press, 1999), 88–115.

5. Nelly Oudshoorn, *Beyond the Natural Body: An Archeology of Sex Hormones* (London: Routledge, 1994); and Merriley Borell, "Organotherapy and the Emergence of Reproductive Endocrinology," *Journal of the History of Biology* 18 (1985): 1–30.

6. The definitive indices to all medical literature, *Index Medicus* and *The Quarterly Cumulative Index* served as my entry points into the literature. I supplemented this core material with a review of approximately thirty gynecology textbooks to determine what physicians were taught to think about menopause and when (and if) the new medical theories proposed in the medical journals became medical orthodoxy.

7. Even then, it merely referred the reader to "menstruation, cessation." It was not until 1927, when *Index Medicus* merged with *The Quarterly Cumulative Index,* that menopause became a subject apart from menstruation. *The Quarterly Cumulative Index,* established in 1916, had always listed menopause separately.

8. The *Index Catalogue of the Library of the Surgeon General's Office,* vol. 7, 3rd series (1928), listed fewer than twenty articles about menopause published in American medical journals and more than fifty articles about "painful menstruation."

9. See George Erety Shoemaker, "Fallacies Concerning the Menopause," *Philadelphia Medical Journal* 7 (1901): 72; George Richter, "On the Physiology and Pathology of the Menopause," *Medical Record* 91 (1917): 446; Marion Craig Potter, "A New Standard of Health for the Menopause," *Medical Woman's Journal* 34 (1927): 158; Edgar A. Dulin, "The Menopause," *Medical Herald* 27 (1908): 154; and Alexander H. P. Leuf, *Gynecology, Obstetrics, Menopause* (Philadelphia: Philadelphia Medical Council, 1902), v.

10. Sara E. Greenfield, "The Dangers of the Menopause," *Woman's Medical Journal* 12 (1902): 183.

11. Emma F. Drake, *What a Woman of Forty-Five Ought to Know* (Philadelphia: Vir Publishing Co., 1902), v.

12. Grace Loucks Elliott, *Women after Forty: The Meaning of the Last Half of Life* (New York: Henry Holt, 1936), viii. See also Herman F. Strongin, "Woman—Her Critical Decade, *American Medicine* (November 1933): 532.

13. James Lewis Ellis, "The Menopause," *Mobile Medical and Surgical Journal* 4 (1902): 389. See also Leuf, *Gynecology,* 272.

14. E. Von Graff, "Climacteric Changes," *Journal of the Iowa State Medical Society* 22 (1932): 185.

15. The full title of the revised edition was *The Change of Life in Health and Disease: A Practical Treatise on the Nervous and Other Affections Incidental to Women at the Decline of Life.*

16. Information about the various versions of Tilt's work comes from Joel Wilbush, "Tilt, E. J., and the Change of Life (1857)—The Only Work on the Subject in the English Language," *Maturitas* 2 (1980): 259–267.

17. Edward J. Tilt, *Elements of Health and Principles of Female Hygiene* (Philadel-

phia, 1853), 326. For more on the nineteenth-century assessment of meno-pause, see Carroll Smith-Rosenberg, "Puberty to Menopause: The Cycle of Femininity in Nineteenth-Century America," in *Disorderly Conduct: Visions of Gender in Victorian America* (New York: Oxford University Press, 1985), 182–196.

18. For examples of the critical period, see Mary Wood-Allen, *Marriage: Its Duties and Privileges* (New York: Revell, 1901), 217; Henry S. Lott, "The Principles of Gynecology," *American Journal of Obstetrics and Diseases of Women and Children* 73 (1916): 112–121; John N. Upshur, "The Meno-pause," *New York Medical Journal* 82 (1905): 650; and George Engelmann, "The President's Address," *Transactions of the American Gynecological Society* 25 (1900): 10–11. For examples of a "kinder gentler menopause," see Palmer Findley, *A Treatise on the Diseases of Women for Students and Practitioners* (Philadelphia: Lea and Febiger, 1913), 73; Edith Belle Lowry, *The Woman of Forty* (Chicago: Forbes and Co., 1919), 71–74; and Strongin, "Woman," 533.

19. Quote in George Wythe Cook, "Some Observations on the Menopause," *American Journal of Obstetrics* 45 (1903): 384. See, for example, Drake, *Woman of Forty-Five*, 83; M. C. M'Gannon, "The Menopause," *Transactions of the Medical Society of Tennessee* 69 (1902): 199; C. S. Carr, "The Meno-pause or Change of Life," *Physical Culture* 32 (1914): 525; and John Cooke Hirst, *A Manual of Gynecology*, vol. 2 (Philadelphia: W. B. Saunders, 1925), 367.

20. Medical Women's Federation, "An Investigation of the Menopause in One Thousand Women," *Lancet* 111 (1933): 107.

21. Kate Campbell Hurd-Mead, "The Middle-Aged Woman: What Can Be Done to Increase Her Efficiency," *WMCP Alumnae Transactions* (1913): 106; Bernarr Aldolphus MacFadden, *Womanhood and Marriage* (New York: Physical Culture Corp., 1918), 355. See also William John Fielding, *What the Woman Past Forty Should Know* (Girard, KS: Haldeman Julius Co., 1925), 5; Florence Dressler, *Feminology: A Guide for Womankind* . . . (Chicago: by the author, 1903), 484; Angenette Parry, "Care of the Health during the Men-strual Period and the Menopause," *New York Medical Journal* 95 (1912): 1367; Howard R. Masters, "Nervous, Mental and Endocrine Manifestations in Menopause," *Virginia Medical Monthly* 50 (1923): 320; Mary D. Rushmore, "Menopause," *Woman's Medical Journal* 21 (1911): 273; and Martin V. Meddaugh, "The Menopause: Its Significance, with Deductions Therefrom," *Detroit Medical Journal* 2 (1902): 648.

22. Fielding, *Woman Past Forty Should Know*, 12. See also Lyman Beecher Sperry, *Husband and Wife: A Book of Information and Advice for the Married and Marriageable* (Chicago: Fleming H. Revell, 1900), 220; MacFadden, *Womanhood and Marriage*, 356; and Lowry, *The Woman of Forty*, 74.

23. Pye Henry Chavasse, *Advice to a Wife and Advice to a Mother on the Manage-ment of Her Own Health, and on the Treatment of Children* . . . , 20th century

ed. (New York: Popular Publishing Co., 1907), 105. For the same quote, see Monfort B. Allen and Amelia C. McGregor, *The Woman Beautiful: Or Maidenhood, Marriage, and Maternity, Containing Full Information on All the Marvelous and Complex Matters Pertaining* (St. Paris, OH: Cornerstone Publishing Co., 1901), 93.

24. Drake, *Woman of Forty-Five,* 62. See also Mary Scharlieb, *Change of Life: Its Difficulties and Dangers* (Chicago: Chicago Medical Book Co., 1912), 74. Although her book was published in the United States, Scharlieb, a prominent physician and eugenicist, was British.

25. For the connection in the late eighteenth century between menopausal suffering and luxurious habits, see John Leake, *Medical Instruction towards the Prevention of Chronic Diseases Peculiar to Women,* 5th ed. (London, 1781), 90–91; and Alexander Hamilton, *The Female Family Physician; Or a Treatise on the Management of Female Complaints and Children in Early Infancy,* 1st Worcester ed. (Worcester, MA, 1792), 90, 99.

26. For examples of the onset of illnesses, see Shoemaker, "Fallacies," 73; see also Ellis, "Menopause," 389; Dulin, "Menopause," 156; T. J. Beattie, "Disturbances of Various Kinds Coincident with the Menopause," *Medical Herald* 27 (1908): 111; Richter, "On the Physiology," 450; W. Londes Peple, "The Menopause," *New York Medical Journal* 82 (1905): 64; Miles J. Breuer, "The Change of Life," *Hygeia,* May 1931, 435–436; and Parry, "Care of Health," 1368. For examples of advice on visiting physicians, see Fielding, *Woman Past Forty Should Know,* 30–31; John H. J. Upham, "The Woman of Middle Age and Some of Her Health Problems," *Hygeia,* April 1927, 187; Breuer, "Change of Life," 437; Edward Podolsky, *Young Woman past Forty: A Modern Sex and Health Primer of the Critical Years* (New York: National Library Press, 1934), 140, 149; William Easterly Ashton, *A Text-Book on the Practice of Gynecology for Practitioners and Students,* 3rd ed. (Philadelphia: W. B. Saunders, 1907), 717; and Charles C. Norris, "The Menopause: An Analysis of Two Hundred Cases," *American Journal of Obstetrics and Diseases of Women and Children* 80 (1919): 77.

27. Quote in Anna M. Galbraith, *The Four Epochs of a Woman's Life: A Study in Hygiene* (Philadelphia: W. B. Saunders, 1904), 197; see also Shoemaker, "Fallacies," 73; M'Gannon, "Menopause," 202; Rushmore, "Menopause," 273; Parry, "Care of Health," 1368; Hirst, *Manual of Gynecology,* vol. 2, 367; George Gellhorn, *Non-Operative Treatment in Gynecology,* Gynecological and Obstetrical Monographs (New York: D. Appleton, 1923), 163; T. J. Marshall, "Abnormal Menopause," *Kentucky Medical Journal* 23 (1925): 377; Potter, "New Standard of Health," 159; Harry Sturgeon Crossen and Robert James Crossen, *Diseases of Women* (St. Louis: C. V. Mosby, 1930), 831; and Ernest Z. Wanous, "The Uterus at the Menopause," *Minnesota Medicine* 3 (1920): 283. Quote in Strongin, "Woman," 534; see also Shoemaker, "Fallacies," 73; Cook, "Some Observations," 385; Win-

throp A. Risk, "The Menopause: Natural and Artificial," *Providence Medical Journal* 2 (1901): 133–134; Crofford, quoted in M'Gannon, "Menopause," 203–204; Andre Crotti, "Hemorrhages of the Menopause and Cancer," *Ohio State Medical Journal* (1913): 370; and A. Ernest Gallant, "Delayed Menopause: Its Dangers and Therapeutic Indications," *New York Medical Journal* 91 (1910): 1283–84.

28. For examples of women failing to see a physician, see Peple, "Menopause," 641; Marshall, "Abnormal Menopause," 377; Potter, "New Standards of Health," 158; and Drake, *Woman of Forty-Five*, 83. Quote in Podolsky, *Young Woman past Forty*, 149; see also Gladys H. Groves and Robert A. Ross, *The Married Woman: A Practical Guide to Happy Marriage* (New York: Blue Ribbon Books, 1936), 264; and Scharlieb, *Change of Life*, 115, Risk, "Menopause," 133–134; Shoemaker, "Fallacies," 73; M'Gannon, "Menopause," 201; Emil Novak, *Menstruation and Its Disorders*, 2nd ed., Gynecological and Obstetrical Monographs (New York: Appleton and Co., 1931), 145.

29. Ellis, "Menopause," 381.

30. Shoemaker, "Fallacies," 72. See also Marshall, "Abnormal Menopause," 377; Von Graff, "Climacteric Changes," 183; Carr, "Menopause," 521; Daniel H. Craig, "The Menopause," *JAMA* 51 (1908): 1507; and Crotti, "Hemorraghes," 370.

31. Von Graff, "Climacteric Changes," 183.

32. Findley, *Treatise*, 76–77; and Crotti, "Hemorraghes," 370.

33. Peple, "Menopause," 644. See also S. Pancoast and William Wesley Cook, *Pancoast's Tokology and Ladies Medical Journal* (Thompson and Thomas, 1901), 275–276; Finley, *Treatise*, 77; Upshur, "The Menopause," 652; and Brooke M. Anspach, *Gynecology*, 2nd ed. (Philadelphia: J. B. Lippincott, 1924), 594.

34. Emil Novak, *The Woman Asks the Doctor* (Baltimore: Williams and Wilkins, 1935), 97–98. See also Rae Thornton La Vake, *A Handbook of Clinical Gynecology and Obstetrics* (St. Louis: C. V. Mosby, 1928), 149.

35. Woods A. M. Hutchinson, "Nature's Mothers' Pension," *Good Housekeeping* (April 1912): 530.

36. La Vake, *Handbook*, 149. See also Rushmore, "Menopause," 273; Craig, "The Menopause," 1507–8; and Mary Ries Melendy, *Perfect Womanhood for Maidens—Wives—Mothers: A Book Giving Full Information on All the Mysterious and Complex Matters Pertaining to Women* (Chicago: Monarch Book Co., 1903), 175.

37. William J. Robinson, *The Menopause or Change of Life; Its Dangers and Disorders, their Prevention and Treatment* (New York: Eugenics Publishing Co., 1923), 36–37.

38. Craig, "The Menopause," 1508.

39. Strongin, "Woman," 522. See also Gellhorn, *Non-Operative Treatment*, 166;

Robinson, *The Menopause,* 26; Mary O'Malley, "Mental Health in Middle Life," *Hygeia,* October 1925, 558; and William J. Fielding, *Sex and the Love-Life* (Garden City, NJ: Dodd, Mead, and Co., 1927), 78.

40. Robinson, *The Menopause,* 37. See also Greenfield, "Dangers," 183; and Dercum, quoted in Hurd-Mead, "Middle-Age Woman," 112.

41. For sources of lifestyle advice see Ashton, *Text-Book on the Practice of Gynecology,* 717; Fielding, *Woman Past Forty Should Know,* 50–52; Galbraith, *Four Epochs of Woman's Life,* 212–214; Clelia Duel Mosher, *Health and the Woman Movement* (New York: The Woman's Press, 1918), 41–42; George B. Norberg, *Golden Rules of Gynecology: Aphorisms, Observations, and Precepts on the Proper Diagnosis and Treatment of Diseases of Women,* Golden Rule Series (St. Louis: C. V. Mosby, 1913), 201–202; Podolsky, *Young Woman past Forty,* 147; Gellhorn, *Non-Operative Treatment,* 164–165.

42. See, for example, Greenfield, "Dangers," 184; Dulin, "The Menopause," 157; Rushmore, "Menopause," 273; and Frank A. Craig, ed., *Diseases of Middle Life: The Prevention, Recognition and Treatment of the Morbid Processes of Special Significance in this Critical Life Period,* vol. 2 (Philadelphia: F. A. Davis Co., 1924), 366.

43. See, for example, Howard A. Kelly, *Medical Gynecology* (New York: D. Appleton and Co., 1908), 89–90; and Findley, *Treatise,* 77. Findley recommended a "sanitarium."

44. The preparation of active follicular and corpus luteum extracts came earlier: in 1923 for the estrogenic substance and in 1929 for the progestational substance. See John G. Gruhn and Ralph R. Kazer, *Hormonal Regulation of the Menstrual Cycle: The Evolution of Concepts* (New York: Plenum Medical Books, 1989), 43–77; Howard Speert, *Gynecologic and Obstetric Milestones, Illustrated* (New York: Parthenon Publishing Group, 1996), 640–644; Edgar Allen, Charles H. Danforth, and Edward A. Doisy, *Sex and Internal Secretions,* 2nd ed. (Baltimore: William and Wilkins, 1939), 846–849, 903–907; Diana Long Hall and Thomas F. Glick, "Endocrinology: A Brief Introduction," *Journal of the History of Biology* 9 (1976): 229–233; and A. S. Parkes, "The Rise of Reproductive Endocrinology, 1926–1940," *Journal of Endocrinology* 34 (1966): 20–33.

45. For more on the history of hormone research, see Oudshoorn, *Beyond the Natural Body;* Borell, "Organotheraphy"; Diana Long Hall, "Biology, Sexism and Sex Hormones in the 1920s," in *Women and Philosophy,* ed. M. Wartofsky and C. Could (New York: Putnam, 1975), 81–96; Diana Long, "Moving Reprints: A Historian Looks at Sex Research Publications of the 1930s," *Journal of the History of Medicine and Allied Sciences* 45 (1990): 452–468; Julia Rechter, "The Glands of Destiny: A History of Popular, Medical and Scientific Views of the Sex Hormones in the 1920s" (Ph.D. diss., University of California, Berkeley, 1997).

46. "To Combat the Annoying Symptoms of the Menopause," *New York Medical Journal* 91 (1910): 756.

47. Barbara Seaman, *The Greatest Experiment Ever Performed on Women: Exploding the Estrogen Myth* (New York: Hyperion, 2003), 10.
48. "To Combat," 756. See also Kelly, *Medical Gynecology*, 89.
49. Amniotin—Squibb, Theelin—Parke Davis, and Progynon—Schering.
50. Alison Li, "Marketing Menopause: Science and the Public Relations of Premarin," in *Women, Health, and Nation: Canada and the United States Since 1945* (Montreal: McGill-Queen's University Press, 2003), 103.
51. In her dissertation, Joy Webster Barbre claims that physicians "were feeding menopausal women ground-up animal ovaries, and injecting women with ovarian extracts, and were asserting, without substantiating scientific evidence, that the therapy was an effective means for managing menopause." Joy Webster Barbre, "From 'Goodwives' to Menoboomers: Reinventing Menopause in American History" (Ph.D. diss., University of Minnesota, 1994), 99.
52. K. I. Sanes, "The Vertigo of the Menopause," *American Journal of Obstetrics and Diseases of Women and Children* 79 (1919): 10–12.
53. Emil Novak, "The Management of the Menopause," *American Journal of Obstetrics and Gynecology* 40 (1940): 592.
54. "Oral Use of Ovarian Products in Menopause Not Established," *JAMA* 95 (1930): 1119. See also Kelly, *Medical Gynecology*, 89; Hans Lisser, "Organotherapy: Present Achievement and Future Prospects," *Endocrinology* 9 (1925): 1–20.
55. Jean Paul Pratt, "Ovarian Therapy," *Endocrinology* 16 (1932): 45–51; Jean Paul Pratt and W. L. Thomas, "The Endocrine Treatment of Menopausal Phenomena," *JAMA* 109 (1937): 1875–1880. See also John P. Seward and Georgene H. Seward, "Psychological Effects of Estrogenic Hormone Therapy in the Menopause," *Journal of Comparative Psychology* 24 (1937): 389.
56. Roy Hoskins, *The Tides of Life: The Endocrine Glands in Bodily Adjustment* (New York: W. W. Norton, 1933), 287. See also Von Graff, "Climacteric Changes," 185.
57. Seward and Seward, "Psychological Effects," 389; Pratt, "Ovarian Therapy," 48; and Charles Dunn, quoted in Pratt and Thomas, "Endocrine Treatment," 1879.
58. Ten Teachers, *Diseases of Women by Ten Teachers*, 5th ed. (Baltimore: William Wood, 1934), 62; Kelly, *Medical Gynecology*, 89; John Osborn Polak, *A Manual of Gynecology*, 3rd ed. (Philadelphia: Lea and Febiger, 1927), 31; and Von Graff, "Climacteric Change," 185.
59. Hurd-Mead, "Middle-Age Woman," 106.
60. Ludwig A. Emge, "Some Certain Considerations in Treating the Menopause," *California and Western Medicine* 26 (1927): 70.
61. Masters, "Nervous, Mental and Endocrine," 320; John Nottingham Upshur, "Menopause and the Climacteric," *Virginia Medical Monthly* 51 (1925): 623; William P. Graves, "Ovarian Therapy," *JAMA* 89 (1927): 1311. See also Elmer L. Sevringhaus and Joseph S. Evans, "Clinical Observations on

the Use of an Ovarian Hormone: Amniotin," 178 (1929): 638–644; Frank A. Craig, *Diseases of Middle Life*, 366; Raphael Kurzrok, *The Endocrines in Obstetrics and Gynecology* (Baltimore: Williams and Wilkins, 1937), 372–380; and Anspach, *Gynecology*, 594.

62. Hirst, *Manual*, 367; and Harold Swanberg, "The Control of Menopausal Symptoms," *Illinois Medical Journal* 72 (1937): 442–443.

63. Emil Novak, "An Appraisal of Ovarian Therapy," *Endocrinology* 6 (1922): 614–615. Such endorsements led Barbre to claim that Novak "strongly recommended organotherapy." Barbre, "From 'Goodwives,'" 98.

64. Emil Novak, *The Woman Asks the Doctor*, 97.

65. Craig, *Diseases of Middle Life*, 366; Anspach, *Gynecology*, 594; and Hirst, *Manual*, 367.

66. Howard Aronson, "The Menopause," *Dallas Medical Journal* 22 (1936): 91–95; and La Vake, *Handbook*, 149.

67. Graves, "Ovarian Therapy," 1308.

68. Strongin, "Woman," 536.

69. "Use of Ovarian Preparations in Artificial Menopause," *JAMA* 96 (1931): 2056.

70. See, for example, Edmund D. Pellegrino, "The Sociocultural Impact of Twentieth-Century Therapeutics," in *The Therapeutic Revolution: Essays in the Social History of American Medicine,* ed. Morris Vogel and Charles E. Rosenberg (Philadelphia: University of Pennsylvania Press, 1979), 245–266; Charles E. Rosenberg, "The Therapeutic Revolution: Medicine, Meaning, and Social Change in Nineteenth-Century America," in *Therapeutic Revolution,* 3–25; Lester S. King, *Transformation in American Medicine* (Baltimore: Johns Hopkins University Press, 1991); and Joel D. Howell, *Technology in the Hospital: Patient Care in the Early Twentieth Century* (Baltimore: Johns Hopkins University Press, 1995).

71. "For Women Only," Vitae-Ore Company (n.d.); "Home Treatment for Female Diseases and Piles," The Miller Company (Kokomo, IN, n.d.), 1–3.

72. "Home Treatment for Female Diseases and Piles," 15.

73. "For Women Only," 2.

74. Peter G. Filene, *Him/Her/Self: Sex Roles in Modern America,* 2nd ed. (Baltimore: Johns Hopkins University Press, 1986), 29.

75. For more about the New Woman, see Estelle B. Freedman, "The New Woman: Changing Views of Women in the 1920s," *Journal of American History* 61 (1974): 372–393; Louise Michele Newman, "The 'New Woman' (1890–1915)," in *Men's Ideas/Women's Realities: Popular Science, 1870–1915* (New York: Pergamon Press, 1985), 298–303; and Smith-Rosenberg, "The New Woman as Androgyne: Social Disorder and Gender Crisis, 1870–1936," in *Disorderly Conduct,* 245–296.

76. The physicians whose writings were examined for this study who feared women's increased presence in public life voiced their anxieties within the context of menopause's mental symptoms, which will be discussed in Chapter 2.

77. Smith-Rosenberg, "Puberty to Menopause," 182–196.
78. Samuel Wyllis Bandler, *The Endocrines* (Philadelphia: W. B. Saunders Co., 1921), 168; Lott, "Principles of Gynecology," 113; Craig, *Diseases of Middle Life*, 363; and Findley, *Treatise*, 73.
79. Cook, "Some Observations," 384.
80. J. T. R. Clark, *The Ills of Womankind. A Treatise on Chronic, Special and Private Ailments of Women* (Kansas City, MO: by the author, 1910), 157.
81. Richter, "Physiology and Pathology," 448–449.
82. Craig, *Diseases of Middle Life*, 363.
83. Hutchinson, "Nature's Mothers' Pension," 532.
84. Groves refers to Anton Nemilov, a Russian physician, whose work was translated into English in 1932.
85. Ernest R. Groves, *Marriage* (New York: Henry Holt and Co., 1933), 477. See also W. Béran Wolfe, *A Woman's Best Years: The Art of Staying Young* (New York: Emerson Books, 1935), 9–10.
86. See, for example, Parry, "Care of the Health," 1368; Scharlieb, *Change of Life*, 32; and Edward B. Foote, *Dr. Foote's Plain Home Talk: A Cyclopedia of Popular Medical, Social and Sexual Science . . .* (New York: Murray Hill, 1917), 544. For histories of birth control, see Janet Farrell Brodie, *Contraception and Abortion in Nineteenth-Century America* (Ithaca: Cornell University Press, 1994); and Andrea Tone, *Devices and Desires: A History of Contraceptives in America* (New York: Hill and Wang, 2001).
87. Filene, *Him/Her/Self*, 11, 55.
88. Engelmann, "President's Address," 10. See also Fielding, *Sex and the Love-Life*, 166.
89. Peple, "The Menopause," 640. See also Ellis, "The Menopause," 381; Parry, "Care of Health," 268; Pancoast, *Tokology*, 278; MacFadden, *Womanhood and Marriage*, 336; Craig, "The Menopause," 1508; and Foote, *Plain Home Talk*, 544.
90. This interpretation differs from that presented by Margaret Morganroth Gullette. Gullette claims that society viewed midlife women as a social problem. She argues that social commentators, including fiction writers and physicians, regarded these women as social "parasites" whose idleness offended and menaced society. Margaret Morganroth Gullette, "Inventing the 'Postmaternal' Woman, 1898–1927: Idle, Unwanted and Out of a Job," *Feminist Studies* 21 (1995): 221–253.
91. Sarah Trent, *Women over Forty* (New York: Macauley, 1934), 52; and Groves and Ross, *Married Woman*, 259.
92. Drake, *Woman of Forty-Five*, 32.
93. Drake, *Woman of Forty-Five*, 44–45; Lowry, *The Woman of Forty*, 144–145; Fielding, *Woman Past Forty Should Know*, 28–29; Carl Ramus, *Outwitting Middle Age* (New York: The Century Co., 1926), 109–110; Podolsky, *Young Woman past Forty*, 28–29; and Trent, *Women over Forty*, 172–184.
94. Olga Knopf, *The Art of Being a Woman* (Boston: Little, Brown, 1932), 239; James L. M. Segall, *Sex Life in America, Its Problems, and Their Solutions*

(New York: Bernard Marks, 1934), 149–151; Wolfe, *Woman's Best Years,* 168; Henry Coe, "Address of the President: Pathology the Basis of Gynecology," *Transactions of the American Gynecological Society* 38 (1913): 18. For discussion of women's emancipation, see Podolsky, *Young Woman past Forty,* 24; Trent, *Women over Forty,* 14; Wolfe, *Woman's Best Years,* 11; and Fielding, *Sex and the Love-Life,* 85.

95. Wolfe, *Woman's Best Years,* 185. See also J. H. Greer, *True Womanhood or Woman's Book of Knowledge* (Chicago: Columbia Publishing House, 1902), 114; Knopf, *Art of Being a Woman,* 239–240; and Trent, *Women over Forty,* 52.

96. Lowry, *The Woman of Forty,* 179; Fielding, *Woman Past Forty Should Know,* 62; MacFadden, *Womanhood and Marriage,* 360; and Wood-Allen, *Marriage,* 220. See also Sperry, *Husband and Wife,* 226; Dercum, quoted in Hurd-Mead, "Middle-Age Woman," 110.

97. Strongin, "Woman," 535. See also Emily Mary Hyde, *The Cycle of Life: Or, the Mystic Seven* (Denver: by the author, 1928), 113.

98. Lowry, *The Woman of Forty,* 179–180.

99. In earlier eras, women used the terms the "cult of true womanhood" and "Republican motherhood" in much the same way.

100. Seth Koven and Sonya Michel, "Womanly Duties: Maternalist Politics, and the Origins of Welfare States in France, Germany, Great Britain, and the United States, 1880–1920," *American Historical Review* 95 (1990): 1079. For more about the feminist deployment of maternalism, see Molly Ladd-Taylor, *Mother-Work: Women, Child Welfare and the State, 1890–1930* (Chicago: University of Illinois Press, 1994), 104–132.

101. Drake, *Woman of Forty-Five,* 24–25. For more on the progressive era, see Paula Baker, "The Domestication of Politics: Women and American Political Society, 1780–1920," *American Historical Review* 89 (1984): 620–649.

102. Nancy Cott, *Grounding of Modern Feminism* (New Haven: Yale University Press, 1987), 29–30; Filene, *Him/Her/Self,* 36–38; and Sara M. Evans, *Born for Liberty: A History of Women in America* (New York: The Free Press, 1989), 152–155.

103. Parry, "Care of Health," 1367.

104. Joseph Tenenbaum, *The Riddle of Sex: The Medical and Social Aspects of Sex, Love and Marriage* (New York: The Macauley Co., 1929), 48.

105. Regina Markell Morantz-Sanchez, *Sympathy and Science: Women Physicians in American Medicine* (New York: Oxford University Press, 1985), 22. In her discussion of women and mental illness in the nineteenth century, Nancy Theriot claims that women physicians created medical knowledge about female patients based on their particular position "in the medial and gender power structures." Nancy M. Theriot, "Women's Voices in Nineteenth-Century Medical Discourse: A Step toward Deconstructing Science," *Signs* 19 (1993): 15. For the influence of gender on medical practice, see also Ellen S. Moore, *Restoring the Balance: Women Physicians and the Profession of Medicine, 1850–1995* (Cambridge, MA: Harvard University Press, 1999), 42–69.

106. Morantz-Sanchez, *Sympathy and Science,* 220. By contrast, Barbre, in her 1994 dissertation, found no difference between male and female physician's attitudes toward menopause. Barbre, "From 'Goodwives,'" 101.

107. Mary Roth Walsh, *Doctors Wanted: No Women Need Apply: Sexual Barriers in the Medical Profession, 1835–1975* (New Haven: Yale University Press, 1977), 107–108, 185–186; Morantz-Sanchez, "Physicians," *Women, Health, and Medicine in America: A Historical Handbook,* ed. Rima Apple (New Brunswick: Rutgers University Press, 1990), 233–234; and Gloria Moldow, *Women Doctors in Gilded-Age Washington: Race, Gender, and Professionalization* (Chicago: University of Illinois Press, 1987), 15.

108. Quoted in Filene, *Him/Her/Self,* 42. See also George Wythe Cook, "Puberty in the Girl," *American Journal of Obstetrics and Diseases of Women and Children* 46 (1902): 804–807.

109. Upshur, "The Menopause," 650.

110. Vern Bullough and Martha Voght, "Women, Menstruation and Nineteenth-Century Medicine," *Bulletin of the History of Medicine* 47 (1973): 66–82.

111. Kelly, *Medical Gynecology,* 88; M'Gannon, "Menopause," 201; Norberg, *Golden Rules,* 200; Marion Edward Clark, *Diseases of Women: A Manual of Gynecology Designed for the Use of Osteopathic Students and Practitioners* (Kirksville, MO: Journal Printing Office, 1904), 384; and Tenenbaum, *Riddle of Sex,* 46.

112. Robinson, *The Menopause,* 40; Masters, "Nervous, Mental and Endocrine," 318; and Anspach, *Gynecology* (1924), 82.

113. Galbraith, *Four Epochs of Woman's Life,* 187–189.

114. Greenfield, "Dangers," 184. It is worth noting that Greenfield (born in 1874), unlike most of the women physicians, was probably not near the age of menopause when she wrote the cited article.

115. Rushmore, "Menopause," 272.

116. Lowry, *The Woman of Forty,* 71–72. While Lowry was trained by the "eclectic" medical sect at Bennett Medical College, her entry in the *American Medical Directory* and *Polk's Medical Register* indicates that she considered herself a "regular" physician. (Eclectic medicine was an alternative to regular or allopathic medicine, relying primarily on concentrated botanical treatments.)

117. Drake, *Woman of Forty-Five,* 29. Drake is clearly responding to Tilt here.

118. Mosher, cited in Helen McKinstry, "The Hygiene of Menstruation," *Mary Hemenway Alumnae Association Bulletin* (1916): 21.

119. Meddaugh, "The Menopause," 648; Engelmann, "President's Address," 9–10. See also Frederic Damrau, *The Menopause: A Clinical Study of Its Nervous Systems* (St. Louis: Dios Chemical Company, 1936), 3.

120. Scharlieb, *Change of Life,* 123; and Drake, *Woman of Forty-Five,* 56.

121. Lowry, *The Woman of Forty,* 74.

122. See Scharlieb, *Change of Life,* 31; Parry, "Care of Health," 1368; Rushmore, "Menopause," 273; and Rachel Lynn Palmer and Sarah K. Greenberg, *Facts and Frauds in Woman's Hygiene: A Medical Guide against Misleading Claims and Dangerous Products* (New York: Vanguard Press, 1936), 105.

123. Drake, *Woman of Forty-Five,* 71; for further discussions of self-control, see Scharlieb, *Change of Life,* 7; Mosher, *Health,* 32; Hurd-Mead, "Middle-Age Woman," 100; and Wood-Allen, *Marriage,* 218. Quote in Dressler, *Feminology,* 486. For further discussions of mind over matter, see Trent, *Woman over Forty,* 41, 50. Trent, however, was not a physician. Quotes in Rushmore, "Menopause," 273; and Galbraith, *Four Epochs in Woman's Life,* 232. For further discussions of women's responsibility for their health, see Theriot, "Women's Voices," 16.

124. Quotes in James King, "Endocrine Influence, Mental and Physical, in Women," *American Journal of Obstetrics and Gynecology* 1 (1921): 328; and Groves, *Marriage,* (1933), 481. For further discussions of medical advice concerning female self-control, see Peple, "The Menopause," 644; Findley, *Treatise,* 77; Gellhorn, *Non-Operative Treatment,* 164; Hirst, *Manual,* 367; Tenenbaum, *Riddle of Sex,* 48–51; and Podolsky, *Young Woman past Forty,* 211. The only exception to this that I have discovered is Upshur, who, in "Menopause and Climacteric," 624–625, claimed that it was important to teach menopausal women self-control but also maintained that a period exists when this might not be possible.

125. Drake, *Woman of Forty-Five,* 42. See also Lowry, *The Woman of Forty,* 14, 85, 179–180; and A. Helena Goodwin, quoted in Hurd-Mead, "Middle-Age Woman," 110.

126. Palmer and Greenberg, *Facts and Frauds,* 103.

127. See, for example, Palmer and Greenberg, *Facts and Frauds,* 104; and Mosher, *Health,* 43–45.

128. Bertha Stuart Dyment, *Health and Its Maintenance: A Hygiene Text for Women* (Stanford: Stanford University Press, 1931), 395.

129. O'Malley, "Mental Health," 559.

130. Lowry, *The Woman of Forty,* v.

131. Galbraith, *Four Epochs in Woman's Life,* 210.

132. Mosher, *Health,* 34–35. See also A. Helena Goodwin, quoted in Hurd-Mead, "Middle-Age Woman," 110.

133. Theriot, "Women's Voices," 12–13.

134. Marie Carmichael Stopes, *Change of Life in Men and Women* (London: Putnam, 1936).

2. "Endocrine Perverts" and "Derailed Menopausics"

1. Bernarr MacFadden, *Womanhood and Marriage* (New York: Physical Culture Corp., 1918), 358–359.

2. William Henry, "Incidents of the Menopause," *St. Louis Medical and Surgical Journal* 35 (1903): 250–251.

3. Indeed, into the early twentieth century women were often institutionalized for menopausal complications. For evidence of this practice, see Records of the Mendota State Mental Hospital, Wisconsin State Historical Society.

4. Ann Douglas Wood, "'The Fashionable Diseases': Women's Complaints and

Their Treatment in Nineteenth-Century America," *Journal of Interdisciplinary History* 4 (1973): 25–52. See also G. J. Barker-Benfield, *The Horror of the Half-Known Life: Male Attitudes toward Women and Sexuality in Nineteenth-Century America* (New York: Harper and Row, 1976).

5. See, for example, Joan Jacobs Brumberg, *Fasting Girls: The History of Anorexia Nervosa* (New York: Plume Books, 1988); Carroll Smith-Rosenberg, "The Hysterical Woman: Sex Roles and Role Conflict in Nineteenth-Century America," *Social Research* 39 (1972): 652–678; Barbara Sicherman, "The Uses of a Diagnosis: Doctors, Patients, and Neurasthenia," *Journal of the History of Medicine and Allied Sciences* 32 (1977): 33–54. Elaine Showalter challenges this model in *The Female Malady: Women, Madness, and English Culture, 1830–1980* (New York: Pantheon, 1985).

6. Elizabeth Lunbeck, *The Psychiatric Persuasion: Knowledge, Gender, and Power in Modern America* (Princeton: Princeton University Press, 1994); Nancy M. Theriot, "Women's Voices in Nineteenth-Century Medical Discourse: A Step toward Deconstructing Science," *Signs* 19 (1993): 1–31.

7. Owsei Tempkin, *The Falling Sickness: A History of Epilepsy from the Greeks to the Beginning of Modern Neurology*, 2nd ed. (Baltimore: Johns Hopkins University Press, 1960), 279–280.

8. Anna Galbraith, *The Four Epochs of a Woman's Life: A Study in Hygiene* (Philadelphia: W. B. Saunders, 1904), 207. See also Alexander H. P. Leuf, *Gynecology, Obstetrics, Menopause* (Philadelphia: Medical Council, 1902), 301; James Lewis Ellis, "The Menopause," *Mobile Medical and Surgical Journal* 4 (1904): 389; John Nottingham Upshur, "The Menopause," *New York Medical Journal* 82 (1905): 651; Edward Reynolds, "The Menopause in Fable and Fact," *Therapeutic Gazette* 30 (1906): 228; and Upshur, "Menopause and Climacteric," *Virginia Medical Monthly* 51 (1925): 622.

9. Clara Dercum, "The Nervous Disorders in Women Simulating Pelvic Disease," *JAMA* 52 (1909): 848. See also Henry Coe, "Pathology, the Basis of Gynecology," *Transactions of the American Gynecological Society* 38 (1913): 9; Francis M. Barnes, "Psychiatry and Gynecology," *Surgery, Gynecology and Obstetrics* 22 (1916): 590–591.

10. See, for example, Martin V. Meddaugh, "The Menopause—Its Significance, with Deductions Therefrom," *Detroit Medical Journal* (1902): 645–648; Samuel Wyllis Bandler, "What Is the Climacterium?" *Medical Record* 69 (1906): 209–212; and Alexander H. P. Leuf, "On the Change of Life in Women," *Medical Council* 3 (1898): 822–825, and 4 (1899): 5–9.

11. See, for example, Karl M. Bowman and Lauretta Bender, "The Treatment of Involutional Melancholia with Ovarian Hormone," *American Journal of Psychiatry* 11 (1932): 867–893.

12. Mary O'Malley, "Mental Health in Middle-Life," *Hygeia*, October 1925, 558.

13. Clelia Duel Mosher, *Health and the Woman Movement* (New York: The Woman's Press, 1918), 31. See also Lyman Beecher Sperry, *Husband and Wife: A Book of Information and Advice for the Married and Marriageable* (Chicago: Fleming H. Revell, 1900), 220; Edith Belle Lowry, *Herself: Talks*

with Women Concerning Themselves (Chicago: Forbes and Co., 1911), 30; C. S. Carr, "The Menopause or Change of Life," *Physical Culture* 32 (1914): 522; William John Fielding, *What the Woman past Forty Should Know* (Girard, KS: Haldeman-Julius Co., 1925), 12, 43; C. B. Farrar and Ruth Maclachlan Franks, "Menopause and Psychoses," *American Journal of Psychiatry* 10 (1931): 1043–44.

14. See, for example, Frank Norbury and Albert Dollear, "The Menopause from the Standpoint of Mental Disorder," *Illinois Medical Journal* 34 (1918): 80; Farrar and Franks, "Menopause and Psychoses," 1043; Ernest Groves, *Marriage* (New York: Holt, 1933): 485; and Mosher, *Health,* 32.

15. See, for example, W. Londes Peple, "The Menopause," *Carolina Medical Journal* 53 (1905): 640–644; August Hoch and John T. MacCurdy, "Prognosis of Involutional Melancholia," *American Journal of Psychiatry* 1 (1922): 433–473; Mary D. Rushmore, "Menopause," *Woman's Medical Journal* 21 (1911): 273; William Easterly Ashton, *A Text-Book on the Practice of Gynecology for Practitioners and Students* 3rd ed., (Philadelphia: W. B. Saunders, 1907), 716; and Howard A. Kelly, *Medical Gynecology* (New York: Appleton and Co., 1908), 88.

16. Ellis, "The Menopause," 382. See also Mary Scharlieb, *Change of Life: Its Difficulties and Dangers* (Chicago: Chicago Medical Book Company, 1912), 32; Galbraith, *Four Epochs,* 204–205; S. Pancoast and William Wesley Cook, *Pancoast's Tokology and Ladies Medical Guide* (Chicago: Thompson and Thomas, 1901), 266; Leuf, *Gynecology,* 277; M. C. M'Gannon, "The Menopause," *Transactions of the Medical Society of Tennessee* 69 (1902): 199.

17. Ellis, "The Menopause," 381. See also Upshur, "The Menopause," 650–653; Galbraith, *Four Epochs,* 204; and Leuf, *Gynecology,* 277.

18. John B. Chapin, "The Psychoses of the Menopause," *Proceedings of the Philadelphia County Medical Society* 21 (1900): 146.

19. See, for example, James Cornelius Wilson, "The Symptomology and Complications of the Menopause," *Proceedings of the Philadelphia County Medical Society* 21 (1900): 135.

20. See, for example, Emil Novak, *Menstruation and Its Disorders* (New York: D. Appleton and Co., 1931), 146; and Upshur, "Menopause and the Climacteric," 622.

21. Norbury and Dollear, "The Menopause," 81.

22. See, for example, W. A. Jones, "Psychoses Incidental to the Climacteric," *Journal-Lancet, MN,* 43 (1923): 222; Farrar and Franks, "Menopause and Psychoses" 1031–44; Novak, *Menstruation,* 146; Edward Podolsky, *Young Woman past Forty: A Modern Sex and Health Primer of the Critical Years* (New York: National Library Press, 1934), 149.

23. William J. Robinson, *The Menopause or Change of Life: Woman's Critical Age, Its Dangers and Disorders, Their Prevention and Treatment* (New York: Critic and Guide Co., 1923), 114–115.

24. Frank P. Norbury, "The Climacteric Period from the Viewpoint of Mental

Disorders," *Medical Record* (1934): 607. This statement was first published in Norbury and Dollear, "The Menopause," 80.

25. Robinson, *The Menopause,* 120.

26. Gerald Jameison and James Wall, "Mental Reactions at the Climacterium," *American Journal of Psychiatry* 11 (1932): 903–906.

27. Jones, "Psychoses," 222.

28. Farrar and Franks, "Menopause and Psychoses," 1041.

29. A. B. Brill, "Discussion of Papers by Jameison and Wall, Stevenson and Montgomery, and Saunders," *American Journal of Psychiatry* 11 (1932): 951.

30. Nathan G. Hale, Jr., *The Rise and Crisis of Psychoanalysis in the United States: Freud and the Americans, 1917–1985,* vol. 2 (New York: Oxford University Press, 1995), 1–167. John C. Burnham, "The Influence of Psychoanalysis upon American Culture," in *Paths into American Culture: Psychology, Medicine and Morals* (Philadelphia: Temple University Press, 1987), 96–110; and John D'Emilio and Estelle B. Freedman, *Intimate Matters: A History of Sexuality in America* (New York: Harper and Row, 1988), 223–226.

31. Peter G. Filene, *Him/Her/Self: Sex Roles in Modern America,* 2nd ed. (Baltimore: Johns Hopkins University Press, 1986), 40–41; Steven Mintz and Susan Kellogg, *Domestic Revolutions: A Social History of American Family Life* (New York: The Free Press, 1988), 108–113; Christina Simmons, "Women's Power in Radical Challenges to Marriage in the Early-Twentieth-Century United States," *Feminist Studies* 23 (2003): 168–198; Ellen Kay Trimberger, "Feminism, Men and Modern Love in Greenwich Village, 1900–1925," in *The Powers of Desire: The Politics of Sexuality,* ed. Christina Simmons, Ann Snitnow and Sharon Thompson (New York: New Feminist Library, 1983), 131–152.

32. Filene, *Him/Her/Self,* 120.

33. For psychiatrists' reactions to the companionate marriage, see Lunbeck, *The Psychiatric Persuasion,* 269–275. For a more general discussion of companionate marriage, see Nancy Cott, *The Grounding of Modern Feminism* (New Haven: Yale University Press, 1987), 154–164; D'Emilio and Freedman, *Intimate Matters,* 265–274; and Christina Simmons, "Modern Sexuality and the Myth of Victorian Repression," in *Passion and Power: Sexuality in History,* ed. Kathy Peiss and Christina Simmons (Philadelphia: Temple University Press, 1989), 157–177.

34. For more about the politicized domesticity and maternalist politics, see Paula Baker, "The Domestication of Politics: Women and American Political Society, 1780–1920," *American Historical Review* 89 (1984): 620–649; Seth Koven and Sonya Michel, "Womanly Duties: Maternalist Politics and the Origins of Welfare States in France, Germany, Great Britain, and the United States, 1880–1920," *American Historical Review* 95 (1990): 1076–1108; and Molly Ladd-Taylor, *Mother-Work: Women, Child Welfare, and the State, 1890–1930* (Urbana: University of Illinois Press, 1994).

35. *U.S. Statutes at Large,* XLII, Pt. 1 (April 1921–March 1923), 224–226.
36. Richard Meckel, *"Save the Babies": American Public Health Reform and the Prevention of Infant Mortality, 1850–1929* (Baltimore: Johns Hopkins University Press, 1990), 209–210.
37. Ladd-Taylor, *Mother-Work,* 170.
38. The women active in the campaign for Sheppard-Towner included Lillian Wald, born 1867; Julia Lathrop, born 1858; Grace Abbott, born 1878; Florence Kelly, born 1859; and S. Josephine Baker, born 1873.
39. Massachusetts Civic Alliance, "Doctor Write Your Senators and Congressmen at Once Opposing the Sheppard-Towner Maternity Bill Now in Congress," *Illinois Medical Journal* 39 (1921): 143.
40. *Congressional Record* 61. 67th Cong., 1st Sess; June 29, 1921. Cited in Ladd-Taylor, *Mother-Work,* 81.
41. Joseph Tenenbaum, *The Riddle of Sex. The Medical and Social Aspects of Sex, Love and Marriage* (New York: The Macaulay Co., 1929), 329–330.
42. W. F. Robie, *Rational Sex Ethics: A Physiological and Psychological Study of the Sex Lives of Normal Men and Women* . . . (Boston: Richard G. Badger, 1918), 292.
43. William T. Sedgwick, *The New York Times,* January 18, 1914, 2. See also Robert Holland, "The Suffragette," *Sewanee Review* 17 (July 1909), 275, cited in Aileen S. Kraditor, *The Ideas of the Woman Suffrage Movement, 1890–1920* (New York: Columbia University Press, 1965), 36–37.
44. Sylvanus Stall, *What a Man of Forty-Five Ought to Know* (Philadelphia: Vir Publishing Co., 1901), 248–250. See also Frederick M. Rossiter, *A Practical Guide to Health: A Popular Treatise on Anatomy, Physiology and Hygiene, with a Scientific Description of Diseases, Their Causes and Treatment* (Washington, D.C.: Review and Herald Publishing Assn., 1908), 433; Edward B. Foote, *Dr. Foote's Plain Home Talk: A Cyclopedia of Popular Medical. Social and Sexual Science:* . . . (New York: Murray Hill, 1917), 817; Podolsky, *Young Woman past Forty,* 139–140.
45. Nelly Oudshoorn, *Beyond the Natural Body: An Archeology of Sex Hormones* (London: Routledge, 1994), 22.
46. Samuel Wyllis Bandler, *The Endocrines* (Philadelphia: W. B. Saunders, 1921), 161; and Norbury and Dollear, "The Menopause," 79.
47. George Richter, "On the Physiology and Pathology of the Menopause," *Medical Record* 91 (1917): 449; Norbury and Dollear, "The Menopause," 79; Robert T. Frank, *The Female Sex Hormone* (Springfield, IL: Charles C. Thomas, 1929), 19; and Roy Hoskins, *The Tides of Life: The Endocrine Glands in Bodily Adjustment* (New York: W. W. Norton, 1933), 285.
48. Prosser Harrison Picot, "The Physiology of the Climacteric Symptomology," *Virginia Medical Monthly* 64 (1937): 208.
49. James L. Segall, *Sex Life in America: Its Problems and Their Solutions* (New York: Bernard Marks, 1934), 31–32.
50. Jameison and Wall, "Mental Reactions," 898–899.

51. See, for example, Stall, *Man of Forty-Five,* 231; Mary Wood-Allen, *Marriage. Its Duties and Privileges* (New York: Revell, 1901), 217, 219; and Bernard S. Talmey, *Woman: A Treatise on the Normal and Pathological Emotions of Feminine Love* (New York: The Stanley Press Corp., 1906), 71.

52. Mary Melendy, *Perfect Womanhood for Maidens—Wives—Mothers: A Book Giving Full Information on All the Mysterious and Complex Matters Pertaining to Women* (Chicago: Monarch Book Co., 1903), 178; Upshur, "The Menopause," 653; Edgar A. Dulin, "The Menopause," *Medical Herald* 27 (1908): 156; M. E. Clark, *Diseases of Women: A Manual of Gynecology Designed for the Use of Osteopathic Students and Practitioners,* 2nd ed. (Kirksville, MO: Journal Printing Office, 1904), 387.

53. William Walling, *Sexology,* 2nd ed. (Philadelphia: Puritan Publishing Co., 1904), 76.

54. Pancoast and Cook, *Tokology,* 268; Carey Culbertson, "A Study of the Menopause with Special Reference to Its Vasomotor Disturbances," *Surgery, Gynecology and Obstetrics* 23 (1916): 668; and Daniel H. Craig, "The Menopause," *JAMA* 51 (1908): 1509.

55. Dulin, "The Menopause," 156.

56. Pancoast and Cook, *Tokology,* 273–274.

57. See, for example, C. B. S. Evans, *Sex Practice in Marriage,* 2nd ed. (New York: Emerson Books Inc., 1935), 48–49; Hannah H. Stone and Abraham Stone, *A Marriage Manual: A Practical Guide-Book to Sex and Marriage,* revised ed. (New York: Simon and Schuster, 1935), 224–225; W. Béran Wolfe, *A Woman's Best Years: The Art of Staying Young* (New York: Emerson Books, 1935), 37; Theodore Hendrik Van de Velde, *Ideal Marriage: Its Physiology and Technique* (New York: Random House, 1930), 111–112; Tenenbaum, *Riddle of Sex,* 55; and Robinson, *The Menopause,* 47–49.

58. Podolsky, *Young Woman past Forty,* 213. See also Eleanora B. Saunders, "Mental Reactions Associated with the Menopause," *Southern Medical Journal, Nashville* 25 (1932): 270.

59. Robinson, *The Menopause,* 73–74.

60. Podolsky, *Young Woman past Forty,* 148. See also Fielding, *Woman past Forty,* 59.

61. Richter, "Physiology and Pathology," 449.

62. Coyne H. Campbell, "Mental Aspects of the Menopause," *Journal of the Oklahoma State Medical Association* 30 (1937): 12–13.

63. John Osborne Polak, *A Manual of Gynecology,* 3rd ed. (Philadelphia: Lea and Febiger, 1927), 29.

64. Edith Belle Lowry, *Woman of Forty* (Chicago: Forbes and Co., 1919), 23–24, 75; William John Fielding, *Sex and the Love-Life* (Garden City, NY: Dodd, Mead and Co., 1927; reprint, Dodd and Mead, 1952), 179–180; and Emily Mary Hyde, *The Cycle of Life: Or the Mystic Seven* (Denver: by the author, 1928), 35–42.

65. Tenenbaum, *Riddle of Sex,* 50.

66. Robinson, *The Menopause,* 128.
67. G. H. Stevenson and S. R. Montgomery, "Paranoid Reactions Occurring in Women of Middle Age," *American Journal of Psychiatry* 11 (1932): 918.
68. Robinson, *The Menopause,* 146.
69. Ibid., 147.
70. Podolsky, *Young Woman past Forty,* 151, 153.
71. Robinson, *The Menopause,* 137–138. See also Jameison and Wall, "Mental Reactions," 902.
72. Robinson's fairly tolerant attitude was reinforced by nonmedical writers. See Sarah Trent, *Women over Forty* (New York: Macauley, 1934), 92–93; and Grace Loucks Elliott, *Woman after Forty: The Meaning of the Last Half of Life* (New York: Henry Holt, 1936), 114.
73. Erin G. Carlston, "'A Finer Differentiation'": Female Homosexuality and the Medical Community, 1926–1940," in *Science and Homosexualities,* ed. Vernon A. Rosario (New York: Routledge, 1997), 177–196; Jennifer Terry, *An American Obsession: Science, Medicine, and Homosexuality in Modern Society* (Chicago: University of Chicago Press, 1999).
74. Norbury and Dollear, "The Menopause," 83; and Frank A. Craig, ed. *Diseases of Middle Life: The Prevention, Recognition and Treatment of the Morbid Processes of Special Significance in This Critical Life Period,* vol. 2 (Philadelphia: F. A. Davis Co., 1924), 365.
75. Robinson, *The Menopause,* 49.
76. Elliott, *Woman after Forty,* 21.
77. Jones, "Psychoses," 221–222.
78. Sperry, *Husband and Wife,* 224.
79. Fielding, *Woman past Forty,* 61. See also Stall, *Man of Forty-Five,* 265.
80. Jameison and Wall, "Mental Reactions," 898. See also Jones, "Psychoses," 222; Howard R. Masters, "Nervous, Mental and Endocrine Manifestations in Menopause," *Virginia Medical Monthly* 50 (1923): 318–319; Upshur, "Menopause and the Climacteric," 624; Saunders, "Mental Reactions," 267; and Stall, *Man of Forty-Five,* 265.
81. Norbury and Dollear, "The Menopause," 80.
82. Norbury, "The Climacteric Period," 607.
83. Stevenson and Montgomery, "Paranoid Reactions," 919.
84. Emma F. Drake, *What a Woman of Forty-Five Ought to Know* (Philadelphia: Vir Publishing Co., 1902), 65.
85. Bowman and Bender, "Treatment of Involutional Melancholia," 886.
86. Upshur, "The Menopause," 653. See also Stevenson and Montgomery, "Paranoid Reactions," 915; and G. Reginald Siegel, "Endocrine Therapy in the Climacteric," *Journal of the Arkansas Medical Society* 31 (1935): 196.
87. Norbury and Dollear, "The Menopause," 81.
88. MacFadden, *Womanhood and Marriage,* 360.
89. See, for example, Trent, *Women over Forty,* 54.
90. Lowry, *Woman of Forty,* 78.

91. Galbraith, *Four Epochs,* 218.
92. Joseph H. Greer, *True Womanhood or Woman's Book of Knowledge* (Chicago: Columbia Publishing House, 1902), 290. See also Stall, *Man of Forty-Five,* 224–225.
93. Theriot suggests that selfishness indicated mental illness in the nineteenth century as well (Theriot, "Women's Voices," 17).
94. Margaret Deland, "The Change in the Feminine Ideal," *Atlantic Monthly* 105 (1910): 289–302. See also Filene, *Him/Her/Self,* 42–43.

3. "Consider the Patient as a Woman and Not a Group of Glands"

1. Dorothy Hamilton Brush and Heather Hoffman, "An Anonymous Questionnaire on Your Second Adolescence," 1950, Dorothy Brush Papers, Sophia Smith Collection, Smith College, Northampton, Massachusetts: Brush, "Questionnaire," #72. All names used in this book are pseudonyms that I have assigned.
2. Susan E. Bell, "Gendered Medical Science: Producing a Drug for Women," *Feminist Studies* 21 (1995): 469–500.
3. See, for example, Robert Ross, "The Involutional Phase of the Menstrual Cycle (Climacteric)," *American Journal of Obstetrics and Gynecology* 45 (1943): 504; Paul de Kruif, "New Help for Women's Change of Life," *Readers' Digest,* January 1948, 11; Robert T. Frank, "The Treatment of the Disorders of the Menopause," *Bulletin of the New York Academy of Medicine* 17 (1941): 860–861; and "Management of the Menopause," *American Journal of Medicine* 10 (1951): 95.
4. Edmund D. Pellegrino, "The Sociocultural Impact of Twentieth-Century Therapeutics," in *The Therapeutic Revolution: Essays in the Social History of American Medicine,* ed. Morris Vogel and Charles Rosenberg (Philadelphia: University of Pennsylvania Press, 1979), 245–266.
5. Bell, "Gendered Medical Science," 480.
6. *Index Medicus* provided the starting point for my examination of the medical literature, and I attempted to locate every article indexed under menopause between 1938 and 1962. My search then radiated from these original sources until, in the end, I had examined more than 130 articles and monographs by more than 110 authors. The articles included those published in the leading medical journals, such as the *Journal of the American Medical Association (JAMA)* and the *American Journal of Obstetrics and Gynecology,* as well as those from regional publications such as *Rhode Island Medical Journal.*
7. For examples of medical musings, see David M. Farell, "Dangers in the Management of the Menopause," *Medical Clinics of North America* 32 (1948): 1523–32; and Lucious E. Burch, "The Medical Aspects of the Menopause," *Journal of the Tennessee State Medical Society* 33 (1940): 208–212. For examples of retrospective analysis, see C. L. Buxton, "Medical Therapy during

the Menopause," *Journal of Clinical Endocrinology* 4 (1944): 591–596. See also L. K. Hawkinson, "The Menopausal Syndrome: One Thousand Consecutive Patients Treated with Estrogen," *JAMA* 111 (1938): 390–393. For examples of therapeutic research, see Mildred Vogel, Thomas H. McGavack, and Joseph Mellow, "Effects of Various Estrogenic Preparations," *American Journal of Obstetrics and Gynecology* 60 (1950): 168–173; and William H. Perloff, "Treatment of Menopause," *American Journal of Obstetrics and Gynecology* 61 (1950): 670–671.

8. Ida Davidoff and Marjorie Platt, "Two Generation Study of Postparental Women," data set, Henry A. Murray Research Center, Radcliffe College, Cambridge, MA. I have supplemented these major contributions with a few letters written to the Children's Bureau and, indirectly, material taken from the popular literature itself.

9. Frank, "Treatment," 858. See also J. P. Pratt, "The Treatment of Menopause," *Southern Medical Journal* 31 (1938): 566; B. P. Watson, "The Menopausal Patient," *Journal of Clinical Endocrinology* 4 (1944): 571; W. P. Devereux, "Management of the Menopause and Climacteric," *Texas State Journal of Medicine* 42 (1947): 683–684; R. F. Farquharson, "The Menopausal Patient," *Medical Record and Annals* 49 (1955): 199; and Joseph Rogers, "Current Status of the Therapy of the Menopause," *JAMA* 175 (1961): 1167.

10. Emil Novak, "The Management of the Menopause," *American Journal of Obstetrics and Gynecology* 40 (1940): 592; David A. Bickel, "The Menopause," *Indiana Medical Association* 33 (1941): 297; Sprague Gardiner, "The Menopause," *Public Health Nursing* 33 (1941): 282; Buxton, "Medical Therapy," 593; Roland Bieren, "Treatment of the Menopause," *Medical Annals of the District of Columbia* 20 (1951): 479; Ralph A. Reis, "The Menopause, Causes, Symptoms, and Treatment," *Trained Nurse and Hospital Review* 112 (1944): 270; and Mary DeWitt Pettit, "Management of the Menopause," *Medical Clinics of North America* 39 (1955): 1727.

11. In 1959, only 21.7 percent of people aged forty-five to fifty-four had health insurance that covered doctors' visits. *Health Statistics From the U.S. National Health Survey: Interim Report on Health Insurance. United States, July–December 1959*, Series B, No. 26 (1960), 46.

12. Brush, "Questionnaire," #52.

13. Peter Temin, *Taking Your Medicine: Drug Regulation in the United States* (Cambridge, MA: Harvard University Press, 1980), 4.

14. Advertisement copy, No. 2031, Job C-3812. Planned for 1944 newspapers. The Lydia Pinkham Collection, The Schlesinger Library, Radcliffe College, Cambridge, MA. Into the 1950s, the Lydia Pinkham Company continued to sponsor clinical trials of their product on menopausal women. Box 111, folder 2173, Lydia Pinkham Collection.

15. James Scott, "You Need Not Fear the Menopause," *Ladies' Home Journal*, March 1946, 190. See also Mario Castallo and Cecilia L. Schulz, *Woman's*

Inside Story (New York: Macmillan, 1948), 97; Miriam Lincoln, *You'll Live Through It: Facts about the Menopause* (New York: Harper, 1950), 85; Elmer Sevringhaus, "A Woman Faces Forty," *Hygeia,* August 1939, 753; Adolph Fredrick Niemoeller, *Feminine Hygiene in Marriage* (New York: Harvest House, 1938), 154–155; and Carl Hartman, "Sex Education for the Woman at Menopause," *Hygeia,* September 1941, 747.

16. For more on the struggle, see James Harvey Young, *Medical Messiahs: A Social History of Quackery in Twentieth-Century America* (Princeton, NJ: Princeton University Press, 1967). Some of the condemnation of self-medication may have been directed at refilling prescription drugs. Not until 1948 did the FDA move toward the regulation of prescription refills. In other words, before this time women could decide whether or not they should continue treatment. Young, *Medical Messiahs,* 273.

17. Stanley Joel Reiser, "The Emergence of the Concept of Screening for Disease," *Milbank Memorial Fund Quarterly* 56 (1978): 406; and Paul K. J. Han, "Historical Changes in the Objectives of the Periodic Health Exam," *Annals of Internal Medicine* 126 (1997): 910–917.

18. Fred Brown and Rudolph T. Kempton, *Sex: Questions and Answers; A Guide to Happy Marriage* (New York: McGraw-Hill, 1950), 116. See also Bernadine Bailey, "Fair, Fit and Forty," *Hygeia,* December 1947, 931; Edwin Hamblen, *Facts about the Change of Life* (Springfield, IL: C. C. Thomas, 1949), 51–53; Abner I. Weisman, *Woman's Change of Life* (New York: Renbayle House, 1951), 2; Lincoln, *You'll Live,* 86; and Albert Q. Maisel, "Promise For Happiness," *Woman's Home Companion,* September 1954, 98.

19. Maxine Davis, *Facts about the Menopause* (New York: McGraw-Hill, 1951), 49. See also William C. Danforth, *A Woman's Health* (New York: Farrar and Rinehart, 1941), 370–371; and Castallo and Schulz, *Woman's Inside Story,* 100–101.

20. Davidoff "Two Generation Study," #19, #18, and #2. (The responses received in this study were labeled using two different sets of numbers. Unless otherwise noted, the number cited refers to the second set. The names used in this book are pseudonyms, which I supplied, in keeping with the strong sense of the personalities revealed by the responses.)

21. *Health in California* (State of California, Department of Public Health, 1956): 33.

22. Brush, "Questionnaire," #78; see also #62. Davidoff, "Two Generation Study," #3 and #1.

23. In the Davidoff data, six of the twenty-five original women had had hysterectomies, which had brought on their menopause. The percentage of women in the Brush sample was similar; 25 of 125 of the Brush sample had had a hysterectomy. This roughly reflects the national scene. Between 1960 and 1962, approximately 25 percent of white women between forty-five and sixty-four had experienced operative menopause, and the percentage of black women was significantly higher. Brian MacMahon and Jane Worcester, "Age

at Menopause, United States, 1960–1962," (Washington, D.C.: U.S. Department of Health, Education, and Welfare, 1966): 3–4.

24. July 4, 1941 letter to the Children's Bureau, Box 741, Folder 4–5–7–5–3, National Archives and Records Administration, College Park, MD.

25. Davidoff, "Two Generation Study," #53.

26. Ibid., #19; see also #55.

27. Brush, "Questionnaire," #13.

28. Charles Frederic Fluhmann, *Menstrual Disorders: Pathology, Diagnosis and Treatment* (Philadelphia: W. B. Saunders, 1939), 306. See also Ephraim Shorr, "The Menopause," *Bulletin of the Academy of Medicine* 16 (1940): 456; Earl Conway Smith, "Estrogen Therapy of the Climacteric: An Analysis of Seventy-Seven Personal Cases," *Surgery, Gynecology and Obstetrics* 71 (1940): 745–746; Edwin Crowell Hamblen, "The Female Climacteric," *Virginia Medical Monthly* 67 (1940): 27; John B. Montgomery, "The Menopause," *Medical Clinics of North America* 29 (1945): 1417–18; Elmer L. Sevringhaus, "Therapy of the Patient in the Menopause: Endocrine Methods," *Journal of Clinical Endocrinology* 4 (1944): 597; J. C. Donovan, "Menopausal Syndrome: A Study of Case Histories," *American Journal of Obstetrics and Gynecology* 62 (1951): 1290; and Paul O. Klingensmith, "The Care of the Menopausal Patient," *Pennsylvania Medical Journal* 57 (1954): 427.

29. On the order of treatment, see Watson C. Finger, "Management of the Menopause," *Journal of the South Carolina Medical Association* 49 (1953): 310; Buxton, "Medical Therapy," 595–596; Foster Coleman, "The Menopause," *Kentucky Medical Journal* 45 (1947): 208; Farell, "Dangers," 1525; Robert A. Ross, "Female Climacterium," *Medical Record and Annals* 46 (1952): 806; Alvin F. Goldfarb, "Physiology and Management of the Climacteric," *Journal of the American Medical Women's Association* 9 (1954): 78; E. Stewart Taylor, "The Use of Sex Hormones in the Menopause," *Geriatrics* 9 (1954): 225; Farquharson, "Menopausal Patient," 202; and S. Leon Israel, "The Menopause," *Postgraduate Medicine* 30 (1961): 420–421.

30. "Management of the Menopause," *New York State Journal of Medicine* 41 (1941): 2345. See also Gardiner, "The Menopause," 282; Emil Novak, "Some Misconceptions and Abuses in Gynecological Organotherapy," *Pennsylvania Medical Journal* 48 (1945): 772; Chloe O. Fry, "The Rational Use of Estrogens," *Journal of the American Medical Women's Association* 4 (1949): 51; and Willard R. Cooke, "The Practical Application of Psychology in Gynecic Practice," *Nebraska State Medical Journal* 35 (1950): 376.

31. Novak, "Management of the Menopause," 589. See also Arthur H. Squires and Douglas E. Cannell, "The Menopausal Patient," *Medical Clinics of North America* 36 (1952): 515; and Joseph Rogers, "The Menopause," *New England Journal of Medicine* 254 (1956): 699.

32. W. O. Johnson, "Menopause from the Viewpoint of the Gynecologist," *Kentucky Medical Journal* 45 (1947): 212; and Fry, "Rational Use," 51.

33. Frank, "Treatment," 859. See also Pettit, "Management," 1725.

34. Watson, "Menopausal Patient," 571, 573–574. See also Rogers, "The Menopause," 699; John C. Weed, "Management of the Postmenopausal Woman," *Postgraduate Medicine* 14 (1953): 370; and Buxton, "Medical Therapy," 591, 593; Edwin N. Nash, "The Climacteric and the Menopause," *Illinois State Medical Journal* 79 (1941): 472, 484; and Robert N. Rutherford, "Therapy During the Menopause—a Review," *Western Journal of Surgery and Gynecology* 53 (1945): 17; Robert B. Greenblatt, "Metabolic and Psychosomatic Disorders in Menopausal Women," *Geriatrics* 10 (1955): 165; and Ephraim Shorr, "Problems of Mental Adjustment at the Climacteric," *Public Health Report, Supplement* (1942): 129.

35. Cooke, "Practical Application," 373–374.

36. See, for example, Ann Douglas Wood, "'The Fashionable Diseases': Women's Complaints and Their Treatment in Nineteenth-Century America," *Journal of Interdisciplinary History* 4 (1973): 25–52; and G. J. Barker-Benfield, *The Horror of the Half-Known Life* (New York: Harper and Row, 1976).

37. See, for example, Richard H. Young, "Relationships of Nervous Disorders to the Menopause," *American Journal of Obstetrics and Gynecology* 38 (1939): 115; Emil Novak, "The Menopause and Its Management," *JAMA* 110 (1938): 621; Devereux, "Management," 685; Johnson, "Menopause," 211; Farell, "Dangers," 1525; Gertrude Flint Jones, "The Physiology and Management of the Climacteric," *California Medicine* 71 (1949): 346; Donovan, "Menopausal Syndrome," 1290; Ross, "Psychosomatic Approach to the Climacterium," *California Medicine* 74 (1951): 241; Taylor, "Use of Sex Hormones," 225; Harry Friedlander, "Education and Sedation in Menopause," *Postgraduate Medicine* 18 (1955): 94–98; Hamblen, "The Female Climacteric," 28–29; Robert N. Creadick, "Menopause," *Texas State Journal of Medicine* 54 (1958): 710–711; Trevor Owen, "The Medical View of the Menopause," *American Journal of Psychiatry* 101 (1945): 759; and E. T. Engle, "The Menopause—An Introduction," *Journal of Clinical Endocrinology and Metabolism* 4 (1944): 569.

38. Farquharson, "Menopausal Patient," 202. See also Coleman, "The Menopause," 208, and Johnson, "Menopause," 210, who cite Novak's claim that he could talk 50 percent of women out of their symptoms.

39. Squires and Cannell, "Menopausal Patient," 523; and Ross, "The Involutional Phase," 502.

40. Donovan, "Menopausal Syndrome," 1290.

41. Ross, "A Psychosomatic Approach," 241. See also R. G. Hoskins, "The Psychological Treatment of the Menopause," *Journal of Clinical Endocrinology and Metabolism* 4 (1944): 608; Charles H. Birnberg, *Female Sex Endocrinology* (Philadelphia: J. B. Lippincott, 1949), 91–92; Donovan, "Menopausal Syndrome," 1290; Squires and Cannell, "Menopausal Patient," 523; Weed, "Management," 373; Finger, "Management," 310; Farquharson, "Menopausal Patient," 202; and Rogers, "The Menopause," 700, 750.

42. Friedlander, "Education," 98.

43. Ibid., 96.
44. Cooke, "Practical Application," 372.
45. Pratt, "Treatment," 567.
46. Greenhill, quoted in Nash, "Climacteric," 476.
47. Pellegrino, "Sociocultural Impact," 255; and Joel D. Howell, *Technology in the Hospital: Transforming Patient Care in the Early Twentieth Century* (Baltimore: Johns Hopkins University Press, 1995), 3; Stanley Joel Reiser, *Medicine and the Reign of Technology* (Cambridge, UK: Cambridge University Press, 1978), esp. 227–231.
48. Frank, "Treatment," 854. See also Nash, "Climacteric," 472; Fluhmann, *Menstrual Disorders,* 306; Maurice H. Greenhill, "A Psychosomatic Evaluation of the Psychiatric and Endocrinological Factors in the Menopause," *Southern Medical Journal, Nashville* 39 (1946): 791; Novak, "Management of the Menopause," 589; S. Charles Freed, "The Menopausal Syndrome," *Journal of Insurance Medicine* 5 (Sept.–Nov. 1950): 23; Esther Loring Richards, "Psychological Aspects of the Menopause," *Public Health Nursing* 33 (1941): 345; Montgomery, "The Menopause," 1417–18; Louis M. Foltz, "Psychiatric Aspects of Menopause," *Kentucky Medical Journal* 45 (1947): 212–213; and H. E. Chamberlain, "Psychiatric Aspects of the Menopause," *Medical Record and Annals* 41 (1947): 133.
49. Farell, "Dangers," 1524.
50. Richards, "Psychological Aspects," 345. See also Bickel, "The Menopause," 296; and Ross, "The Involutional Phase," 501.
51. Shorr, "Problems of Mental Adjustment," 129.
52. Creadick, "Menopause," 710. See also Benjamin Blackman, "The Treatment of the Climacterium," *Illinois Medical Journal* 113 (1958): 228; Farquharson, "Menopausal Patient," 198; Young, "Relationship of Nervous Disorders," 113; and Farell, "Dangers," 1524.
53. Squires and Cannell, "Menopausal Patient," 522. See also Farquharson, "Menopausal Patient," 202; and Creadick, "Menopause," 710.
54. Herbert W. Coone and Roberto Escamilla, "Oral Estrogen Therapy in the Menopause Syndrome: Some Comparison of Products of Synthetic and Natural Origin," *American Practitioner and Digest of Treatment* 2 (1951): 54.
55. Hoskins, "Psychological Treatment," 609.
56. Buxton, "Medical Therapy," 591–594; Rita S. Finkler, "The Use and Misuse of Estrogens in Menopause," *Medical Woman's Journal* 52 (1945): 28; and Devereux, "Management," 686.
57. Novak, "The Menopause," 576; Coone and Escamilla, "Oral Estrogen Therapy," 54. See also Squires and Cannell, "Menopausal Patient," 518; Creadick, "Menopause," 710; Buxton, "Medical Therapy," 593; Isracl, "The Menopause," 420; Bickel, "The Menopause," 296; Blackman, "Treatment," 227–228; Ross, "Involutional Phase," 501; and Nash, "Climacteric," 472.
58. Nancy A. Walker, *Shaping Our Mother's World: American Women's Magazines* (Jackson, MS: University of Mississippi Press, 2000), 160n232.

59. For advocates of sedation, generally before hormones, see Fluhmann, *Menstrual Disorders,* 313; Burch, "Medical Aspects," 211; Hamblen, "Female Climacteric," 27; Nash, "Climacteric," 475; Bickel, "The Menopause," 296; Frank, "Treatment," 855; Buxton, "Medical Therapy," 595–596; Rutherford, "Therapy During the Menopause,"17; Owen, "Medical View," 759; Montgomery, "The Menopause," 1421; Coleman, "The Menopause," 208; Devereux, "Management," 685; Johnson, "Menopause," 210; Farell, "Dangers," 1525; Birnberg, *Female Sex Endocrinology,* 91–92; Freed, "Menopausal Syndrome," 23; Bieren, "Treatment," 479; "Management," (1951), 94; Squires and Cannell, "Menopausal Patient," 524; Robert A. Ross, "The Care of the Female in the Climacteric," *Journal of the Medical Association of Georgia* 41 (1952): 286; Klingensmith, "Care," 427; Taylor, "Use of Sex Hormones," 225; Farquharson, "Menopausal Patient," 202; Creadick, "Menopause," 711; Blackman, "Treatment," 229–230; Novak, "Management of the Menopause," 593; Goldfarb, "Physiology," 78; and Pettit, "Management," 1728. This is still the standard dosage for mild sedation. To put it in perspective, physicians currently recommend 100 to 200 milligrams at bedtime to induce sleep and 60 to 250 milligrams to prevent seizures. James J. Rybacki and James W. Long, *The Essential Guide to Prescription Drugs,* 1998 ed. (New York: Harper and Collins, 1998), 761–767.

60. Friedlander, "Education," 96–97.

61. Ibid., 96; and Bickel, "The Menopause," 296.

62. C. L. Buxton, "The Menopause," *Medical Clinics of North America* 35 (1944): 888; and Allan C. Barnes, "The Menopause," *Clinical Obstetrics and Gynecology* 1 (1958): 209.

63. See Kevin Koumjian, "The Use of Valium as a Form of Social Control," *Social Science and Medicine* 15 (1981): 245–249.

64. See, for example, Young, "Relationship of Nervous Disorders," 115; Farquharson, "Menopausal Patient," 202; and Barnes, "The Menopause," 210.

65. When physicians recommended hormone therapy, they generally had in mind estrogen treatments. Throughout this period, androgens were also given to menopausal women, but despite an increasing popularity, they remained on the margins of medical orthodoxy. Androgens generally did not prove more beneficial than estrogen alone, and they caused unwanted side effects such as unwanted facial hair.

66. Joy Webster Barbre claims that during the postwar period medical discussion about HRT "faded into the background." Discussion of HRT, however, continued to dominate the medical literature on menopause, even if recommendations in the literature downplayed hormones' usefulness. Joy Webster Barbre, "From 'Goodwives' to Menoboomers: Reinventing Menopause in American History" (Ph.D. diss., University of Minnesota, 1994), 178.

67. Friedlander, "Education," 94; David N. Danforth, "The Climacteric," *Medical Clinics of North America* 45 (1961): 52; Novak, "Management of the

Menopause," 593; Fluhmann, *Menstrual Disorders,* 311; Hamblen, "Female Climacteric," 27–28; Frank, "Treatment," 858; Watson, "Menopausal Patient," 571; Reis, "The Menopause," 270; Montgomery, "The Menopause," 1418–20; Coleman, "The Menopause," 208; Finger, "Management," 309; Novak, "The Menopause," 575–576; and Rogers, "The Menopause," 698.

68. Novak, "Some Misconceptions," 772. There were very few physicians who believed that most women benefited from hormone treatment. See, for example, Robert B. Greenblatt, "Newer Concepts in the Management of the Menopause," *Geriatrics* 7 (1952): 266.

69. See, for example, Buxton, "Medical Therapy," 591; Buxton, "The Menopause," 879; Novak, "Some Misconceptions," 772; Fry, "Rational Use," 51; Novak, "The Menopause," 576; Rogers, "The Menopause," 699; Danforth, "The Climacteric," 51; Rogers, "Current Status," 1167; and Hamblen, quoted in Ross, "The Involutional Phase," 505.

70. Hamblen, "Female Climacteric," 28. See also Shorr, "The Menopause," 461; Novak, "Management of the Menopause," 591; Montgomery, "The Menopause," 1421; Devereux, "Management," 685; Farquharson, "Menopausal Patient," 202; and Danforth, "Climacteric," 52.

71. See, for example, Devereux, "Management," 685; Birnberg, *Female Sex Endocrinology,* 91; and Ross, "Psychosomatic Approach," 241.

72. Devereux, "Management," 686; and Franklin L. Payne, "The Postmenopausal Patient," *Journal of the Medical Association of the State of Alabama* 22 (1952): 32. See also, for example, Klingensmith, "Care," 427; Friedlander, "Education," 94–95; Jones, "Physiology," 347; and Coleman, "The Menopause," 208.

73. Watson, "Menopausal Patient," 572.

74. Bieren, "Treatment," 478, 481. See also Klingensmith, "Care," 427; Novak, "Some Misconceptions," 773; Coleman, "The Menopause," 208; Johnson, "Menopause," 212; and Danforth, "The Climacteric," 52.

75. See, for example, J. W. Cook and E. C. Dodds, "Sex Hormones on Cancer-Producing Compounds," *Nature* 137 (1933): 205–209; W. V. Gardner, "Tumors in Experimental Animals Receiving Steroid Hormones," *Surgery* 16 (1944): 8–14; and I. H. Perry and L. L. Ginzton, "The Development of Tumor in Female Mice Treated with 1:2:5:6: Dibenzanthracone and Theelin," *American Journal of Cancer* 29 (1937): 680–682.

76. S. H. Geist and U. J. Salmon, "Are Estrogens Carcinogenic in the Human Female?" *American Journal of Obstetrics and Gynecology* 41 (1941): 29. This paper was originally presented before the Third International Cancer Congress, Atlantic City, NJ, in 1939.

77. Edgar Allen, "Ovarian Hormone and Female Genital Cancer," *JAMA* 114 (1940): 2107.

78. Saul B. Gusberg, "Precursors of Corpus Carcinoma: Estrogens and Adenomatous Hyperplasia," *American Journal of Obstetrics and Gynecology* 54 (1947): 905.

79. Hamblen, "Female Climacteric," 28.

80. Rogers, "Menopause," 753. See also Rogers, "Current Status," 1169; Shorr, "The Menopause," 468–469; Nash, "Climacteric," 475; "Management," 1941, 2342; Coone and Escamilla, "Oral Estrogen Therapy," 54–55; W. H. Masters, "Menopause and Thereafter," *Minnesota Medicine* 41 (1958): 3; and E. Kost Shelton, "The Use of Estrogen after the Menopause," *Journal of the American Geriatrics Society* 2 (1954): 630–631.

81. Jones, "Physiology," 347. See also Bickel, "The Menopause," 297–298; Montgomery, "The Menopause," 1421; and Fry, "Rational Use," 54.

82. Novak, "Management of the Menopause," 594; Robert N. Rutherford, "Recent Advances in Medical Gynecology," *Western Journal of Surgery and Gynecology* 53 (1945): 17; Finkler, "Use and Misuse," 29; Devereux, "Management," 686; Johnson, "Menopause," 211–212; Payne, "Postmenopausal Patient," 32; Alvin F. Goldfarb and E. Edward Napp, "Use of Methallenestril (Vallestril) in Control of Menopausal Symptoms," *JAMA* 161 (1956): 618; and Danforth, "The Climacteric," 51.

83. Hamblen, "The Female Climacteric," 24. See also Buxton, "The Menopause," 891; Mathew Ross, "Current Concepts of the Climacterium," *American Practitioner and Digest of Treatment* 2 (1951): 956; Ross, "The Involutional Phase," 497; Robert A. Ross, "The Care of the Female," 285; and Edmund R. Novak, "The Menopause," *JAMA* 156 (1954): 577.

84. Montgomery, "The Menopause," 1416; and Farell, "Dangers," 1523; Captain Paul Peterson, "Management of the Climacteric," *Military Medicine* 116 (1955), 348.

85. Minnie B. Goldberg, *Medical Management of the Menopause, Modern Medical Monographs,* vol. 17 (New York: Grune and Stratton, 1959), 64; Elmer Sevringhaus, "Therapy of the Patient," 597; Sevringhaus's comment cited in S. J. Glass and M. R. Shapiro, "Androgen-Estrogen Treatment in the Menopause," *GP* 3 (1951): 39; Novak, "Some Misconceptions," 772; and Fluhmann, *Menstrual Disorders,* 311.

86. Bell, "Gendered Medical Science," 480–481; Kathleen I. MacPherson, "Menopause as Disease: The Social Construction of a Metaphor," *Advances in Nursing Science* 3 (1981): 105; Geri L. Dickson, "Metaphors of Menopause: The Metalanguage of Menopause Research," in *Menopause: A Midlife Passage,* ed. Joan C. Callahan (Bloomington: Indiana University Press, 1993), 37–41; and Margaret Morganroth Gullette, "Menopause as Magic Marker: Discursive Consolidation in the United States and Strategies for Cultural Combat," in *Reinterpreting Menopause: Cultural and Philosophical Issues,* ed. Paul Komesaroff, Philipa Rothfield, and Jeanne Daly (New York: Routledge, 1997), 176–199.

87. George N. Papanicolaou and Ephraim Shorr, "The Action of Ovarian Follicular Hormone in the Menopause, as Indicated by Vaginal Smears," *American Journal of Obstetrics and Gynecology* 31 (1936): 823.

88. Shorr, "The Menopause," 462; "Management," (1941), 2339; Johnson, "Menopause," 210; "Management," (1951), 95; Goldfarb, "Physiology," 78; and Finkler, "Use and Misuse," 28.

89. Novak, "Management of the Menopause," 590; Ross, "Psychosomatic Approach," 241; Reis, "The Menopause," 271; Greenblatt, "Newer Concepts," 269; and Pettit, "Management," 1727.

90. Goldberg, *Medical Management,* 64.

91. Susan Bell explained this refusal to rely on a diagnostic test as a political strategy by medical clinicians to "protect their cultural authority" from impingement by laboratory scientists. This strategy supported clinical judgment rather than diagnostic tests as the defining feature of patient treatment. While Bell's interpretation nicely illuminates the professional struggles within medical institutions, she glosses over an equally significant point, that women and their subjective experiences mattered in the diagnosis and treatment of menopause. Bell, "Changing Ideas: The Medicalization of Menopause," *Social Science and Medicine* 24 (1987): 537; and Bell, "Gendered Medical Science," 481–483.

92. Goldberg, *Medical Management,* 67.

93. Greenblatt, "Newer Concepts," 266. See also August A. Werner, "Management of the Menopause," *Postgraduate Medicine* 9 (1951): 158–159; Allan C. Barnes, "Is Menopause a Disease?" *Consultant* 2 (1962): 22–24; and Hawkinson, "Menopausal Syndrome," 392.

94. Taylor, "Use of Sex Hormones," 224.

95. Fuller Albright, Patricia H. Smith, and Anna Richardson, "Postmenopausal Osteoporosis: Its Clinical Features," *JAMA* 116 (1941): 2474.

96. Philip H. Henneman and Stanley Wallach, "The Use of Androgens and Estrogens and Their Metabolic Effects: A Review of the Prolonged Use of Estrogens and Androgens in Postmenopausal and Senile Osteoporosis," *AMA Archives of Internal Medicine* 100 (1957): 715.

97. Henneman and Wallach, "Use of Androgens," 721. See also Stanley Wallach and Philip H. Henneman, "Prolonged Estrogen Therapy in Postmenopausal Women," *JAMA* 171 (1959): 1637–42.

98. J. H. Wuerst, Jr., T. J. Dry, and J. E. Edwards, "Degree of Coronary Atherosclerosis in Bilaterally Oophorectomized Women," *Circulation* 7 (1953): 801–809; A. U. Rivin and S. P. Dimitroff, "Incidence and Severity of Atherosclerosis in Estrogen Treated Males and in Females with Hypoestrogenic or Hyperestrogenic State," *Circulation* 9 (1954): 533–539; R. W. Robinson, N. Higano, and W. D. Cohen, "Increased Incidence of Coronary Heart Disease in Women Castrated Prior to Menopause," *AMA Archives of Internal Medicine* 104 (1959): 908–913; and Robinson, et al., "Estrogen Replacement Therapy in Women with Coronary Atherosclerosis," *Annals of Internal Medicine* 48 (1958): 95–101. See also Rogers, "Current Status," 1167–70.

99. Shelton, "Use of Estrogen," 629.

100. Ibid., 632.

101. Masters, "Menopause and Thereafter," 4. See also William H. Masters, "Rationale of Sex Steroid Replacement in the 'Neutral Gender,'" *Journal of the American Geriatrics Society* 3 (1955): 389–395; William H. Masters, "Estrogen-Androgen Substitution Therapy in the Aged Female," *Obstetrics*

and Gynecology 2 (1953): 139–147. Other physicians also claimed that estrogen therapy could be used to "slow the aging process." See Noel Bailey, "Postmenopausal Medical Gynecology," *Texas State Journal of Medicine* 53 (1957): 836–839.

102. Barnes, "Is Menopause a Disease?" 22–24.

103. Coleman, "The Menopause," 207; Edmund Novak, "The Menopause," 576. See also Ross, "Involutional Phase," 497; Finkler, "Use and Misuse," 28; Devereux, "Management," 686; Johnson, "Menopause," 209; Farell, "Dangers," 1525–6; Novak, "Management of the Menopause," 595; Smith, "Estrogen Therapy," 745; Blackman, "Treatment," 229; Payne, "Postmenopausal Patient," 31–32; Klingensmith, "Care," 246; and Rogers, "The Menopause," 750.

104. Farell, "Dangers," 1525–26. See also Payne, "Postmenopausal Patient," 31–32; Cooke, "Practical Application," 376; Klingensmith, "Care," 426; Rogers, "The Menopause," 699; and Fry, "Rational Use," 51.

105. Fry, "Rational Use," 51.

106. Frank, "Treatment," 855; and Ross, "Care of the Female," 285.

107. Emil Novak, *Gynecology and Female Endocrinology* (Boston: Little and Co., 1941), 465. Menopausal women received more than hormones from their doctors; evidence suggests that they also received sedatives. Although sedatives did not play as large a role in the therapeutic experience as did hormones, 29 percent (31 of 125) of the Brush women did receive some sort of "nerve pills." This indicates that while the medical literature suggested that sedatives should be deployed before hormones, physicians in their medical practices—perhaps convinced by their patients—relied first on estrogen replacement for the relief of menopausal difficulties.

108. The exact percentage is difficult to determine. One reckoning shows that 46 of the 125 women (37 percent) who returned Brush surveys indicated that they received hormone replacement therapy, as did 9 of 25 of the women (36 percent) in the Davidoff sample. Some women, however, claimed that they received "gland treatments," but they did not indicate that they had had hormone treatments. This indicates that women may not have always known what they received from their physicians.

109. The medical literature recommended hormone therapy for only 5 to 10 percent of all cases.

110. Margaret Lock, "Models and Practice in Medicine: Menopause as Syndrome or Life Transition?" *Culture, Medicine and Psychiatry* 6 (1982): 261–280. Lock's study examines Canadian physicians' views of menopause in the early 1980s.

111. Temin, *Taking Your Medicine,* 58–87; Young, *Medical Messiahs,* 260–281; Pellegrino, "Sociocultural Impact," 261; and C. Muller, "The Overmedicated Society: Forces in the Marketplace for Medical Care," *Science* 16 (1972): 488.

112. Temin, *Taking Your Medicine,* 82–87.

113. "In the menopause . . . transition without tears," *American Journal of Obstet-*

rics and Gynecology 78 (1959): 29; and "At the menopause . . . that feeling of well-being," *JAMA* 129 (1945): 23.

114. "Of course, women like 'Premarin'," *Journal of the Maine Medical Association* 50 (1959), n.p.

115. Elina Hemminki, "Review of Literature on the Factors Affecting Drug Prescribing," *Social Science and Medicine* 9 (1975): 111–112.

116. Milton Silverman and Philip R. Lee, *Pills, Profits, and Politics* (Berkeley: University of California Press, 1974); and Temin, *Taking Your Medicine,* 85.

117. Novak, "Some Misconceptions," 771. See also Rogers, "The Menopause," 699.

118. Silverman and Lee, *Pills,* 21.

119. Pellegrino, "Sociocultural Impact," 261. See also Muller, "Overmedicated Society," 488.

120. Silverman and Lee, *Pills,* 22–23; Hemminki, "Review," 113.

121. Rogers, "The Menopause," 699. Physicians generally preferred oral administration to intramuscular injections, condemning both the high cost of "shots" and the estrogen spikes that followed weekly or biweekly injections. Indeed, many physicians argued that injections, and the office visits they required, unnecessarily tethered women to their physicians. One physician likened the shot regimen to "slavery" and condemned it soundly.

122. Samuel R. Meaker, *A Doctor Talks to Women: What They Should Know about the Normal Functions and Common Disorders of the Female Organs* (New York: Simon and Schuster, 1954), 36; Leonard Biskind, *Health and Hygiene for the Modern Woman* (New York: Harper and Brothers, 1957), 117.

123. Frederic Loomis, *Consultation Room* (New York: Alfred A. Knopf, 1939), 234; Lawrence Galton, "What Every Husband Should Know about the Menopause," *Better Homes and Gardens,* July 1950, 127. See also Edith M. Stoney, "The Menopause," *Today's Health,* August 1952, 38.

124. Weisman, *Woman's Change of Life,* 88; Watson, "Menopausal Patient," 571. See also Montgomery, "The Menopause," 1418; and Hamblen, *Facts About the Change,* 86.

125. Goldberg, *Medical Management,* 64. We should not immediately accept patient demand as the driving force behind the use of hormone therapy. As John B. McKinlay suggests in "From 'Promising Report' to 'Standard Procedure': Seven Stages in the Career of a Medical Innovation," *Milbank Memorial Fund Quarterly/Health and Society* 59 (1981), 385–387, drug companies and medical professionals have used "public demand" to legitimate their promotion or prescription of medical innovations before the innovation exhibited any proven benefits. In the case of HRT, however, evidence of patient demand from both physicians and women themselves emerged well after HRT had been proven effective for at least some menopausal symptoms.

126. Barbre claims that the popular literature seldom included recommendations for HRT. It is difficult to understand this claim. See Barbre, "From 'Goodwives,'" 193.

127. Loomis, *Consultation Room,* 232.
128. Maxine Davis, "Menopause," *Good Housekeeping,* July 1943, 30; and Davis, *Facts About the Menopause,* 44. See also Maxine Davis, *Woman's Medical Problems,* 2nd ed. (New York: McGraw-Hill, 1948), 214.
129. Maisel, "Promise," 41.
130. Sevringhaus, "A Woman Faces Forty," 753. See also Helen Haberman, "Help for Women Over 40," *Hygeia,* November 1941, 898–899; and Ernest Grafenberg, "Personal Hygiene of Women," in *Every Woman's Standard Medical Guide* (New York: Greystone Press, 1948), 94.
131. Haberman, "Help," 899.
132. Bailey, "Fair, Fit and Forty," 931, 959.
133. Carl G. Hartman, "Sex Education at Menopause," *Hygeia,* September 1941, 747.
134. Lincoln, *You'll Live,* 46.
135. Emil Novak, *Gynecology and Female Endocrinology* (Boston: Little, Brown and Company, 1941), 485.
136. Brush, "Questionnaire," #255.
137. Ibid., #258.
138. Ibid., #107.
139. Ibid., #259.
140. Ibid., #78.
141. Frances B. McCrea, "The Politics of Menopause: The 'Discovery' of a Deficiency Disease," *Social Problems* 31 (1983): 113; Pauline B. Bart and Marilyn Grossman, "Menopause," *Women and Health* 1 (1973): 3; and MacPherson, "Menopause as Disease," 96.
142. Brush, "Questionnaire," unnumbered survey; and Brush, "Questionnaire," #10.
143. Ibid., #76.
144. Ibid., #65.
145. Harold Maurice Imerman, *What Women Want to Know: A Noted Gynecologist's Guide to the Personal Problems of Women's Health* (New York: Crown, 1958), 225–226.
146. Brush, "Questionnaire," #23.
147. Ibid., #79. See also Brush, "Questionnaire," #59, #267, and #82, responses from women who found that hormones did not work for their symptoms.
148. Davidoff, "Two Generation Study," #12.
149. Brush, "Questionnaire," #108.
150. Davidoff, "Two Generation Study," #15.
151. Brush, "Questionnaire," #62.

4. "The Change Emancipates Women"

1. Edwin Crowell Hamblen, *Facts about the Change of Life* (Springfield, IL: C. C. Thomas, 1949), 2.

2. Susan M. Hartmann, *The Homefront and Beyond: American Women in the 1940s* (Boston: Twayne Publishers, 1982), 15–29; and Nancy Woloch, *Women and the American Experience* (New York: Knopf, 1984), 439.

3. Elaine Tyler May, *Homeward Bound: American Families in the Cold War Era* (Basic Books, 1988), 102.

4. See, for example, May, *Homeward Bound*, 183–207.

5. Jessica Weiss, *To Have and to Hold: Marriage, the Baby Boom, and Social Change* (Chicago: University of Chicago Press, 2000), 184.

6. Peter G. Filene, *Him/Her/Self: Sex Roles in Modern America*, 2nd ed. (Baltimore: Johns Hopkins University Press, 1986), 168; and Alice Kessler-Harris, *Out to Work: A History of Wage-Earning Women in the United States* (New York: Oxford University Press, 1982), 302.

7. Joanne Meyerowitz, "Beyond the *Feminine Mystique:* A Reassessment of Postwar Mass Culture, 1946–1958," in *Not June Cleaver: Women and Gender in Postwar America, 1945–1960,* ed. Joanne Meyerowitz (Philadelphia: Temple University Press, 1994), 234, 241–245.

8. Elizabeth Hawes, *Why Women Cry: Or Wenches with Wrenches* (Cornwall, NY: Cornwall Press, 1943); and Eva Moskowitz, "'It's Good to Blow Your Top': Women's Magazines and a Discourse of Discontent, 1945–1965," *Journal of Women's History* 8 (1996): 66–98.

9. Weiss, *To Have and to Hold*, 49–81.

10. Susan M. Hartmann, "Women's Employment and the Domestic Ideal in the Early Cold War Years," in Meyerowitz, ed., *Not June Cleaver*, 84–100.

11. Kessler-Harris, *Out to Work*, 296–297.

12. Ibid., 30; Weiss, *To Have and to Hold*, 51.

13. Kessler-Harris, *Out to Work*, 302.

14. See, for example, "American Woman's Dilemma," *Life*, June 16, 1947, 101–116. For the discussion of the "dilemma," see William H. Chafe, *The American Woman: Her Changing Social, Economic, and Political Roles, 1920–1970* (New York: Oxford University Press, 1972), 199–225; Evans, *Born for Liberty: A History of Women in America* (New York: The Free Press, 1989), 235–237; and Woloch, *Women*, 500–502.

15. Margaret Mead, "What Women Want," *Fortune*, December 1946, 173, quoted in Evans, *Born for Liberty*, 235.

16. Ferdinand Lundberg and Marynia F. Farnham, *Modern Woman: The Lost Sex* (New York: Harper and Brothers Publishers, 1947), v, 235–236. For similar positions, see Helene Deutsch, *The Psychology of Women: A Psychoanalytic Approach*, 2 vols. (New York: Grune and Stratton, 1944–45); Edward A. Strecker and Vincent T. Lathbury, *Their Mothers' Daughters* (New York: J. B. Lippincott, 1956).

17. See Mirra Komarovsky, *Women and the Modern World* (Boston: Little and Brown, 1953), cited in Woloch, *Women*, 500.

18. For references to puberty in reverse, see, for example, Florence Shutt Edsall, *Change of Life: A Modern Woman's Guide* (New York: Grosset and Dunlap,

1949), 22; Marion Hilliard, "Woman's Greatest Blessing," *A Woman Doctor Looks at Love and Life* (New York: Doubleday, 1957), 149; Miriam Lincoln, *You'll Live through It: Facts about the Menopause* (New York: Harper, 1950), 30; and James C. Janney, "Sexual Hygiene," in *Every Woman's Standard Medical Guide* (New York: Greystone Press, 1948), 164.

19. Carl G. Hartman, "Sex Education for the Woman at Menopause," *Hygeia*, September 1941, 699; and Maxine Davis, *Facts about the Menopause* (New York: McGraw Hill, 1951), 43. For statistics about how many women suffer or for claims that "only a few women suffer" see, for example, Maxine Davis, "Menopause," *Good Housekeeping*, July 1943, 147; Bernadine Bailey, "Fair, Fit, and Forty," *Hygeia*, December 1947, 931; Edith M. Stoney, "The Menopause," *Today's Health*, August 1952, 37; and Leonard Biskind, *Health and Hygiene for the Modern Woman* (New York: Harper and Brothers, 1957), 116.

20. Madeline Gray, *The Changing Years: How to Stop Worrying about the Menopause* (Garden City, New York: Doubleday, 1956, reprint of Country Life Press, 1951), 56.

21. Edsall, *Change of Life*, 27; Ernest Grafenberg, "Personal Hygiene of Women," in *Every Woman's Standard Medical Guide* (New York: Greystone Press, 1948), 93.

22. Maxine Davis, *Woman's Medical Problems*, 2nd ed. (New York: McGraw-Hill Book Co., 1948), 211; and Lincoln, *You'll Live*, 44–45, 47.

23. Janney, "Sexual Hygiene," 164; Edsall, *Change of Life*, 22; and Hilliard, "Woman's Greatest Blessing," 149.

24. Lincoln, *You'll Live*, 71–72.

25. Harold Shryock, "Why Nervousness at 45?" *Hygeia*, March 1947, 206.

26. Gray, *The Changing Years*, 57; Joseph Rety, *Transition Years: The Modern Approach to "the Change" in Womanhood* (New York: Greenberg, 1940), 124. See also Hamblen, *Facts about the Change of Life*, 64–65; Davis, *Facts about the Menopause*, 39; Edsall, *Change of Life*, 57; Hartman, "Sex Education," 747; Helen Haberman, "Help for Women Over 40," *Hygeia*, November 1941, 899; and Ruth Brecher and Edward Brecher, "The Facts About the Menopause," *Reader's Digest*, July 1958, 79.

27. Edward Stieglitz, *The Second Forty Years* (New York: J. B. Lippincott, 1946), 193.

28. Davis, *Woman's Medical Problems*, 210–211. See also Fred Brown and Rudolph Kempton, *Sex: Questions and Answers: A Guide to Happy Marriage* (New York: McGraw-Hill, 1950), 114; Anna Kleegman Daniels, "Change of Life," in *Every Woman's Standard Medical Guide* (New York: Greystone Press, 1948), 254; Paul de Kruif, "New Help for Women's Change of Life," *Reader's Digest*, January 1948, 11; Julie E. Miale, "Easing Those Difficult Years," *Today's Health*, February 1956, 29; Lawrence Galton, "What Every Husband Should Know About the Menopause," *Better Homes and Gardens*, July 1950, 54; and Davis, *Facts about the Menopause*, 6.

29. Hamblen, *Facts about the Change,* 66–67.
30. Samuel Lewin and John Gilmore, *Sex After Forty* (New York: Medical Research Press, 1952), 30. See also William C. Danforth, *A Woman's Health* (New York: Farrar and Rinehart, 1941), 373; Leland Ellis Glover, *Sex Life of the Modern Adult* (New York: Belmont Books, 1961), 61; and Miale, "Easing," 31.
31. De Kruif, "New Help," 12. See also Mario A. Castallo and Celilia L. Schulz, *Woman's Inside Story* (New York: Macmillan, 1948), 95; Maxine Davis, *Woman's Medical Problems,* 212; Hamblen, *Facts about the Change,* 68; Edward F. Griffith, *A Sex Guide to a Happy Marriage* (New York: Emerson, 1956), 246; Carl Leonard Anderson, *Physical and Emotional Aspects of Marriage* (St. Louis: C. V. Mosby, 1953), 178; and Goodrich C. Schauffler, "Tell Me Doctor," *Ladies' Home Journal,* April 1959, 37.
32. Rety, *Transition Years,* 125; Stieglitz, *Second Forty,* 198; Grafenberg, "Personal Hygiene," 94.
33. Gray, *The Changing Years,* 160.
34. David O. Cauldwell, *What Women Should Know about the Menopause: Prevention of Suffering through an Understanding of the Hygiene of Life's Natural Changes* (Girard, KS: Haldeman-Julius, 1947), 3; Edsall, *Change of Life,* 70; Laura Hutton, "The Unmarried," in *Sex in Social Life,* ed. Sybil Neville-Rolfe (New York: W. W. Norton, 1950), 449; and Castallo and Schulz, *Woman's Inside Story,* 99.
35. Bailey, "Fair, Fit, and Forty," 931, 959. See also Elmer L. Sevringhaus, "A Woman Faces Forty," *Hygeia,* August 1939, 687; Rety, *Transition Years,* 121; Foster Kennedy, "Don't Fear the Change of Life," *Woman's Home Companion,* November 1944, 24; Hamblen, *Facts about the Change,* 66; and Stella Applebaum and Nadine Kavinoky, *Understanding Your Menopause* (New York: New York Public Affairs Committee, 1956), 15.
36. Galton, "Every Husband," 126; Lincoln, *You'll Live,* 123; Davis, *Facts about the Menopause,* 7; and Madeline Gray, *The Changing Years,* 159–160.
37. Stoney, "The Menopause," 39.
38. For more on the effect of menopause on family relations, see Chapter 5.
39. This, of course, need not be the case. Motherhood includes the rearing of children, not just their bearing.
40. Biskind, *Health,* 114. See also James Scott, "You Need Not Fear the Menopause," *Ladies' Home Journal,* March 1946, 33.
41. Davis, *Facts about the Menopause,* 160. See also Ida Bailey Allen, *Youth after Forty* (Garden City, NY: Halcyon House, 1950), 13.
42. See Elizabeth Dawson, *Menopause: Is It a Change of Life?* (Springfield, IL: State of Illinois, Department of Public Health, 1955), 12.
43. Applebaum and Kavinoky, *Understanding,* 20.
44. Gray, *The Changing Years,* 100.
45. Edsall, *Change of Life,* 18.
46. See, for example, Danforth, *Woman's Health,* 382; and Lincoln, *You'll Live,* 178.

47. Gray, *The Changing Years,* 100; and Lincoln, *You'll Live,* 178.

48. Edsall, *Change of Life,* 104–108. Davis, *Facts about the Menopause* notes that it may be a time of financial worries (131), but she also claims that it should be a time of fewer financial worries (160). See also Lena Levine and Beka Doherty, *The Menopause* (New York: Random House, 1952), 194–196.

49. Daniels, "Change of Life," 253.

50. Emily Martin, *The Woman in the Body: A Cultural Analysis of Reproduction* (Boston: Beacon Press, 1987), 27–53.

51. Abner Weisman, *Woman's Change of Life* (New York: Renbayle House, 1951), 24.

52. Daniels, "Change of Life," 256–257.

53. Lincoln, *You'll Live,* 1, 3.

54. May, *Homeward Bound,* 141–142.

55. Ibid., 136.

56. Filene, *Him/Her/Self,* 166.

57. May, *Homeward Bound,* 100.

58. See, for example, Filene, *Him/Her/Self,* 158–159; John D'Emilio and Estelle Freedman, *Intimate Matters: A History of Sexuality in America* (New York: Harper and Row, 1988), 248–249.

59. Hamblen, *Facts about the Change,* 44, 54.

60. Edward Podolsky, *Sex Today in Wedded Life* (New York: Simon Publications, 1943), 186.

61. Hutton, "The Unmarried," 431.

62. Weisman, *Woman's Change of Life,* 25. See also Edsall, *Change of Life,* 116–117; and Rety, *Transition Years,* 116–117.

63. Lincoln, *You'll Live,* 144.

64. Harold M. Imerman, *What Women Want to Know: A Noted Gynecologist's Guide to the Personal Problems of Women's Health* (New York: Crown, 1958), 225–226.

65. Cauldwell, *What Women Should Know,* 11.

66. Moskowitz, "'Blow Your Top,'"66–91.

67. Levine and Doherty, *The Menopause,* 57.

68. Rety, *Transition Years,* 157. See also Davis, *Facts about the Menopause,* 154; Hamblen, *Facts about the Change,* 45; and Daniels, "Change of Life," 256.

69. Frederic Loomis, *Consultation Room* (New York: Alfred A. Knopf, 1939), 236.

70. Galton, "Every Husband," 55.

71. Samuel A. Lewin, *Sex Without Fear* (New York: Medical Research Press, 1952), 178–179.

72. Stieglitz, *Second Forty,* 193.

73. Fred Trevitt and Freda Dunlop White, *How to Face the Change of Life with Confidence: A Practical Guide for Mature Living* (New York: Exposition Press, 1955), 14. See also Levine and Doherty, *The Menopause,* 6; and Castallo and Schulz, *Woman's Inside Story,* 91.

74. Cauldwell, *What Women Should Know,* 13; and Stieglitz, *Second Forty,* 193.

75. Lois Mattox Miller, "Changing Life Sensibly," *Independent Woman,* September 1939, 311. See also Milton L. Miller, "Facts About the Menopause," *Hygeia,* August 1940, 740; and Lincoln, *You'll Live,* 149.

76. Trevitt and White, *How to Face the Change,* 26.

77. Jessamyn Neuhaus, "The Importance of Being Orgasmic: Sexuality, Gender, and Marital Sex Manuals in the United States, 1920–1963," *Journal of the History of Sexuality* 9 (2000): 447–473; and Lori Rostoff, *Love on the Rocks: Men, Women, and Alcohol in Post–World War II America* (Chapel Hill: University of North Carolina Press, 2002).

78. Evans, *Born for Liberty,* 245.

79. Lincoln, *You'll Live,* 2; and Charles A. Clinton, *Sex Behavior in Marriage* (New York: Pioneer Publication, 1944), 72.

80. Miller, "Change Life Sensibly," 311.

81. Miller, "Facts about the Menopause," 740.

82. Castallo and Schulz, *Woman's Inside Story,* 103; Frank Caprio, *The Modern Woman's Guide to Sexual Maturity* (New York: Grove Press, 1959), 178–184.

83. For a look at selfishness and women, see Wini Breines, *Young, White, and Miserable: Growing Up Female in the Fifties* (Boston: Beacon Press, 1992).

84. Danforth, *Woman's Health,* 382; and Castallo and Schulz, *Woman's Inside Story,* 103. Joy Webster Barbre, in "From 'Goodwives' to Menoboomers: Reinventing Menopause in American History," (Ph.D. diss., University of Minnesota, 1994), also stressed the importance of keeping busy.

85. See, for example, Rety, *Transition Years,* 194; and Weisman, *Woman's Change of Life,* 40.

86. Miale, "Easing," 31; Edsall, *Change of Life,* 98–102, Shryock, "Why Nervousness," 209; Louisa R. Church, "No Time for Tears," *American Home,* June 1945, 17.

87. Biskind, *Health,* 120.

88. Danforth, *Woman's Health,* 381.

89. Anderson, *Physical,* 180. See also Church, "No Time," 17.

90. Lincoln, *You'll Live,* 109. See also Virginia Stitzenberger, "Silent House or Second Chance," *Today's Health,* April 1958, 30.

91. See Evans, *Born for Liberty,* 246–247, on domesticity and community service.

92. Rety, *Transition Years,* 60. See also Danforth, *Woman's Health,* 382.

93. Hamblen, *Facts about the Change,* 43–44.

94. Levine and Doherty, 113.

95. Biskind, *Health,* 108.

96. Stitzenberger, "Silent House," 30. See also Trevitt and White, *How to Face the Change,* 61; Davis, *Facts about the Menopause,* 160–164; and Lincoln, *You'll Live,* 107.

97. Cauldwell, *What Women Should Know,* 10. See also Miale, "Easing," 3; Shryock, "Why Nervousness," 210; and Imerman, *What Women Want,* 233.

98. "American Woman's Dilemma," 101–116; quotations on page 109.

99. Levine and Doherty, *The Menopause,* 163.

100. Miller, "Changing Life Sensibly," 297.

101. Davis, *Women's Medical Problems,* 217.

102. Polly Allison, "You're In It—You're Facing It—or You're Through It—You Hope!" *Independent Woman,* February 1954, 49. See also Dawson, 14.

103. Gray, *The Changing Years* (1951), 112. See also Dawson, Menopause, 14; and Levine and Doherty, *The Menopause,* 194–195.

104. Jacqueline Jones, *Labor of Love, Labor of Sorrow: Black Women, Work, and the Family from Slavery to the Present* (New York: Basic Books, 1985).

105. Caprio, *Modern Woman's Guide,* 187.

5. "Casting an Evil Spell over Her Once Happy Home"

1. Oliver Butterfield, *Sex Life in Marriage* (New York: Emerson Books, 1949), 158–159.

2. Fred Trevitt and Freda Dunlop White, *How to Face the Change of Life with Confidence: A Practical Guide for Mature Living* (New York Exposition Press, 1955), 12.

3. Elmer L. Sevringhaus, "A Woman Faces Forty," *Hygeia,* August 1939, 752.

4. James Scott, "You Need Not Fear the Menopause," *Ladies' Home Journal,* March 1946, 191.

5. Mario A. Castallo and Cecilia A. Schulz, *Woman's Inside Story* (New York: Macmillan, 1948), 95. See also Leonard Biskind, *Health and Hygiene for the Modern Woman* (New York: Harper and Brothers, 1957), 118; and Edward Stieglitz, *The Second Forty Years* (New York: J. B. Lippincott, 1946), 264.

6. Florence Shutt Edsall, *Change of Life: A Modern Woman's Guide* (New York: Grosset and Dunlap, 1949), 68.

7. Miriam Lincoln, *You'll Live Through It: Facts About the Menopause* (New York: Harper, 1950), 107. See also Joseph Rety, *Transition Years: The Modern Approach to "the Change" in Womanhood* (New York: Greenberg, 1940), 84; Carl Gottfried Hartman, "Sex Education for Women at Menopause," *Hygeia,* September 1941, 747; Castallo and Schulz, *Woman's Inside Story,* 95; Ida Bailey Allen, *Youth after Forty* (Garden City, NY: Halcyon House, 1950), 11–12; Trevitt and White, *How to Face,* 12.

8. Lois Mattox Miller, "Changing Life Sensibly," *Independent Woman,* September 1939, 311; and Trevitt and White, *How to Face,* 45.

9. Lincoln, *You'll Live,* 148.

10. Edsall, *Change of Life,* 65.

11. Marion Hilliard, "Women's Greatest Blessing," in *A Woman Doctor Looks at Love and Life* (New York: Doubleday, 1957), 160–162.

12. Lena Levine and Beka Doherty, *The Menopause* (New York: Random House, 1952), 58.

13. See, for example, Frank Caprio, *Sexually Adequate Female* (New York: The Citadel Press, 1953), 213.

14. Leland Ellis Glover, *Sex Life of the Modern Adult* (New York: Belmont Books,

1961), 60. See also Lawrence Galton, "What Every Husband Should Know About the Menopause," *Better Homes and Gardens,* July 1950, 128.

15. Edith M. Stoney, "The Menopause," *Today's Health,* August 1952, 36.

16. Anna Kleegman Daniels, "Change of Life," in *Every Woman's Standard Medical Guide* (New York: Greystone Press, 1948), 258.

17. Galton, "Every Husband," 54.

18. Edwin C. Hamblen, *Facts about the Change of Life* (Springfield, IL: C. C. Thomas, 1949), 55.

19. Abner I. Weisman, *Woman's Change of Life* (New York: Renbayle House, 1951), 63.

20. Frederic Loomis, *Consultation Room* (New York: Alfred A. Knopf, 1939), 234. See also Galton, "Every Husband," 127; Weisman, *Woman's Change of Life,* 63.

21. Nora Preddy, *Minnie Pauses to Reflect* (San Antonio: The Naylor Co., 1950), 23.

22. "The Upset Family" [advertisement], Eli Lilly and Company, in *JAMA* 142 (1950): 34.

23. Emil Novak, "The Management of the Menopause," *American Journal of Obstetrics and Gynecology* 40 (1940): 589.

24. Miller, "Changing Life," 297.

25. Paul de Kruif, "New Help for Women's Change of Life," *The Reader's Digest,* January 1948, 14.

26. Samuel A. Lewin, *Sex Without Fear* (New York: Medical Research Press, 1951), 184.

27. Scott, "You Need Not Fear," 191; and Rety, *Transition Years,* 91.

28. Jessica Weiss, *To Have and to Hold: Marriage, the Baby Boom, and Social Change* (Chicago: University of Chicago Press, 2000), 148.

29. Lori Rotskoff, *Love on the Rocks: Men, Women, and Alcohol in Post–World War II America* (Chapel Hill: University of North Carolina Press, 2002), 172–182; Hartmann, "Sex Education," 169; and Elaine Tyler May, *Homeward Bound: American Families in the Cold War Era* (New York: Basic Books, 1988), 14.

30. Maxine Davis, *Facts about the Menopause* (New York: McGraw Hill, 1951), 72. See also Madeline Gray, *The Changing Years: What to Do About the Menopause* (Garden City, NY: Doubleday, 1951), 124–125; Lincoln, *You'll Live,* 143; Julie E. Miale, "Easing Those Difficult Years," *Today's Health,* February 1956, 29; and Biskind, *Health,* 114–115.

31. James C. Janney, "Sexual Hygiene," in *Every Woman's Medical Guide,* 164.

32. Levine and Doherty, *The Menopause,* 34–35.

33. See, for example, Milton L. Miller, "Facts about the Menopause," *Hygeia,* August, 1940, 694; Edward Podolsky, *Sex Today in Wedded Life* (New York: Simon Publications, 1943), 177; and Stieglitz, *Second Forty,* 197.

34. Daniels, "Change of Life," 260.

35. David O. Cauldwell, *What Women Should Know about the Menopause: Preven-*

Notes to Pages 122–124   283

tion of Suffering through an Understanding of the Hygiene of Life's Natural Changes (Girard, KS: Haldeman-Julius, 1947), 10–11. See also Edward F. Griffith, *A Sex Guide to a Happy Marriage* (New York: Emerson, 1956), 246; and Allen, *Youth after Forty,* 12.

36. Hamblen, *Facts,* 45.

37. Charles A. Clinton, *Sex Behavior in Marriage* (New York: Pioneer Publications, 1944), 65; and Edsall, *Change of Life,* 83. See also Harold Maurice Imerman, *What Women Want to Know: A Noted Gynecologist's Guide to the Personal Problems of Women's Health* (New York: Crown, 1958), 228; Samuel R. Meaker, *A Doctor Talks to Women: What They Should Know about the Normal Functions and Common Disorders of the Female Organs* (New York: Simon and Schuster, 1954), 236; Hilliard, "Women's Greatest Blessing," 162; and Biskind, *Health,* 115.

38. Caprio, *Sexually Adequate Female,* 213.

39. Lena Levine and David Loth, *The Frigid Wife: Her Way to Sexual Fulfillment* (New York: Julian Messner, 1962), 184–185. See also Hamblen, *Facts,* 44.

40. Hilliard, "Women's Greatest Blessing," 156.

41. May, *Homeward Bound,* 114–134.

42. Linda Gordon, *Woman's Body, Woman's Right: Birth Control in America,* rev. and updated ed. (New York: Penguin Books, 1990), 365–385. See also Janice Irvine, *Disorders of Desire: Sex and Gender in Modern American Sexology* (Philadelphia: Temple University Press, 1990); and John D'Emilio and Estelle Freedman, *Intimate Matters: A History of Sexuality in America* (New York: Harper and Row, 1988), 239–325.

43. Gordon, *Woman's Body,* 381. Many others view sex education of the period as a means to family stability. See, for example, Wini Breines, *Young, White, and Miserable: Growing Up Female in the Fifties* (Boston: Beacon Press, 1992), 55; Barbara Ehrenreich and Deirdre English, *For Her Own Good: 150 Years of the Experts' Advice to Women* (Garden City, NY: Anchor Press, 1978), 217–222.

44. Jessamyn Neuhaus, "The Importance of Being Orgasmic: Sexuality, Gender, and Marital Sex Manuals in the United States, 1920–1963," *Journal of the History of Sexuality* 9 (2000): 447–473.

45. Ibid., 467.

46. Sarah Evans, *Born for Liberty: A History of Women in America* (New York: The Free Press, 1989), 248. See also May, *Homeward Bound,* 145; and Weiss, *To Have and to Hold,* 153–156.

47. Ferdinand Lundberg and Marynia F. Farnham, *Modern Woman: The Lost Sex* (New York: Harper and Brothers, 1947), 265.

48. Butterfield, *Sex Life,* 160.

49. Podolsky, *Sex Today,* 190 and 186.

50. Daniels, "Change of Life," 257. See also Elizabeth Dawson, *Menopause: Is It a Change of Life?* (Springfield, IL: State of Illinois Department of Public Health, 1955), 12.

51. Castallo and Schulz, *Woman's Inside Story,* 99; and Clinton, *Sex Behavior,* 66.

52. Caprio, *Sexually Adequate Female,* 217.

53. Cauldwell, *Women Should Know,* 26. See also Lincoln, *You'll Live,* 143, 194; Meaker, *A Doctor Talks,* 36; and Stieglitz, *Second Forty,* 194.

54. Butterfield, *Sex Life,* 159–160.

55. Trevitt and White, *How to Face,* 17.

56. Samuel Lewin and John Gilmore, *Sex after Forty* (New York: Medical Research Press, 1952), 162.

57. Frank Caprio, *The Modern Woman's Guide to Sexual Maturity* (New York: Grove Press, 1959), 232–233. See also Rety, *Transition Years,* 144–146.

58. Bernadine Bailey, "Fair, Fit, and Forty," *Hygeia,* December 1947, 960.

59. Caprio, *Modern Woman's Guide,* 230. Rety, *Transition Years,* 67.

60. Neuhaus, "Importance," 463–468.

61. Allen, *Youth after Forty,* 12.

62. I. M. Hotep [pseud.], *Love and Happiness: Intimate Problems of the Modern Woman* (New York: Alfred Knopf, 1938), 179.

63. Rety, *Transition Years,* 146–147.

64. Imerman, *Women Want to Know,* 227.

65. Daniels, "Change of Life," 258. See also Dorothy Baruch and Hyman Miller, *Sex in Marriage: New Understandings* (New York: Harper and Brothers, 1962), 237–238.

66. Imerman, *Women Want to Know,* 227.

67. Laura Hutton, "Sex in Middle Age," in *Sex in Social Life* (New York: W. W. Norton, 1950), 447–448.

68. Weisman, *Woman's Change of Life,* 110.

69. Rety, *Transition Years,* 149–150. See also Caprio, *Modern Woman's Guide,* 232–233.

70. Georgene H. Seward, *Sex and the Social Order* (New York: McGraw-Hill, 1946), 224.

71. Podolsky, *Sex Today,* 181.

72. About the national obsession with male perversion, see Estelle Freedman, "'Uncontrolled Desires': The Response to the Sexual Psychopath, 1920–1960," in *Passion and Power: Sexuality in History,* ed. Kathy Peiss and Christina Simmons (Philadelphia: Temple University Press, 1989), 199–225; and John D'Emilio, "The Homosexual Menace: The Politics of Sexuality in Cold War America," in Peiss and Simmons, eds., *Passion and Power,* 226–240.

73. May, *Homeward Bound,* 89; see also Stephen Robertson, "Separating the Men From the Boys: Masculinity, Psychosexual Development, and Sex Crime in the United States, 1930–1960s," *Journal of the History of Medicine* 56 (2001): 3–35.

74. For more about women and sexuality in 1940s' and 1950s' films, see Hartman, "Sex Education," 201–203, and Breines, *Young, White, and Miserable,* 102.

75. For the explosive potential of female sexuality, see May, *Homeward Bound,* 109–112.

76. Imerman, *Women Want to Know,* 230.

77. Hotep, *Love,* 180.

78. Ibid., 181–182. See also Edsall, *Change of Life,* 117.

79. Alfred Kinsey, et al., *Sexual Behavior in the Human Female* (Philadelphia: W. B. Saunders, 1953), 735–736.

80. "An Anonymous Questionnaire on Your Second Adolescence," 1950, Dorothy Brush Papers, Sophia Smith Collection, Smith College, Northampton, Massachusetts. Names used in this book are pseudonyms, which I assigned. Brush, "Questionnaire," #75. See also #64.

81. Ibid., #53. The phrase "frigid" comes from the survey itself. The woman merely checked a box.

82. Brush, "Questionnaire," #113.

83. Ida Davidoff and Marjorie Platt, "Two Generation Study of Postparental Women," data set, Henry A. Murray Research Center, Radcliffe College, Cambridge, Massachusetts. Davidoff and Platt revisited these women—and interviewed thirty others—in 1978. Names used in this book are pseudonyms, which I assigned. Davidoff #19. See also Brush, "Questionnaire," #64 and #15.

84. June 1952 letter responding belatedly to the Brush survey. See also Brush, "Questionnaire," #88.

85. Davidoff, "Two Generation Study," #17 and #18.

86. Brush, "Questionnaire," #263.

87. Ibid., #83.

88. Brush, "Questionnaire," #262, cited in Joy Webster Barbre, "From 'Goodwives' to Menoboomers: Reinventing Menopause in American History," (Ph.D. diss., University of Minnesota, 1994), 213–214.

89. Brush, #58.

90. Ibid.

91. Ibid., #75. See also #51, in which the writer claimed that one couldn't lose interest in one's appearance "when a girl has to hold down a job."

92. Peter Laipson, "'Kiss Without Shame for She Desires It': Sexual Foreplay in American Medical Advice Literature, 1900–1925," *Journal of Social History* 29 (1996): 507–525; and Neuhaus, "Importance," 451–461.

6. "Why All the Fuss?"

1. Dorothy Hamilton Brush and Heather Hoffman, "An Anonymous Questionnaire on Your Second Adolescence," 1950, Dorothy Brush Papers, Sophia Smith Collection, Smith College, Northampton, Massachusetts. The responses to the questionnaire were numbered in two ways. One set was numbered "FJG" followed by a number. (One of the "FJG" questionnaires was not followed by a number.) The other set was numbered without any prefix. Names used in the text are pseudonyms, which I assigned.

2. Brush, "Questionnaire," #71, #61, #83, and #67.

3. Brush, "Anonymous Questionnaire" and #65.
4. Ida Davidoff and Marjorie Platt, "Two Generation Study of Postparental Women" data set, Henry A. Murray Research Center, Radcliffe College, Cambridge, Massachusetts. Davidoff and Platt revisited these women—and interviewed thirty others—in 1978. Names cited in the text are pseudonyms, which I assigned.
5. I supplement these archival sources with the published work of Bernice Neugarten and her colleagues. Neugarten devised the "Attitudes Toward Menopause Checklist" to gauge the perspectives on menopause of 267 women. One hundred of these women were between forty-five and fifty-five years of age in 1962, and sixty-five were between fifty-six and sixty-five. Their years of birth thus ranged from 1897 and 1917. All of the women were married and had at least one child; 35 percent had one or more years of college, and 65 percent had a high school diploma or less. Bernice L. Neugarten et al., "Women's Attitudes Toward the Menopause," *Vita Humana* 6 (1963): 140–151.
6. Hellman, quoted in Susan Ware, *Beyond Suffrage: Women in the New Deal* (Cambridge, MA: Harvard University Press, 1981), 19–20.
7. Davidoff, "Two Generation Study," #6, #7, and #13.
8. Brush, "Questionnaire," #102. See also the letter from Madge Liston, Andover, Massachusetts.
9. Brush, "Questionnaire," #61. See also #207.
10. Ibid., #68. See also #212.
11. Ibid., #67. Brush #FJG3 claimed that doctors had mostly invented menopause. See also #65 and #250, and Davidoff, "Two Generation Study," #10.
12. Brush, "Questionnaire," #76.
13. Ibid., #81. See also #51.
14. Ibid., #207 and #102; and Davidoff, "Two Generation Study," #8, #10, #17, and #18. See also undated letter from MJL, Brush papers, "Correspondence about the book."
15. Joanne Meyerowitz, "Women, Cheesecake, and Borderline Material: Responses to Girlie Pictures in the Mid-Twentieth Century," *Journal of Women's History* 8 (1996): 9–35.
16. Brush, "Questionnaire," #75, #86, #90, #101, #266, and #FJG.
17. Davidoff, "Two Generation Study," #10. See also Brush, "Questionnaire," #102 and #2.
18. Neugarten, "Women's Attitudes," 146.
19. Brush, "Questionnaire," #83. See also #113; Davidoff, "Two Generation Study," #16 and Neugarten, "Women's Attitudes," 146.
20. Brush, "Questionnaire," #64.
21. Ibid., #53.
22. E. A. to *Parent's Magazine* and forwarded to Edwin Dailey of the Children's Bureau, October 10, 1940, Box 741, File 4–5–7–5–3, National Archives and Records Administration, College Park, MD; and Davidoff, "Two Generation Study," #51.

23. Brush, "Questionnaire," #101.

24. Ibid., #FJG4. See also #76.

25. Neugarten, "Women's Attitudes," 141.

26. Brush, "Questionnaire," #88.

27. Ibid., #FJG4. See also #51; and Davidoff, "Two Generation Study," #15 and #19.

28. Brush, "Questionnaire," #13.

29. Davidoff, "Two Generation Study," #5. One of the Brush respondents claimed to know a woman who went insane at menopause, but she attributed this in part to her tuberculosis and kidney stones. Brush letter June 10, 1952.

30. Brush, "Questionnaire," #350.

31. Ibid., #113.

32. Ibid., #101. See also #90, #108, and #88.

33. Neugarten, "Women's Attitudes," 141. Ellipses in original.

34. Brush, "Questionnaire," #90; Davidoff, "Two Generation Study," [old] #3 and #2.

35. Brush, "Questionnaire," #72.

36. Davidoff, "Two Generation Study," #12, #13, and #17.

37. Ibid., #14.

38. Brush, "Questionnaire," #52.

39. Ibid., #FJG4.

40. Ibid., #266.

41. Ibid., #88.

42. Davidoff, "Two Generation Study," #9.

43. Brush, "Questionnaire," #75.

44. Ibid., #57.

45. Davidoff, "Two Generation Study," #9. Davidoff #1 was in Silver Hill for two months. Silver Hill was a Connecticut institution dedicated to the treatment of "psychoneurosis."

46. Brush, Questionnaire," #101. See also #59; and Davidoff, "Two Generation Study," #2, #1, and #5.

47. Davidoff, "Two Generation Study," #9.

48. Brush, "Questionnaire," #262 and #210, cited in Joy Webster Barbre, "From 'Goodwives' to Menoboomers: Reinventing Menopause in American History," (Ph.D. diss., University of Minnesota, 1994), 206.

49. Brush, "Questionnaire," #204, #52, #53, #260, and #268.

50. Ibid., #73.

51. Ibid., #260.

52. Ibid., #262. See also Brush #FJG, who experienced "precarious" finances at menopause "due to job change at the end of the war." Brush #89 lost everything at the beginning of the Depression and never recovered. See also Brush, "Questionnaire," #65 and #71.

53. Ibid., #81. See also #12.

54. Ibid., #55. See also #90.

55. Ibid., #202. See also #208; and Davidoff, "Two Generation Study," #17,

#14, #16, and #10. Two of the Davidoff women didn't discuss menopause with female friends because they had none; see Davidoff, "Two Generation Study," #12 and #6.

56. A whopping 80 percent of the women aged forty-five to fifty-five surveyed by Bernice Neugarten agreed with the statement, "Women often use the change of life as an excuse for getting attention." Neugarten, "Women's Attitudes," 146.

57. Brush, "Questionnaire," #69, #65, and #79. See also #63; and Davidoff, "Two Generation Study," #10.

58. Brush, "Questionnaire," #65.

59. Neugarten, "Women's Attitudes," 142.

60. Davidoff, "Two Generation Study," #2 and #15. See also Brush, "Questionnaire," #15, #58, #52, and #75; and Davidoff, "Two Generation Study," #18, #8, and #3.

61. Brush, "Questionnaire," #76.

62. Ibid., #52.

63. Ibid., #FJG4 and #78.

64. Ibid., #78.

65. For a sense of the variety of pastimes enjoyed by the Brush women, see Brush, "Questionnaire," #88, #58, #68, #109, #101, and #75.

66. Ibid., #59.

67. See, for example, Brush, "Questionnaire," #58 and #78.

68. Ibid., #51.

69. Ibid., #69. See also #265.

70. Young Women's Christian Association YWCA, Women in Midstream, Manuscripts and University Archives, University of Washington, Seattle (hereafter cited as WIM). This refers to a response to a questionnaire written by WIM. WIM, #168.

71. Brush, "Questionnaire," #68.

72. Ibid., #101 and #109.

73. Ibid., #108, unnumbered survey, and #78. See also #66.

74. Neugarten, "Women's Attitudes," 145.

75. Brush, "Questionnaire," #83.

76. Ibid., #108, #207, and #252. See also #109 and #66.

77. Ibid., #266 and #109. See also #78 and #87.

78. Ibid., #259.

79. Ibid., #258.

80. Ibid., unnumbered survey.

81. Ibid., #61 and #259.

7. Feminine Forever

1. Robert A. Wilson and Thelma A. Wilson, "The Fate of the Nontreated Postmenopausal Woman: A Plea for the Maintenance of Adequate Estrogen

from Puberty to the Grave," *Journal of the American Geriatrics Society* 11 (1963): 347–362.

2. Wilson and Wilson, 347, 351, 352, 353, 359. Last two quotes from Robert A. Wilson, *Feminine Forever* (New York: M. Evans and Company, 1966), dust jacket.

3. Frances B. McCrea, "The Politics of Menopause: The 'Discovery' of a Deficiency Disease," *Social Problems* 31 (1983): 111–123; Sandra Coney, *The Menopause Industry: How the Medical Establishment Exploits Women* (Alameda, CA: Hunter House, 1994), 69–77; Kathleen I. MacPherson, "Menopause as Disease: The Social Construction of a Metaphor," *Advances in Nursing Science* 3 (1981): 106–107; and Renate Klein and Lynette Dumble, "Disempowering Midlife Women: The Science and Politics of Hormone Replacement Therapy (HRT)," *Women's Studies International Forum* 17 (1994): 327–342.

4. See Robert A. Wilson, "The Roles of Estrogen and Progesterone in Breast and Genital Cancer," *JAMA* 182 (1962): 327–333.

5. Wilson Research Foundation Mission Statement, undated (probably before 1970). Wilson Research Foundation, AMA, Department of Investigation, AMA Archive, Chicago (hereafter cited as AMA archive). To protect the privacy of those who wrote to the AMA, I have used pseudonyms.

6. Morton Mintz and Victor Cohn, "Hawking the Estrogen Fix," *The Progressive*, September 1977, 24.

7. WRF to "Colleague," November 16, 1970, AMA archive.

8. WRF to B. L. Johnson, June 1969, AMA archive.

9. *WRF Bulletin: Newsletter of the Wilson Research Foundation*, Winter 1971, 2; *WRF Bulletin*, Winter 1972, 3; and *WRF Bulletin*, Spring 1973, 4; all AMA archive.

10. See, for example, *The Complete Woman* (New York: Wilson Research Foundation, 1964); *Feminine . . . For Life* (New York: Wilson Research Foundation, 1964); *Mistrust Without Logic* (New York: Wilson Research Foundation, 1964); and *WRF Bulletin*, Fall 1971, 2; all AMA archive.

11. Barbara Seaman and Gideon Seaman, *Women and the Crisis in Sex Hormones* (New York: Rawson Associates Publishers, 1977), 289.

12. Frank Chappell of the AMA News Department to Doyle Taylor, Director of Investigations, August 15, 1966, AMA archive.

13. "No More Menopause," *Newsweek*, January 13, 1964, 53; "Durable, Unendurable Women," *Time*, October 16, 1964, 72; "How to Live Young at Any Age," *Vogue*, August 1965, 61–64; Sherwin A. Kaufman, "The Truth about Female Hormones," *Ladies' Home Journal*, January 1965, 22–23; "Oh, What a Lovely Pill!" *Cosmopolitan*, July 1965, 33–37; Ann Walsh, "Pills to Keep Women Young," *McCall's*, October 1965, 104–105; and "No More Menopause," *Pageant*, August 1964.

14. Ann Walsh, *E.R.T.: The Pills to Keep Women Young* (New York: Bantam, 1965).

15. See, for example, "Doctors Discuss Female Sex Hormones," *The Atlanta*

Journal, May 11, 1964, 33; Opal Crandall, "Science Paints Bright Future for Older Women," *The San Diego Union,* December 13, 1964, D14; and Henry W. Pierce, "Hormones Found Aid to Bones," *Pittsburgh Post-Gazette,* November 10, 1964, 25.

16. Wilson, *Feminine Forever,* 18. See, for example, his attack on Maxine Davis for suggesting that menopause was as "normal as morning and evening, normal as summer after spring." Wilson, *Feminine Forever,* 170–171, 105.

17. Ibid., 52–53.

18. Ibid., 43, 44, 40, 89.

19. Ibid., 103.

20. Ibid., 42, 40, 42, 51.

21. Ibid., 95–97.

22. Ibid., 69–70.

23. Ibid., 27, 62, 54.

24. Ibid., 40–50, 43.

25. Ibid., 116–117.

26. Ibid., 120.

27. Ibid., 119–129; quote, 126. This "planned bleed" should not be understood as menstruation, as the menstrual cycle is a process that depends on ovulation. With menopausal hormones, as with contraceptive hormones, the endometrial shedding is a response to pharmaceutical manipulation of hormones rather than the "natural" consequences of ovulation without fertilization.

28. Ibid., 207, 67–68. See also *Mistrust without Logic* and *Feminine for Life,* AMA archive.

29. Wilson, *Feminine Forever,* 181.

30. John D'Emilio and Estelle Freedman, *Intimate Matters: A History of Sexuality in America* (New York: Harper and Row, 1988), 302–306; Peter G. Filene, *Him/Her/Self: Sex Roles in Modern America,* 2nd ed. (Baltimore: Johns Hopkins University Press, 1986), 202–204; and Janice M. Irvine, *Disorders of Desire: Sex and Gender in Modern American Sexology* (Philadelphia: Temple University Press, 1990), 70–71.

31. For histories of the sexual revolution, see David Allyn, *Make Love Not War: The Sexual Revolution: An Unfettered History* (Boston: Little Brown, 2000); Beth L. Bailey, *Sex in the Heartland* (Cambridge, MA: Harvard University Press, 1999), 306–308, 250–251; Elizabeth Siegel Watkins, *On the Pill: A Social History of Oral Contraceptives, 1950–1970* (Baltimore: Johns Hopkins University Press, 1998); and D'Emilio and Freedman, *Intimate Matters,* 306–308, quote on 309.

32. D'Emilio and Freedman, *Intimate Matters,* 330–331; Elaine Tyler May, *Homeward Bound: American Families in the Cold War Era* (New York: Basic Books, 1988), 220–221.

33. Elizabeth Haiken, *Venus Envy: A History of Cosmetic Surgery* (Baltimore: Johns Hopkins University Press, 1997), 155; Susan Sontag, "The Double

Standard of Aging" (1972), reprinted in *Psychology of Women: Selected Readings,* ed. Juanita H. Williams (New York: W. W. Norton and Company, 1979), 465; Marya Mannes, "Of Time and the Woman," *Psychosomatics* 9 (1968): 9.

34. Haiken, *Venus Envy,* 131–174.

35. Filene, *Him/Her/Self,* 177–221; D'Emilio and Freedman, *Intimate Matters,* 331; May, *Homeward Bound,* 220–221; and Jessica Weiss, *To Have and to Hold: Marriage, the Baby Boom, and Social Change* (Chicago: University of Chicago Press, 2000), 177–200.

36. Weiss, *To Have and to Hold,* 177–179, for references to *An American Family* and *The Mary Tyler Moore Show.*

37. Janice Delaney, Mary Jane Lupton, and Emily Toth, *The Curse: A Cultural History of Menstruation,* rev. ed. (Urbana and Chicago: University of Illinois Press, 1988), 218–219; Rosetta Reitz, *Menopause: A Positive Approach* (New York: Chilton Book Company, 1977; reprint, New York: Penguin Books, 1979), 180–185; Frances B. McCrea and Gerald Markle, "The Estrogen Replacement Controversy in the US and the UK: Different Answers to the Same Question?" *Social Studies of Science* 14 (1984): 4; Jacquelyn N. Zita, "Heresy in the Female Body: The Rhetorics of Menopause," in *Menopause: A Midlife Passage,* ed. Joan C. Callahan (Bloomington, IN: Indiana University Press, 1993), 62; and MacPherson, "Menopause as Disease," 106–107.

38. MacPherson, "Menopause as Disease," 107; Connie Bruck, "Menopause," *Human Behavior,* April 1979, 41.

39. Wilson, *Feminine Forever,* 17, 35, 18.

40. Robert B. Greenblatt, introduction to *Feminine Forever,* 12.

41. Wilson, *Feminine Forever,* 62–63, 100.

42. Wilson, *Feminine Forever,* 201–204.

43. Robert B. Hemphill to AMA, May 1, 1968, AMA archive; William D. McCrady to AMA, July 3, 1967, AMA archive; and Helen Hickey, Medical Society of the State of New York to AMA, December 6, 1967, AMA archive. See also Margaret B. Carson to AMA, December 5, 1967 and Augustus H. Hillman to AMA, November 2, 1965, AMA archive.

44. Robert Youngman of the AMA to Arnold V. Gold, May 7, 1964; Kathryn Huss of the AMA to Mrs. Grabin, September 17, 1964; AMA form letter to Frank Smith of the Chemist's Club, NY, June 13, 1966; all AMA archive.

45. Fuller Albright, Patricia H. Smith, and Anna Richardson, "Postmenopausal Osteoporosis: Its Clinical Features," *JAMA* 116 (1941): 2474; Philip H. Henneman and Stanley Wallach, "The Use of Androgens and Estrogens and Their Metabolic Effects: A Review of the Prolonged Use of Estrogens and Androgens in Postmenopausal and Senile Osteoporosis," *AMA Archives of Internal Medicine* 100 (1957): 715; J. H. Wuerst, Jr., T. J. Dry, and J. E. Edwards, "Degree of Coronary Atherosclerosis in Bilaterally Oophorectomized Women," *Circulation* 7 (1953): 801–809; R. W. Robinson, N. Higano, and W. D. Cohen, "Increased Incidence of Coronary Heart Disease in Women

Castrated Prior to Menopause," *AMA Archives of Internal Medicine* 104 (1959): 908–913; Robinson, et al., "Estrogen Replacement Therapy in Women with Coronary Atherosclerosis," *Annals of Internal Medicine* 48 (1958): 95–101; E. Kost Shelton, "The Use of Estrogen after the Menopause," *Journal of the American Geriatrics Society* 2 (1954): 630–631; William H. Masters, "Rationale of Sex Steroid Replacement in the 'Neutral Gender,'" *Journal of the American Geriatrics Society* 3 (1955): 389–395.

46. Wilson, *Feminine Forever,* 37. See also Chapter 3 of this book.

47. Helen Z. Jern, "Hormone Therapy of the Menopause," *Journal of the American Medical Women's Association* 30 (1975): 491, 492.

48. *Menopause and Aging: Summary Report and Selected Papers from a Research Conference on Menopause and Aging, May 23–26, 1971, Hot Springs, Arkansas* (Bethesda: U.S. Department of Health, Education, and Welfare, 1973 or 1971), 3; Robert Greenblatt, "The Management of the Menopause," *Medical Gynaecology and Sociology* 2 (1967): 2–6; and Robert B. Greenblatt, "Reprise," in *The Menopausal Syndrome,* ed. Robert B. Greenblatt, Virendra Mahesh, and Paul G. McDonough (New York: Medcom, 1974), 225.

49. Robert W. Kistner, "The Menopause," *Clinical Obstetrics and Gynecology* 16 (1973): 107, 109; Francis Rhoades, "The Menopause: A Deficiency Disease," *Michigan Medicine,* June 1965, 411.

50. Greenblatt, "Reprise," 227.

51. Herbert S. Kupperman, Ben B. Wetchler, and Meyer H. G. Blatt, "Contemporary Therapy of the Menopausal Syndrome," *JAMA* 171 (1959): 1628; Herbert S. Kupperman, "The Menopausal Woman and Sex Hormones," *Medical Aspects of Human Sexuality,* September 1967, 65.

52. Francis P. Rhoades, "Minimizing the Menopause," *Journal of the American Geriatrics Society* 15 (1967): 346; Silvio Dalla Pria, et al., "Hormone Therapy of the Menopause: A Panel," in *The Menopausal Syndrome* (New York: Medcom, 1974), 209. See also Rhoades, "The Menopause," 411.

53. Allan C. Barnes, "Is Menopause a Disease?" *Consultant* 2 (1962): 24, 22–23.

54. John L. Bakke, "Is the Menopause a Normal Change or Is It a Disease Needing Treatment?" *Western Journal of Surgery, Obstetrics and Gynecology* 71 (1963): 243; and M. Edward Davis, "The Physiology and Management of the Menopause," in *Advances in Obstetrics and Gynecology,* ed. Stewart L. Marcus and Cyril C. Marcus (Baltimore: The Williams and Wilkins Company, 1967), 426.

55. Helen Jern, *Hormone Therapy of the Menopause and Aging* (Springfield: Charles C. Thomas Publishers, 1973), 287. See also "Is Menopause a Disease?," 22–24; Rhoades, "Minimizing," 346–354; Robert B. Greenblatt, "The Menopause and Its Management," *Pituitary Ovarian Endocrinology,* ed. R. I. Dorfman and M. N. Castro (San Francisco: Holden Day, 1963), 159; and Davis, "The Physiology," 419.

56. Davis, "The Physiology," 430–431.

57. Greenblatt, "Management," 6; Herbert Kupperman, "The Climacteric Syn-

drome," *Medical Folio* 15 (1972): 2; and Lawrence S. Sonkin and Eugene J. Cohen, "Treatment of the Menopause," *Modern Treatment* 5 (1968): 547.

58. Identical quote in Greenblatt, "Reprise," 225, and "Management," 3.

59. Rhoades, "Minimizing," 346, 347.

60. Ibid., 347.

61. Davis, quoted in Kistner, "The Menopause," 106.

62. M. E. Davis, "The Therapeutic Role of the Estrogens," *The Surgical Clinics of North America* 23 (1943), 121; Kupperman, "The Menopausal Woman," 68.

63. Norman L. Stahl, "Hormones and Cancer," in *The Menopausal Syndrome*, ed. Robert B. Greenblatt, Virendra Mahesh, and Paul G. McDonough, 116; and Sonkin, 560.

64. Rhoades, "Minimizing," 346–354. See also Greenblatt, "Management," 2–6.

65. M. G. N. Dukes, in "The Menopause and the Pharmaceutical Industry," *Journal of Psychosomatic Obstetrics and Gynecology* 18 (1997): 186, noted that in the 1970s only a small proportion of doctors came down firmly on the side of estrogens.

66. I have not yet found any individual physicians who fall into this category, but they seem to exist both in legend and in reality. The medical and popular literature refer to this group, and, as one survey noted, 10 percent of gynecologists never prescribed hormones for their menopausal patients. David M. Rorvik, "You Can Stop Worrying about Menopause," *McCall's*, October 1971, 103, 160; and Somers H. Sturgis, "Hormone Therapy in the Menopause: Indications and Contraindications," *Medical Aspects of Human Sexuality*, May 1969, 69.

67. "Treating Menopausal Women and Climacteric Men," *Medical World News*, June 28, 1974, 33.

68. Paul D. Saville, "Treatment of Postmenopausal Osteoporosis," *Modern Treatment* 5 (1968): 571–580; Norton Spritz, "Atherosclerosis and the Menopause," *Modern Treatment* 5 (1968): 581–586; Rorvik, "You Can Stop Worrying," 160; Roy Hertz, "The Role of Steroid Hormones in the Etiology and Pathogenesis of Cancer," *American Journal of Obstetrics and Gynecology* 98 (1967): 1013–19; Nathan Kase, "Estrogens and the Menopause" [Editorial], *JAMA* 227 (1974): 318–319; and Edmund R. Novak, Georgeanna Seegar Jones, and Howard Jones, *Gynecology* (Baltimore: Williams and Wilkins, 1975), 387.

69. For citations concerning breast cancer, see J. C. Burch, B. F. Byrd, and W. K. Vaugh, "The Effect of Long-Term Estrogen on Hysterectomized Women," *American Journal of Obstetrics and Gynecology* 118 (1974): 778. For citations concerning gallstones, see Boston Collaborative Drug Surveillance Program, "Surgically Confirmed Gallbladder Disease, Venous Thromboembolism and Breast Tumors in Relation to Postmenopausal Estrogen Therapy," *New Eng-*

land Journal of Medicine 290 (1974): 15. For citations concerning heart disease, see C. H. Bolton, M. Ellwood, and M. Hartog, "Comparison of the Effects of Ethinyl Oestradiol and Conjugated Equine Oestrogens in Oophorectomized Women," *Clinical Endocrinology* 4 (1976): 131; and L. Rosenberg and H. Jick, "Myocardial Infarction and Estrogen Therapy in Postmenopausal Women," *New England Journal of Medicine* 294 (1976): 1256. For citations concerning deep vein thrombosis and thromboembolism, see Boston Collaborative Drug Surveillance Program, "Surgically Confirmed," 15; and J. J. Strangel, J. Innerfield, and V. Reyniak, "The Effects of Conjugated Estrogens on Coagulability in Menopausal Women," *Obstetrics and Gynecology* 49 (1977): 314.

70. Kenneth J. Ryan, "Conference Summary," *Menopause and Aging: Summary Report and Selected Papers from a Research Conference on Menopause and Aging, May 23–26, 1971, Hot Springs, Arkansas* (Bethesda: U.S. Department of Health, Education, and Welfare, 1973), 11; and Kase, "Estrogens and the Menopause," 319.

71. Robert E. Markush and Sarah L. Turner, "Epidemiology of Exogenous Estrogens," *HSMHA Health Reports* 86 (1971): 84.

72. Maragret Lock, *Encounters with Aging: Mythologies of Menopause in Japan and North America* (Berkeley: University of California Press, 1993), 317.

73. Morton Mintz, *The Pill: An Alarming Report* (Greenwich, CT: Fawcett Publications Inc., 1969), 30–31. As late as June 1998, *Feminine Forever* remained in print. *Feminine Forever* was syndicated by King Features. See, for example, *Wisconsin State Journal*, July 1966; Robert A. Wilson, "A Key to Staying Young," *Look*, January 11, 1966, 66–73; and Robert A. Wilson, "Which Hormone to Take and When," *Vogue*, June 1966, 92–95.

74. Kaufert and McKinlay argue that "ERT entered the public domain" only after 1975. This is clearly untrue. Patricia A. Kaufert and Sonja M. McKinlay, "Estrogen Replacement Therapy: The Production of Medical Knowledge and the Emergence of Policy," in *Women, Health, and Healing: Toward a New Perspective*, ed. Ellen Lewin and Virginia Olesen (New York: Tavistock, 1985), 133.

75. "Popular literature" is defined here as materials directed to a lay audience. Magazine articles provide the bulk of this material, but it also includes books and pamphlets. The majority of the magazine articles were gleaned from the *Reader's Guide to Periodical Literature*, although these entries were not exhaustive.

76. Critics have claimed that the popular literature on menopause overwhelmingly followed Wilson's lead by promoting both estrogen therapy and the disease model of menopause. Anita Johnson, "The Risks of Sex Hormones," *Women and Health* 1 (1977): 8–11. See also MacPherson, "Menopause as Disease," 95, 106; Madeline Goodman, "Toward a Biology of Menopause," *Signs: Journal of Women in Culture and Society* 5 (1980): 741; Coney, *The Menopause Industry*, 201–211; Jane Lewis, "Feminism, the Menopause, and

Hormone Replacement Therapy," *Feminist Review* 43 (1993): 48–49; McCrea, "Politics," 114; Bruck, "Menopause," 40, 46; and Reitz, *Menopause,* 182–186.

77. Joanne Meyerowitz, "Beyond the Feminine Mystique: A Reassessment of Postwar Mass Culture, 1946–1958," in *Not June Cleaver: Women and Gender in Postwar America, 1945–1960,* ed. Joanne Meyerowitz (Philadelphia: Temple University Press, 1994), 231.

78. Linda S. Mitteness reached a similar conclusion in her content analysis of the popular coverage of menopause, "Historical Changes in Public Information About the Menopause," *Urban Anthropology* 12 (1983): 161–179.

79. David Reuben, *Everything You Always Wanted to Know about Sex but Were Afraid to Ask* (New York: David McKay Co., 1969), 290.

80. See, for example, Seaman and Seaman, *Women and the Crisis,* 308–309; Bruck, "Menopause," 43; McCrea, "Politics," 114; MacPherson, "Menopause as Disease," 107; Estelle Fuchs, *The Second Season: Life, Love, and Sex—Women in the Middle Years* (Garden City, NY: Doubleday, 1977), 130; and Reitz, *Menopause,* 84.

81. Dabney Rice, "Anti-Aging Pills," *Harper's Bazaar,* August 1975, 76.

82. Alice Lake, "Menopause: Is It Necessary?" *Good Housekeeping,* April 1965, 158.

83. "Change of Life," 12. See also Rorvik, "You Can Stop Worrying," 103; and Bill Davidson, "Menopause: Is There a Cure?" *Saturday Evening Post,* August 26, 1967, 71.

84. Ayerst Laboratories, *The Second Forty Years: A Time of Change and Choice* (New York: Ayerst Laboratories, 1973), 7.

85. Lindsay R. Curtis, *The Menopause: A New Life of Confidence and Contentment* (Bristol, TN: S. E. Massengill Company, 1969), 18.

86. William A. Nolen, "A Doctor's World: What Menopause Is—and Isn't," *McCall's,* May 1972, 40. See also Grace Naismith, "Common Sense and the 'Femininity Pill,'" *Reader's Digest,* September 1966, 100–101. See, for example, Kenneth C. Hutchin, "The Change and What Husbands Should Know About It," *Today's Health,* September 1966, 54–56; Julia Kagan, "Hormone Therapy at Menopause: What Women Doctors Prescribe and Take," *McCall's,* October 1975, 33; and Derek Llewellyn-Jones, *Everywoman and Her Body* (New York: Taplinger Publishing Company, 1971), 296–297; and Kaufman, "Truth," 22.

87. Rorvik, "You Can Stop Worrying," 102; Rice, "Anti-Aging Pills," 128B; and "How to Live Young," 149–150. Other sources that promote estrogen include Kagan, "Hormone Therapy," 33–34; Naismith, "Common Sense," 101–102; Kaufman, "Truth," 22; Lake, "Menopause: Is It Necessary?" 160–164; M. Dorthea Kerr, "Look Better, Feel Better—Can Hormones Help?" *Vogue,* January 1974, 102; and Davidson, "Menopause," 72.

88. "Change of Life," *Good Housekeeping,* September 1967, 19–20; and "The Menopause that Refreshes," *Harper's Bazaar,* August 1973, 87.

89. William H. Cooper, *A Husband's Guide to Menopause* (New York: Essandess Special Edition, 1969), 112. See also Kaufman, "Truth," citing Wilson, 23.

90. Louis Parrish, *No Pause at All* (New York: Reader's Digest Press, 1976), 142–144.

91. "Durable, Unendurable Women," 72.

92. M. Edward Davis and Dona Meilach, *A Doctor Discusses Menopause and Estrogens* (Chicago: Budlong Press, 1969), 45. See also Lake, "Menopause: Is It Necessary?" 158.

93. Kerr, "Look Better," 102–103.

94. Davidson, "Menopause," 71.

95. Lake, "Menopause: Is It Necessary?" 160. See also "No More Menopause," 53; Kaufman, "Truth," 23; and Cooper, *Husband's Guide*, 74.

96. Kerr, "Look Better," 102–103.

97. Earl Ubell, "Are Estrogens Really the Answer to Femininity?" *McCall's*, July 1969, 122.

98. "The Menopause that Refreshes," 87.

99. Arthur Snider, "Cancer—Where Doctors Fail," *Science Digest*, November 1966, 13. See also Wendy Cooper, *Don't Change: A Biological Revolution for Women* (New York: Stein and Day, 1975), 136–137; and Rhoades, "Minimizing," 346–354.

100. Kaufman, "Truth," 22. See also Sherwin Kaufman, *The Ageless Woman: Menopause, Hormones, and the Quest for Youth* (Englewood Cliffs, NJ: Prentice-Hall, Inc., 1967), 44; and "Change of Life," *Good Housekeeping*, September 1967, 16; Lin Root, "Oh What A Lovely Pill!" *Cosmopolitan*, July 1965, 36; and Davidson, "Menopause," 72.

101. Curtis, *The Menopause*, 31.

102. Faye Marley, "Sex and the Older Woman," *Science News*, April 29, 1967, 413; Kerr, "Look Better," 140; Rice, "Anti-Aging Pills," 128B; Helen D. Borel, "The Book that Ends Menopause," *Science Digest* 59 (June 1966): 28; Rorvik, "You Can Stop Worrying," 161; "Live Young," 62; Root, "Lovely Pill," 36; and Walsh, *Pills to Keep Women Young*, 121–122. See also the articles written by Wilson himself; Wilson, "Key to Staying Young," 70; and Wilson, "Which Hormones to Take," 93.

103. Wilson, "A Key to Staying Young," 66–73; Wilson, *Feminine Forever*; and Wilson, "Which Hormones to Take," 92–95.

104. Kerr, "Look Better," 102–103; and Kerr, *The Female Climacteric* (New York: Ayerst Laboratories, 1974). Kerr's role in both was cited in Fuchs, *Second Season*, 131.

105. Seaman and Seaman, *Women and the Crisis*, 289.

106. "Should Hormone Therapy Be Used in Menopause?" *Good Housekeeping*, May 1973, 201. See also Llewellyn-Jones, *Everywoman*, 296, 303; Ubell, "Are Estrogens Really the Answer?" 122; Nolen, "Doctor's World," 36, 40; "Your Doctor: Answers to the Most Frequently Asked Questions," *Good Housekeeping*, February 1974, 180; Kagan, "Hormone Therapy," 34; Shel-

don Cherry, *The Menopause Myth* (New York: Ballantine Books, 1976), 20; Lydia McClean, "The Great Estrogen Controversy," *Vogue,* March 1976, 107; Hutchin, "The Change," 80; and Lawrence R. Wharton, *The Ovarian Hormones: Safety of the Pill; Babies after Fifty* (Springfield, IL: Charles C. Thomas, 1967), 26.

107. Naismith, "Common Sense," 101.

108. Nolen, "Doctor's World," 40. See also Kerr, "Look Better," 103; Rice, "Anti-Aging Pills," 128B; Lila Nachtigall, *Lila Nachtigall Report* (New York: Putnam, 1977), 179–184, 189–191; Parrish, *No Pause,* 21; and Root, "Lovely Pill," 37.

109. Kaufman, *The Ageless Woman,* 64; Lake, "Menopause: Is It Necessary?" 180.

110. See, for example, Kagan, "Hormone Therapy," 33–34; Llewellyn-Jones, *Everywoman,* 299–300; Lake, "Menopause: Is It Necessary?" 162–164; "How to Live Young," 62–63; Naismith, "Common Sense," 100–102; Davidson, "Menopause," 72; Marley, "Sex," 143; and Ruth Carson, *Your Menopause* (New York: Public Affairs Committee, 1970), 8–9.

111. Davidson, "Menopause," 72; and Lake, "Menopause: Is It Necessary?" 162.

112. Kaufman, "Truth," 23.

113. Davidson, "Menopause," 71. See also Lake, "Menopause: Is It Necessary?" 158 (which presents the menopause as disease theory as one side of the debate); and the literature by Wilson.

114. Cherry, *Menopause Myth,* 19–23.

115. Hutchin, "The Change," 54. See also Fuchs, *Second Season,* 128–130; Carson, *Your Menopause,* 1; Naismith, "Common Sense," 100; and Lake, "Menopause: Is It Necessary?" 160–164.

116. Davis and Meilach, *A Doctor Discusses,* 45–46. See also Sally Olds, "Menopause—Something to Look Forward To?"; Mary Neil Dunne, "How I Took the Menace Out of Menopause," *Farm Journal,* March 1965, 101+.

117. "How to Live Young," 61. See also Wilson, "Which Hormones to Take," 93, citing Henry Leis of New York Medical College.

118. Rice, "Anti-Aging Pill," 76.

119. Root, "Lovely Pill," 37. See also Walsh, *Pills to Keep Women Young,* 94–100; Nachtigall, *Report,* 187–188; and Kaufman, "Truth," 23.

120. Both Kupperman and Morton are interviewed in Davidson, "Menopause," 71.

121. Naismith, "Common Sense," 99. See also Kerr, "Look Better," 103; Llewellyn-Jones, *Everywoman,* 297–298; Nachtigall, *Report,* 185; and Elizabeth B. Connell, et al., *Hormones, Sex, and Happiness* (Chicago: Cowles Book Company, 1971), 220.

122. Peter Greenwald, et al., "Endometrial Cancer after Menopausal Use of Estrogens," *Obstetrics and Gynecology* 50 (1977): 239.

123. I. Waldron, "Increased Prescribing of Valium, Librium, and Other Drugs—An Example of the Influence of Economic and Social Factors on the Practice of Medicine," *International Journal of Health Services* 7 (1977): 37–62;

National Prescription Audit: General Information Report, College Edition (Dedham, MA: R. A. Gosselin, 1962); *National Prescription Audit: National Hospital Survey, General Information Report* (Dedham, MA: R. A. Gosselin, 1966); and *National Prescription Audit: General Information Report* (Ambler, PA: IMS America, LTD., 1976).

124. *National Prescription Audit: General Information Report; Ten Year Trend, 1965–1974* (Ambler, PA: IMS America LTD., 1975).

125. Harry K. Ziel and William D. Finkle, "Increased Risk of Endometrial Carcinoma among Users of Conjugated Estrogens," *New England Journal of Medicine* 293 (1975): 1167–70; and Donald C. Smith, et al., "Association of Exogenous Estrogen and Endometrial Carcinoma," *New England Journal of Medicine* 293 (1975): 1164–67.

126. "Estrogen Is Linked to Uterine Cancer," *New York Times,* December 4, 1975, 1, 55. Reports also appeared on the ABC News, December 4, 1975; and NBC News, December 4, 1975.

127. "Estrogens and Endometrial Cancer," *FDA Drug Bulletin* 6 (1976): 18–20. For a history of this package insert, see Elizabeth Siegel Watkins, "'Doctor, Are You Trying to Kill Me?': Ambivalence about the Patient Package Insert for Estrogen," *Bulletin of the History of Medicine* 76 (2002): 84–104.

128. Robert K. Kistner, "Estrogens and Endometrial Cancer," *Obstetrics and Gynecology* 48 (1976): 481.

129. See also Gilbert S. Gordan and Bernard G. Greenberg, "Exogenous Estrogens and Endometrial Cancer—an Invited Review," *Postgraduate Medicine* 59 (June 1976): 66–77.

130. Ralph I. Horwitz and Alvan R. Feinstein, "Alternative Analytic Methods for Case-Control Studies of Estrogens and Endometrial Cancer," *New England Journal of Medicine* 299 (1978): 1089–94. See also L. Rauramo, "Estrogen Replacement Therapy and Endometrial Carcinoma," *Frontiers of Hormone Research* 5 (1977): 117–125.

131. Robert W. Kistner, "Treatment of Premenopausal and Postmenopausal Women," *Journal of Reproductive Medicine* 19 (1977): 108–109.

132. "Unopposed" refers to estrogen-only therapy, in contrast to an estrogen-progestin regimen.

133. See, for example, Thomas M. Mack, et al., "Estrogens and Endometrial Cancer in a Retirement Community," *New England Journal of Medicine* 294 (1976): 1262–67; Noel Weiss, et al., "Increasing Incidence of Endometrial Cancer in the United States," *New England Journal of Medicine* 294 (1976): 1259–62; Layman A. Gray, William M. Christopherson, and Robert N. Hoover, "Estrogens and Endometrial Cancer," *Obstetrics and Gynecology* 49 (1977): 385; Hershel Jick et al., "Replacement Estrogens and Endometrial Cancer," *New England Journal of Medicine* 300 (1979): 218–22; Thomas W. McDonald, et al., "Exogenous Estrogen and Endometrial Carcinoma: Case Control and Incidence Study," *American Journal of Obstetrics and Gynecology* 127 (1977): 572–580. Another researcher also claimed that replacement

estrogens increased the risk of breast cancer. See Robert Hoover, et al., "Menopausal Estrogens and Breast Cancer," *New England Journal of Medicine* 295 (1976): 401–405. There are many reviews of these studies. See, for example, Douglas R. Knab, "Estrogen and Endometrial Cancer," *Obstetrics and Gynecology Survey* 32 (1977): 267–281.

134. McCrea, "Politics," 115. See also U.S. Department of Health, Education, and Welfare, National Institute of Aging, *Summary of Conclusions of the NIH Conference on Estrogen Use and Postmenopausal Women* (Washington, DC: HEW, 1979). Other sources recommended the low dose for a short period. See, for example, Martin M. Quigley and Charles B. Hammond, "Estrogen-Replacement Therapy—Help or Hazard?" *New England Journal of Medicine* 301 (1979): 646–648.

135. G. S. Gordan and C. Vaughan, "Prevention and Treatment of Postmenopausal Osteoporosis," in *The Menopause and Postmenopause: The Proceedings of an International Symposium Held in Rome, June 1979*, ed. N. Pasetto, R. Paoletti, and J. L. Ambrus (Lancaster, England: MTP Press Limited, 1980), 191.

136. Charles B. Hammond, et al., "Effects of Long-Term Estrogen Replacement Therapy: I Metabolic Effects," *American Journal of Obstetrics and Gynecology* 133 (1979): 525–536.

137. Hammond et al., "Effects," 537–547.

138. Quoted in "Estrogens and Endometrial Cancer," 20. This episode is discussed in Seaman and Seaman, *Women and the Crisis,* 292.

139. This letter was published in its entirety in *Majority Report: The Women's Newspaper* 6 (1977): 1.

140. Charles Rodrigues, "Jack Anderson and Les Whitten: PR Firm Suggested Estrogen Hype," *The Washington Post,* May 12, 1977, F23.

141. Mintz and Cohn, "Hawking the Estrogen Fix," 25.

142. McClean, "Great Estrogen Controversy," 177; and Marilyn Mercer, "Can Estrogen Therapy Cause Cancer?" *McCall's,* March 1976, 39. See also Margaret Markham, "The Estrogen Myth," *Harper's Bazaar,* October 1976, 143+; Alice Lake, "Myths of Menopause," *Reader's Digest,* October 1979, 145–148; and Georgeanna S. Jones, "How Safe Are Estrogens?" interview by Walter S. Ross, *Reader's Digest,* November 1978, 261–266.

143. Paula Weideger, "Estrogen: The Rewards and the Risks," *McCall's,* March 1977, 70–79. See also Weideger, "Estrogen: Are the Benefits Worth the Risk?" *McCall's,* May 1979, 65–66; and M.L.S. [Midge Lasky Schildkraut?], "An Updated Look at the Estrogen Scare," *Good Housekeeping,* March 1979, 227–228. For more on Weideger's view of estrogen therapy, see Chapter 9.

144. Marion Steinmann, "Estrogens: Can They Hold Back the Clock?" *Family Health/Today's Health,* May 1977, 26.

145. Melva Weber, "Are Hormones Giving You Cancer?" *Vogue,* February 1976, 114. Emphasis in original.

146. Melva Weber, "Estrogen Replacement—The Late News," *Vogue,* August 1978, 260.
147. "Estrogen Therapy: The Dangerous Road to Shangri-La," *Consumer Reports* 41 (1976), 642–645; and Sidney Wolfe, "Feminine Straight to the Grave," *Mother Jones,* May 1978, 18–19. See also Mintz and Cohen, "Hawking the Estrogen Fix," 24–25.
148. Jane Brody, "Physicians' Views Unchanged on Use of Estrogen Therapy," *New York Times,* December 5, 1975, 55.
149. Nancy Worcester and Mariamne Whatley, "The Selling of HRT: Playing on the Fear Factor," *Feminist Review* (Summer 1992), 4. (The number of prescriptions written in 1989, however, far exceeded those written in 1975.)
150. Beverly H. Pasley, Susan Standfast, and Selig Katz, "Prescribing Estrogen During Menopause: Physician Survey of Practices in 1974 and 1981," *Public Health Reports* 99 (1984): 424–429; and *FDA Drug Bulletin,* February–March 1979, 2–3.

8. "At the Will and Whim of My Hormones"

1. Young Women's Christian Association YWCA, Women in Midstream, Manuscripts and University Archives, University of Washington, Seattle (hereafter cited as WIM), WIM #8.
   The WIM records include correspondence from women as well as two sets of separately numbered (and some unnumbered) questionnaires. One set, printed on blue paper and numbered 1 through 500, included unnumbered responses. These will be referred to in the notes as WIM #00 or WIM [unnumbered survey]. A smaller set of numbered questionnaires (beginning again at 1) was printed on white paper; these will be referred to as WIM #00 (white survey). Names referenced in the text are pseudonyms, which I assigned. All the surveys can be found at ACC 1930-14, Box 11, Surveys.
   Although the woman cited as WIM #8 claimed that Butesin was a "mild nerve pill," this is not supported by the 1975 *Physicians' Desk Reference,* which refers to Butesin as a mild anesthetic useful for treating itching (possibly prescribed for genital itching). Perhaps she was taking Butisol sodium or butizide, suggested as a sedative to ease anxiety and tension. *Physicians' Desk Reference* (Oradell, NJ: Medical Economics Co., 1975).
2. This group was originally the Ad Hoc Committee on Menopause of the University of Washington YWCA. They had switched to the less unwieldy title Women in Midstream by the autumn of 1974.
3. WIM Papers. My claim about class diversity is based on anecdotal evidence. The questionnaires do not inquire about socioeconomic status; on occasion, however, the sources do provide some limited evidence of class diversity. Pauline Bart and Marlyn Grossman, for example, have claimed that these women

were overwhelmingly white, an assertion neither supported nor contradicted by the questionnaires themselves. Bart and Grossman, "Menopause," *Women and Health* 1 (May–June 1976): 8.

4. Wilson Research Foundation, American Medical Association, Department of Investigation, AMA Archive, Chicago (hereafter cited as AMA Archive).

5. Marjorie (Lowenthal) Fiske, Majda Thurnher, and David Chiriboga, Longitudinal Study of Transitions in Four Stages, 1968, data set, Henry A. Murray Research Center, Radcliffe College, Cambridge, Massachusetts (hereafter cited as Fiske). The names used for the women in this data set are pseudonyms provided by the researchers.

6. Susan A. LaRocco and Denise F. Polit, "Women's Knowledge about the Menopause," *Nursing Research* 20 (1980): 10.

7. Boston Women's Health Book Collective, *Our Bodies, Ourselves: A Book by and for Women,* 2nd ed. (New York: Simon and Schuster, 1976), 335. (Hereafter cited as BWHBC. This is the second Simon and Schuster edition; its first was published in 1973. The Boston Women's Health Course Collective had published an edition in 1971.)

8. *Women in Midstream Newsletter,* April 1975, WIM.

9. Fiske 3.2.49.

10. Fiske 3.2.35. See also Fiske 3.2.04.

11. WIM #124 and #324.

12. WIM #423, #407, and #362. See also WIM #124, #126, and #101.

13. WIM [unnumbered survey]; and letter from Katherine Thom, "Menopause Speak-Out," *Prime Time,* April 1974, 9–10. See also Julie Shaffer to WIM, April 1, 1973; Mary Gaines to WIM, 1973; and WIM #45. In order to preserve the anonymity of the correspondents, I have used pseudonyms that preserve the correspondents' initials.

14. WIM #85.

15. WIM #415. See also WIM #293.

16. Julie Schaffer to WIM, April 11, 1973; Beth Cauldwell to WIM, March 16, 1973; and BWHBC, *Our Bodies,* 330. See also Fiske 3.2.41.

17. BWHBC, *Our Bodies,* 231.

18. Fiske 3.2.36; and Fiske [unnumbered], Edith Morrow. (Edith Morrow is a pseudonym assigned by Fiske. Her interview was not assigned a number.)

19. Martha Rice, Wyoming, to WIM, March 31, 1973; and Hester Newman to WIM. See also Ellen Furber to WIM, March 18, 1973.

20. *Women in Midstream Newsletter,* April, 1975, WIM Papers.

21. WIM #346, #356, #147, and #44 (white survey).

22. WIM #403.

23. Alice Stone, Colorado, to WIM, March 18, 1973.

24. Quotes in WIM #307 and #468; statistic taken from April 1975, *Women in Midstream Newsletter.* See also WIM #367, #254, and #129.

25. WIM #395. See also WIM #356.

26. WIM #54. See also WIM #208.
27. Kathleen W. Seegers, "My Dark Journey Through Insanity," *Reader's Digest,* November 1969, 70.
28. Rita White, Fort Collins, Colorado, to WIM, March 21, 1973. (This correspondent may be WIM #7.)
29. WIM #77. See also WIM #254 and Grace Van Bronkhurst, Spokane, Washington, to WIM, March 21, 1973. Bronkhurst's psychiatrist also recommended electric shock, but she declined it.
30. For more on this topic, see Chapter 9.
31. WIM #255, #35, and #45.
32. Judy Bartlett to WIM, October 23, 1976.
33. WIM #66.
34. Fiske 3.3.49 and 3.2.16.
35. Jennifer Stang to WIM, March 16, 1973.
36. WIM #368.
37. WIM #147. See also WIM #44 (white survey) and WIM #460.
38. BWHBC, *Our Bodies,* 335.
39. WIM #223.
40. WIM #232. See also WIM #481, who experienced "sexual problems" in the "husband-wife relationship." WIM #424 and #58 both noted a decline in their libidos.
41. Susan Price to WIM, March 24, 1973.
42. Jessica Weiss, *To Have and to Hold: Marriage, the Baby Boom, and Social Change* (Chicago: University of Chicago Press, 2000), 164.
43. Heidi Hauser to WIM, March 19, 1973.
44. WIM [unnumbered] 1973.
45. Iris Pushkin, Colorado Springs, Colorado, to WIM, March 18, 1973. See also Lucy Draper, to WIM, undated (probably March 1973); WIM #8; Julie Shaffer to WIM, April 11, 1973; Kristine Sterling to WIM, June 24, 1973; and BWHBC, *Our Bodies,* 327.
46. WIM #378.
47. Bernice Trask, Colorado, to WIM, May 5, 1978. See also WIM #304.
48. Diane Bates, Sunnyvale, California, to WIM, June 10, 1973.
49. WIM #395. See also WIM #379.
50. Dorothy Sutter, Denver, Colorado, to WIM, May 22, 1973.
51. Hadley Cantril, ed., *Public Opinion, 1935–1946* (Princeton: Princeton University Press, 1951), 567; and Dennis A. Gilbert, *Compendium of American Public Opinion* (New York: Facts on File, 1988), 25–26.
52. Regina Morantz-Sanchez, in *Conduct Unbecoming a Woman: Medicine on Trial in Turn-of-the Century Brooklyn* (New York: Oxford University Press, 1999), shows that even in the 1890s, women sought out physicians who would provide the treatments they demanded. See also Judith Walzer Leavitt, *Brought to Bed: Childbearing in America, 1750–1950* (New York: Oxford University Press, 1986); Jane Lewis, *The Politics of Motherhood* (London:

Croom Helm, 1980); and Jane Lewis, "Feminism, the Menopause, and Hormone Replacement Therapy," *Feminist Review* 43 (1993): 38–56.

53. B. V. Stadl and N. S. Weiss, "Characteristics of Menopausal Women: A Survey of King and Pierce Counties in Washington, 1973–1974," *American Journal of Epidemiology* 102 (1975): 209–216, cited in Peter Greenwald, et al., "Endometrial Cancer after Menopausal Use of Estrogen," *Obstetrics and Gynecology* 59 (1977): 240. A 1978 survey conducted in Detroit showed that roughly two-thirds of the menopausal women who saw their doctors received estrogen treatments. Mary Dosey and Michael Dosey, "The Climacteric Woman," *Patient Counseling and Health Education* 2 (1980): 14–21, cited in Frances B. McCrea, "Politics of Menopause: The 'Discovery' of a Deficiency Disease," *Social Problems* 31 (1983): 116.

54. See Greenwald, "Endometrial Cancer," 242; "Women and Estrogens," *FDA Consumer* (Washington, D.C.: Government Printing Office, 1976), 5; Virginia Olesen, "Sociological Observations on Ethical Issues Implicated in ERT at Menopause," in *Changing Perspectives on Menopause,* ed. Ann M. Voda, Myra Dinnerstein, and Sheryl R. O'Donnell (Austin: University of Texas Press, 1982), 346–360; and "Estrogen Therapy: The Dangerous Road to Shangri-La," *Consumer Reports,* November 1976, 642. The sources use the term "middle class" quite loosely to mean those not in the working class. Upper-class women are presumably just as likely as middle-class women to receive hormones.

55. WIM letter from Nora Stevens to WIM [undated]. See also Belle Canon, "Menopause: A Deficiency Disease," *Human Ecology* 4 (1973): 8–10.

56. WIM [unnumbered survey].

57. WIM #93. See also Fiske [unnumbered], Edith Morrow. Although she never received hormones, Morrow visited three doctors trying to get a prescription.

58. Nathan Kase, "Estrogens and the Menopause," *JAMA,* 227 (1974): 318.

59. Ann Walsh, *E.R.T.: Pills to Keep Women Young* (New York: Bantam Books, 1965), 8–10.

60. WIM #45.

61. Faye Marley, "Sex and the Older Woman," *Science News,* 29 April, 1967, 413.

62. Bill Davidson, "Menopause: Is There a Cure?" *Saturday Evening Post,* 26 August, 1967, 71.

63. Ibid., 72. See also "Pills to Keep Women Young," *Time,* April 1966, 50; Kenneth Hutchin, "The Change and What Husbands Should Know about It," *Today's Health,* September 1966, 54; and Grace Naismith, "Common Sense and the 'Femininity Pill,'" *Reader's Digest,* September 1966, 99.

64. WIM #9.

65. WIM #8.

66. WIM #387. For other women celebrating HRT, see WIM #93, #457, #395, #254, #367, #368, #424, and #412. See also Rita White to WIM, March 21,

1973; Fiske 3.2.07, Fiske 3.2.19, and Fiske 3.2.43; BWHBC, *Our Bodies,* 232; and Wendy Cooper's collection of letters from women in *Don't Change: A Biological Revolution for Women* (New York: Stein and Day, 1975), 141–156. Although I have no reason to doubt the veracity of her letters, I have no independent evidence that these letters existed.

67. Mrs. Harold Nielson to AMA, October 21, 1965. See also Jane Cross to AMA, April 4, 1968; Mrs. Dennis Blink to AMA, November 9, 1970; Ann Reed, Dearborn, Michigan, to AMA, April 27, 1966; Mrs. Roy Glick, Rego Park, New York, to AMA, August 15, 1966; Mrs. Paul Grant to AMA, September 1, 1966 (telephone message); Mrs. Beth Clark to AMA, September 1, 1966; and Mrs. Mary Stokes, Kennewick, WA to AMA, May 9, 1966. AMA Archive.

68. Judy Finch, Tucson, AZ, to WIM, April 30, 1973; and Dorothy Lynch, Denver, CO, to WIM, March 27, 1973.

69. Barbara Seaman, "The Dangers of Sex Hormones," in *Seizing Our Bodies: The Politics of Women's Health,* ed. Claudia Dreifus (New York: Vintage, 1977), 172.

70. Fiske 3.2.53.

71. Fiske 3.2.04.

72. Fiske 3.2.10.

73. Kathleen MacPherson, "Menopause as a Disease: The Social Construction of a Metaphor," *Advances in Nursing Science* 3 (1981): 106; and Nancy Worcester and Mariamne H. Whatley, "The Selling of HRT: Playing on the Fear Factor," *Feminist Review* (Summer 1992): 3.

74. Sandra Coney, *The Menopause Industry: How the Medical Establishment Exploits Women* (Alameda, CA: Hunter House, 1994), 23–27. See also Renate Klein and Lynette J. Dumble, "Disempowering Midlife Women: The Science and Politics of Hormone Replacement Therapy (HRT)," *Women's Studies International Forum* 17 (1994): 329; and Patricia A. Kaufert and Sonja M. McKinlay "Estrogen Replacement Therapy: The Production of Medical Knowledge and the Emergence of Policy," in *Women, Health, and Healing: Toward a New Perspective,* ed. Ellen Lewin and Virginia Olesen (New York: Tavistock, 1985), 114.

75. Dorothy Nelkin, *Selling Science: How the Press Covers Science and Technology* (New York: W. H. Freeman and Co., 1987), 79–80.

76. Naismith, "Common Sense," 99; Davidson, "Menopause," 71; "How to Live Young at Any Age," *Vogue,* August 1965, 64; and Walsh, *Pills to Keep Women Young,* 50.

77. Fiske 3.2.04.

78. WIM #258.

79. Mrs. Dennis Blink to AMA, November 9, 1970. AMA Archive.

80. Fiske 3.2.08. See also Cooper, *Don't Change,* 141–142 and 154.

81. WIM [unnumbered survey].

82. Elizabeth Siegel Watkins, "Dispensing with Aging: Changing Rationales for

Long-Term Hormone Replacement Therapy, 1960–2000," *Pharmacy in History* 43 (2001): 23–37; Patricia Kaufert and Margaret Lock, "Medicalization of Women's Third Age," *Journal of Psychosomatic Obstetrics and Gynecology* 18 (1997): 86; and Worcester and Whatley, "Selling of HRT," 3.

83. Karen A. Frey, "Middle-Aged Women's Experience and Perceptions of Menopause," *Women and Health* 6 (1981): 25–36.

84. Fiske 3.2.36.

85. WIM #293. For other emphatic claims that menopause was "natural," see WIM #415, #324, and #124.

86. Elizabeth Fuchs, *The Second Season: Life, Love, and Sex: Women in the Middle Years* (Garden City, NJ: Anchor Press, 1977), 142.

87. Lila Nachtigall *The Lila Nachtigall Report* (New York: Putnam, 1977), 94.

88. David M. Rorvik, "You Can Stop Worrying About Menopause," *McCall's,* October 1971, 161.

89. Worcester and Whatley, "Selling of HRT," 3.

90. Melva Weber, "Estrogen Replacement—The Late News," *Vogue,* August 1978, 211. See also Kaufert and McKinlay, "Estrogen Replacement Therapy," 125; and W. J. Baggs, "Publicity Seeking *New England Journal of Medicine,*" *New England Journal of Medicine* 295 (1976): 897–898.

91. Karla Smithers to WIM, October 6, 1976; Carmen Slovnik to WIM, November 1976; and Theresa Sheldon to WIM, November 1976.

92. Linda Rogers to WIM, November 1976.

93. WIM #368.

94. Abigail Barnes to WIM, October 25, 1976.

95. WIM #307.

96. *FDA Drug Bulletin,* February–March 1979, 3; and Ronald Ross, "Breast Cancer and Menopausal Estrogens," in *Estrogens and Cancer,* ed. Steven G. Silverberg and Frances J. Major (New York: Wiley, 1978), 55–65.

9. "What Do These Women Want?"

1. My application of the terms "feminist" and "feminism" is somewhat retrospective. The overwhelming majority of my sources explicitly aligned themselves with the women's movement by publishing in overtly feminist publications, acknowledging membership in feminist organizations, or proposing "women's liberation" as the primary solution to current social ills. There are a few others, however, whose connection to the women's movement is less certain. Nevertheless, I regard as feminists all of the women who see their work on menopause as empowering women to make educated decisions about their health.

2. For histories of second-wave feminism, see Flora Davis, *Moving the Mountain: The Women's Movement in America since 1960* (New York: Simon and Schuster, 1991); Alice Echols, *Daring to Be Bad: Radical Feminism in America, 1967–1975* (Minneapolis: University of Minneapolis Press, 1989); Ruth

Rosen, *The World Split Open: How the Modern Women's Movement Changed America* (New York: Viking, 2000); and Estelle Freeman, *No Turning Back: The History of Feminism and the Future of Women* (New York: Ballantine, 2002).

3. The organization's name was later changed to the Boston Women's Health Book Collective.

4. Helen Marieskind, "The Women's Health Movement," *International Journal of Health Services* 5 (1975): 218.

5. The Boston Women's Health Course Collective (BWHCC), *Our Bodies, Ourselves: A Course by and for Women* (Boston: The Collective, 1970, 1971), 45. This edition came before overwhelming demand persuaded BWHCC to turn publication over to Simon and Schuster in 1973.

6. Sheryl Burt Ruzek, *The Women's Health Movement: Feminist Alternatives to Medical Control* (Praeger: New York, 1978), 190. See also Patricia A. Kaufert and Sonja M. McKinlay, "Estrogen-Replacement Therapy: The Production of Medical Knowledge and the Emergence of Policy," in *Women, Health, and Healing: Toward a New Perspective,* ed. Ellen Lewin and Virginia Olesen (New York: Tavistock, 1985), 132–133; and Myrna I. Lewis and Robert N. Butler, "Why Is Women's Lib Ignoring Old Women?" *Aging and Human Development* 3(1972): 223–231.

7. See, for example, Barbara Ehrenreich and Deirdre English, *Complaints and Disorders: The Sexual Politics of Sickness,* Glass Mountain Pamphlet No. 2 (Old Westbury, NY: The Feminist Press, 1973); and Ehrenreich and English, *Witches, Midwives, and Nurses: A History of Women Healers,* Glass Mountain Pamphlet No. 1 (Old Westbury, NY: The Feminist Press, 1972).

8. Barbara Seaman, "Physician Heel [*sic*] Thyself," *Proceedings for the 1975 Conference on Women and Health* (Boston, MA: April 4–7, 1975), 25–27. For an overview of different feminist health strategies, see Elizabeth Fee, "Women and Health Care: A Comparison of Theories," in *Women and Health: The Politics of Sex in Medicine,* ed. Elizabeth Fee (Farmingdale, NY: Baywood Publishing Co., 1983), 17–34.

9. Ehrenreich and English, *Complaints and Disorders,* 88.

10. See, for example, Frances B. McCrea, "The Politics of Menopause: The 'Discovery' of a Deficiency Disease," *Social Problems* 31 (1983): 111–123; McCrea and Gerald E. Markle, "The Estrogen Replacement Controversy in the USA and UK: Different Answers to the Same Question?" *Social Studies of Science* 14 (1984): 1–26; Judith Posner, "It's All in Your Head: Feminist and Medical Models of Menopause (Strange Bedfellows)," *Sex Roles* 5 (1979): 179–190; Kwok Wei Leng, "Menopause and the Great Divide: Biomedicine, Feminism, and Cyborg Politics," in *Reinterpreting Menopause: Cultural and Philosophical Issues,* ed. Paul Komesaroff, Philipa Rothfield, and Jeanne Daly (New York: Routledge, 1997), 255–272; Jacquelyn N. Zita, "Heresy in the Female Body: The Rhetorics of Menopause," in *Menopause: A Midlife Passage,* ed. Joan C. Callahan (Bloomington, IN: Indiana University Press,

1993), 59–78; and Jane Lewis, "Feminism, the Menopause and Hormone Replacement Therapy," *Feminist Review* 43 (1993): 38–56.

11. Medical sociologist McCrea claims that within a few years of the publication of *Feminine Forever,* "U.S. feminists in the vanguard of an organized women's health movement defined the health care system, including estrogen treatment, as a serious social problem." McCrea, "Politics," 111.

12. In her analysis of feminism and menopause in the United States and Britain, Jane Lewis claims that "there is no one feminist view of menopause." She nevertheless concludes that "feminist literature tends to be universally suspicious of HRT," thus obscuring feminist debates and the shifts in those debates over time. Lewis, "Feminism," 50.

13. Although few feminists or feminist organizations gave menopause significant attention between 1963 and 1975, others mentioned menopause briefly in their larger critique of medicine. See, for example, Mary Daly, *Gyn/Ecology: The Metaethics of Radical Feminism* (Boston: Beacon Press, 1978), 248–250; and Ehrenreich and English, *Complaints and Disorders,* 87–88.

14. Belle Canon, "Menopause: A Deficiency Disease," *Human Ecology* 4 (1973): 8–10.

15. Canon, "Menopause: A Deficiency Disease," 9, 8.

16. Ibid., 10.

17. Citing Cooper as their main example, Gerald Markle and Frances McCrea have argued that the feminist demand for estrogen therapy was a uniquely British response to menopause. But Cooper's work, published both in England and in the United States and reliant upon letters written by American women, also fits within the larger American women's movement. Consequently, Cooper's work should be seen as part of the feminist viewpoint available in America.

18. Wendy Cooper, *Don't Change: A Biological Revolution for Women* (New York: Stein and Day, 1975), 16.

19. Ibid., 12–13.

20. Ibid., 12.

21. Francis P. Rhoades, "Minimizing the Menopause," *Journal of the American Geriatrics Society* 16 (1967): 346–354; quoted in Cooper, *Don't Change,* 136–137.

22. Cooper, *Don't Change,* 20.

23. Paula Weideger, *Menstruation and Menopause: The Physiology and Psychology, the Myth and the Reality* (New York: Alfred A. Knopf, 1976 [1975]), 71.

24. Herbert Kupperman, "The Climacteric Syndrome," *The Medical Folio* 5 (1972): 1–2; quoted in Weideger, *Menstruation and Menopause,* 65.

The belief that medicine had given women "extra years" is a common misconception founded on a misunderstanding of life-expectancy data. A woman born in 1850, for example, had at birth a life expectancy of forty-three years, below the average age of menopause. If she lived to be twenty, however, her life expectancy zoomed to over sixty. In other words, the increase in life expectancy does not reflect extra years added to the end of life, as Weideger and others claim: It primarily describes the decrease in child mortality.

25. Ibid., 69–70.
26. Ibid., 71.
27. Ibid., 67.
28. Ibid., 71.
29. Shulamith Firestone, *The Dialectic of Sex: The Case for Feminist Revolution* (New York: William Morrow, 1970; reprint 1993), 10.
30. Ibid., 8–9.
31. BWHCC, *Our Bodies* (1971), 45.
32. The Boston Women's Health Book Collective, *Our Bodies, Ourselves: A Book by and for Women* (New York: Simon and Schuster, 1973), 229. This is the first Simon and Schuster edition.
33. BWHBC, *Our Bodies* (1973), 230.
34. Ibid., 232.
35. Ibid., 230.
36. Ibid., 229–235. See also the pamphlet *Menopause* (New York: HealthRight, 1975).
37. Frances McCrea points to this article in support of her claim that feminists responded promptly to Wilson and the indiscriminate use of ERT. McCrea, "Politics," 118.
38. Joan Solomon, "Menopause: A Rite of Passage," *Ms.,* December 1972, 16–18.
39. Barbara Seaman, "Examine Your Doctor Thoroughly—For Symptoms of Male Chauvinism and a Propensity for Performing Unnecessary Surgery," *Prime Time,* November 1972, 1–3+.
40. Ibid., 10, 3; and Barbara Seaman, *Free and Female: The Sex Life of the Contemporary Woman* (New York: Coward, McCann and Geoghegan, 1972), 84–92, quote 91.
41. Seaman, "Examine Your Physician," 2.
42. Harry K. Ziel and William D. Finkle, "Increased Risk of Endometrial Carcinoma among Users of Conjugated Estrogens," *New England Journal of Medicine* 293 (1975): 1167–70; and Donald C. Smith, et al., "Association of Exogenous Estrogen and Endometrial Carcinoma," *New England Journal of Medicine* 293 (1975): 1164–67.
43. "Estrogen Is Linked to Uterine Cancer," *New York Times,* December 4, 1975, 1, 55. Reports also appeared on ABC News, December 4, 1975, and NBC News, December 4, 1975.
44. Susan E. Bell, "Changing Ideas: The Medicalization of Menopause," *Social Science and Medicine* 24 (1987): 535–542; and Bell, "Gendered Medical Science: Producing a Drug for Women," *Feminist Studies* 21 (1995): 469–500.
45. Diana B. Dutton, "DES and the Elusive Goal of Drug Safety," in *Worse than the Disease: Pitfalls of Medical Progress* (Cambridge, UK: Cambridge University Press, 1988), 31–90; Roberta J. Apfel and Susan M. Fisher, *To Do No Harm: DES and the Dilemmas of Modern Medicine* (New Haven: Yale Uni-

versity Press, 1984); Robert Meyers, *DES: The Bitter Pill* (New York: Seaview/Putnam, 1983); and Ruzek, *Women's Health Movement,* 38–42.

46. Morton Mintz, *At Any Cost: Corporate Greed, Women, and the Dalkon Shield* (New York: Pantheon, 1985); Susan Perry and Jim Dawson, *Nightmare: Women and the Dalkon Shield* (New York: Macmillan, 1985); and Ruzek, *Women's Health Movement,* 43–44.

47. Rosetta Reitz, *Menopause: A Positive Approach* (New York: Chilton Book Company, 1977; reprint, New York: Penguin Books, 1979), 181. See also Barbara Seaman and Gideon Seaman, *Women and the Crisis in Sex Hormones* (New York: Rawson Associates, 1977), xi; Caroline Derbyshire, *The New Woman's Guide to Health and Medicine* (New York: Appleton Century Croft, 1980), 269; Belita H. Cowan, "Questions and Answers on Menopause," in *Women's Health Care: Resources, Writings, Bibliographies* (Ann Arbor: Anshen Pub., 1977), 22; Cynthia W. Cooke and Susan Dworkin, *The Ms. Guide to a Woman's Health* (Garden City, NY: Doubleday, 1979), 281; and Belle Canon, "Menopause: It's a Disease Says Insurance Company," *Ms.,* March 1977, 22.

48. Reitz, *A Positive Approach,* 26.

49. Ibid., 28.

50. Ibid., 75.

51. Ibid., 180. See also Cowan, "Questions," 22; Fran Moira, "Estrogens Forever: Marketing Youth and Death," *off our backs,* March 1977, 12; Cooke and Dworkin, *Ms. Guide,* 288–293; Rachel Gillett Fruchter, "ERT: A Risky Proposition," *HealthRight* 2 (1976): 7; and Fruchter, "Menopause," *HealthRight* 2 (1976): 9.

52. See, for example, Reitz, "Venerable Vaginas," *Majority Report,* November 26-December 9, 1977, 7; Reitz, "Menopause Questions and Answers," in *Menopause, Resource Guide* 3rd ed. (Washington, D.C.: National Women's Health Network, 1980), 7–19; Reitz, "Love My Menopause? You Must Be Crazy!" *Prime Time,* April 1976, 17–18; and Reitz, "What Doctors Won't Tell You About Menopause," in *Seizing Our Bodies: The Politics of Women's Health,* ed. Claudia Dreifus (New York: Vintage Books, 1977), 209–211.

53. BWHBC, *Our Bodies, Ourselves: A Book by and for Women,* 2nd ed., completely revised and expanded (New York: Simon and Schuster, 1976), 330. Italics in original. The 1977 edition of Weideger's book significantly backed away from her earlier acceptance of ERT. Paula Weideger, *Menstruation and Menopause,* rev. ed. (New York: Delta, 1977).

54. See also Jane Page, *The Other Awkward Age: Menopause* (Berkeley, CA: Ten Speed Press, 1977), 48, 7; and National Women's Health Network, *Menopause Resource Guide.*

55. Irma Levine, unpublished 1978 letter to *Prime Time.* References to WIM are to the Women in Midstream archives of the Young Women's Christian Association (YWCA, Women in Midstream, Manuscripts and University Archives, University of Washington, Seattle [hereafter cited as WIM]). The WIM records include correspondence from women and two sets of separately num-

bered (and some unnumbered) questionnaires. One set, printed on blue paper and numbered 1 through 500 also included unnumbered responses; when referred to in the notes these responses are cited in the form WIM #00 or WIM [unnumbered survey]. A smaller set of numbered questionnaires (beginning again at 1) was printed on white paper; these will be referred in the form WIM #00 (white survey). All the surveys can be found at ACC 1930-14, Box 11, Surveys.

56. BWHBC, *Our Bodies* (1976), 335.
57. Vidal S. Clay, *Women: Menopause and Middle Age* (Pittsburgh: Know Inc., 1977), 2.
58. Ibid., 112. See also BWHBC (1976), 335.
59. See, for example, Pauline B. Bart, "Depression in Middle-Aged Women," in *Female Psychology: The Emerging Self,* ed. Sue Cox (Chicago: Science Research Associates, 1976), 349–367; and Bart and Marlyn Grossman, "Menopause," *Women and Health* 1 (May/June 1973): 3–11.
60. Cooke and Dworkin, *Ms. Guide,* 295. See also "Menopause: Let it Be," *off our backs,* Summer 1971, 12; and Marcha Flint, "The Menopause: Reward or Punishment?" *Psychosomatics* 16 (1975): 163.
61. "And Now, the 'Liberated' Woman Patient," *American Medical News,* October 7, 1974, 14.
62. "Women's Liberation and the Practice of Medicine," *Medical World News,* June 22, 1973, 34. See also "And Now," 14–18; and Barbara L. Kaiser and Irwin H. Kaiser, "The Challenge of the Women's Movement to American Gynecology," *American Journal of Obstetrics and Gynecology* 120 (1974): 652–665.
63. "Women's Liberation," 34.
64. Seaman, "Examine Your Physician," 3.
65. Judith Walzer Leavitt, *Brought to Bed: Childbearing in America, 1750–1950* (New York: Oxford University Press, 1986); and Elizabeth Siegel Watkins, *A Social History of Oral Contraceptives, 1950–1970* (Baltimore: Johns Hopkins University Press, 1998).
66. Robert N. Mayer, *The Consumer Movement: Guardians of the Marketplace* (Boston: Twayne Publishers, 1989).
67. Patty Boland to WIM, October 23, 1976.
68. WIM [unnumbered survey].
69. WIM #120.
70. Lynn Laredo, "Garbage Pail Syndrome," *Prime Time,* May 1974, 5.
71. Annette Henkin Landau, "Some Thoughts on the Menopause Rap," *Newsletter of the Women's Liberation Center of Nassau County, Inc.,* New York, 3 (June 1974): 7.
72. WIM #217. See also Cathy Smith to WIM, October 1976.
73. WIM #364.
74. WIM #441. See also WIM #158, #433, #403, #364, and #383; and Daphne Cryer to WIM, October 1976.

75. WIM #402. See also WIM #12.

76. WIM [unnumbered survey].

77. WIM #257. See also WIM #368 and #460; and Jennifer Stang to WIM, March 16, 1973.

78. Sarah Seidlitz, "Menopause Speak-Out," *Prime Time*, April 1974, 8.

79. WIM #402.

80. WIM #35 (white survey).

81. Florence Rush, "A Woman of that Age," *Prime Time*, April 1976, 3.

Epilogue

1. Phyllis Bogen, "Mixed Estrogen Signals" [letter], *New York Times*, 9 September, 2002, F4.

2. Gina Kolata, with Melody Petersen, "Hormone Replacement Study a Shock to the Medical System," *New York Times*, July 10, 2002, p. A1; "Hormone Therapy Woes" [editorial], *New York Times*, July 11, 2002, A22.

3. Writing Group for the Women's Health Initiative Investigators, "Risks and Benefits of Estrogen Plus Progestin in Healthy Postmenopausal Women," *JAMA* 288 (2002): 321–333.

4. Elizabeth Siegel Watkins, "Dispensing with Aging: Changing Rationales for Long-Term Hormone Replacement Therapy, 1960–2000," *Pharmacy in History* 43 (2001), 33.

5. Karen Scott Collins, et al., *Health Concerns across a Woman's Lifespan: The Commonwealth Fund 1998 Survey of Women's Health* (New York: Commonwealth Fund, 1999). This is a high but often repeated estimate. Other sources place the percentage of postmenopausal women on HRT between 13 and 33 percent.

6. Watkins, "Dispensing," 30–32.

7. Denise Grady and Susan Rubin, "Postmenopausal Hormone Therapy," *Annals of Internal Medicine* 119 (1993): 347–348; "Hormone Replacement Therapy," *International Journal of Gynecology and Obstetrics*, 41 (1993): 194–202; and U.S. Preventative Services Task Force, *Guide to Clinical Preventative Services*, 2nd ed. (Baltimore: Williams and Wilkins, 1996).

8. Barry G. Saver, et al., "Physician Policies on the Use of Preventive Hormone Therapy," *American Journal of Preventive Medicine* 13 (1997): 358–365.

9. Gina Kolata, "Estrogen Question Gets Tougher," *New York Times*, April 6, 2000, A22.

10. Nancy Worcester and Marianne H. Whatley, "The Selling of HRT: Playing on the Fear Factor," *Feminist Review* 41 (1992), 8; National Women's Health Network, *The Truth about Hormone Replacement Therapy: How to Break Free from the Medical Myths of Menopause* (Roseville, CA: Prima Publishing, 2002).

11. *Taking Hormones and Women's Health: Choices, Risks, Benefits* (Washington, DC: National Women's Health Network, 1989). See also Sandra Coney,

The Menopause Industry: How the Medical Establishment Exploits Women (Alameda, CA: Hunter House, 1994), 22.

12. Barbara Seaman, *The Greatest Experiment Ever Performed on Women: Exploding the Estrogen Myth* (New York: Hyperion, 2003). See also National Women's Health Network, *Taking Hormones,* 3.

13. Worcester and Whatley, "Selling of HRT," 9–13. See also Kathleen MacPherson, "Osteoporosis and Menopause: A Feminist Analysis of the Social Construction of a Syndrome," *Advances in Nursing Science* 7 (1985): 11–22.

14. Susan M. Love, with Karen Lindsey, *Dr. Susan Love's Hormone Book: Making Informed Choices about Menopause* (New York: Random House, 1997, paperback edition, 1998), xxii.

15. Quoted in Kate Hunt, "A 'Cure for All Ills'? Construction of the Menopause and the Chequered Fortunes of Hormone Replacement Therapy," in *Women and Health: Feminist Perspectives,* ed. Sue Wilkinson and Celia Kitzinger (London: Taylor and Francis, 1994), 147.

16. Coney, *Menopause Industry,* 18–39; National Women's Health Network, *The Truth about Hormone Replacement Therapy,* 3–22; Worcester and Whatley, "Selling of HRT," 2; Patricia A. Kaufert and Margaret Lock, "Medicalization of Woman's Third Age," *Journal of Psychosomatic Obstetrics and Gynecology* 18 (1997): 86.

17. See Collins, *Health Concerns,* for example.

18. Rayanne S. Berman, Robert S. Epstein, and Eva Lydick, "Compliance of Women in Taking Estrogen Replacement Therapy," *Journal of Women's Health* 5 (1996): 213–220; P. M. Sarrel, *Postmenopausal Hormone Therapy: Solving the Problem of Discontinuance* (Kendall Park, NJ: Interactive Network for Continuing Education, 1996).

19. S. Hurley, et al., "Randomized Trial of Estrogen Plus Progestin for Secondary Prevention of Coronary Heart Disease in Postmenopausal Women," *JAMA* 280 (1998): 605–613; and S. Hurley, et al., "Noncardiovascular Disease Outcomes During 6.8 Years of Hormone Therapy," *JAMA* 288 (2002): 58–66.

20. Jennifer Hays, et al., "Effects of Estrogen Plus Progestin on Health-Related Quality of Life," *New England Journal of Medicine,* 348 (2003): 1–16 (www.nejm.com); and The Women's Health Initiative Steering Committee, "Effects of Conjugated Equine Estrogen in Postmenopausal Women with Hysterectomy: The Women's Health Initiative Randomized Controlled Trial," *JAMA* 291 (2004): 1701–12.

21. Mary Duenwald, "Hormone Therapy: One Size, Clearly, No Longer Fits All," *New York Times,* July 16, 2002, http://www.nytimes.com; Emily Gurnon, "Much Ado about Nothing?" *North Coast Journal Weekly,* December 19, 2002, 1.

22. Gina Kolata, "No Hormones? Seeking New Menopause Approach," *New York Times,* November 10, 2002, A1.

23. Duenwald, "Hormone Therapy"; Nina Morris-Faber, "The Role of Estrogens" [letter], *New York Times,* July 23, 2002; Gina Kolata, "Many Taking Hormone Pills Now Face a Difficult Choice," *New York Times,* July 15, 2002, A1.

24. By May 2005, The U.S. Preventative Services Task Force, The American College of Gynecologists, The American Heart Association, and the North American Menopause Society had all recommended against the use of hormone therapy for the prevention of chronic diseases in postmenopausal women. U.S. Preventive Service Task Force, "Hormone Therapy for the Prevention of Chronic Conditions in Postmenopausal Women: Recommendations from the U.S. Preventive Services Task Force," *Annals of Internal Medicine* 142 (2005): 855–860; and "Management of Menopause-Related Symptoms," *National Institutes of Health State-of-the-Science Conference Statement,* March 23, 2005, 1–31. For the continued role for preventive hormones, see L. Speroff, P. Kenemans, and H. G. Burger, "Practical Guidelines for Postmenopausal Hormone Therapy," *Maturitas* 51 (2005): 4–7; and John C. Stevenson, "Justification for the Use of HRT in the Long-Term Prevention of Osteoporosis," *Maturitas* 51 (2005): 113–126.

25. Watkins, "Dispensing," 27–32; and Margaret Lock, "The Politics of Mid-Life and Menopause: Ideologies for the Second Sex in North America and Japan," in *Knowledge, Power and Practice: The Anthropology of Medicine and Everyday Life,* ed. Shirley Lindenbaum and Margaret Lock (Berkeley: University of California Press, 1993), 342.

26. Lock, "Politics of Mid-Life," 332.

27. Germaine Greer, *The Change: Women, Aging and the Menopause* (New York: Knopf, 1992; reprint of 1991), 9.

28. Germaine Greer, *The Female Eunuch* (New York: McGraw-Hill, 1971).

29. Gail Sheehy, *The Silent Passage: Menopause* (New York: Random House, 1992), 79, 41, 134, 136–137.

30. These are not the only authors who make this claim. See, for example, Deborah Lupton, "Constructing the Menopausal Body: The Discourse on Hormone Replacement Therapy," *Body and Society* 2 (1996): 91–97.

31. Lock, "Politics of Mid-Life," 344.

Index

Abortion, 15, 161, 211
African-American women, 113, 231, 265n23
After Forty (Gorney), 177
Ageless Woman, The (Kaufman), 173, 174
Aging: double standard regarding, 161–162; and estrogen deficiency, 165; hormones as preventing, 75–76, 80, 81, 85–86, 152, 168–169, 171, 177–179, 189, 204; menopause as marker of, 13, 27, 74, 196, 201; not pathological, 77, 210, 231; physicians as capitalizing on women's fears of, 153, 162–163, 172, 180, 196, 204, 232; not preventable, 75, 85; and women's achievements, 29, 30–32, 38. *See also* Appearance; Menopause; Rejuvenation; Youth
Albright, Fuller, 79, 165, 183
Alcohol. *See* Sedatives
Alfie (movie), 160
Allen, Edgar, 76
Allison, Polly, 112
Alzheimer's disease, 233
AMA. *See* American Medical Association
Amenorrhea, 16
American College of Obstetricians and Gynecologists, 182, 185
American Medical Association (AMA), 9, 64, 164–165, 190, 196, 203
Androgens, 269n65
Appearance, of menopausal women, 56, 66, 71, 115, 120, 124–126, 129, 131, 158, 161–162, 166–167, 173–174, 178, 179–180, 205. *See also* Femininity; Masculinity
Applebaum, Stella, 100
Archibald, Elizabeth, 149
Aronson, Howard, 24

Aronson, Shepard, 1–2
Arthritis, 152, 205
Atlantic Monthly (magazine), 108
"Attitudes Toward Menopause Checklist." *See* Neugarten, Bernice
Ayerst (company): on cancer risks of estrogen, 183–184; and Emmenin, 22; marketing by, 155, 174, 177, 231; and Premarin, 59, 155, 231; and Wilson's research, 155

Bailey, Agnes, 146
Bailey, Bernadine, 86, 99, 126
Ball, Lucille, 139
Bandler, Samuel, 50
Barbiturates, 73. *See also* Sedatives
Barbre, Joy Webster, 251n51, 255n106, 269n66, 274n126
Barnes, Allan C., 80, 81, 167–168
Bart, Pauline, 222, 300n3
Bartlett, Judy, 197
Bates, Diane, 200
Battsen, Georgina, 141, 143
Bay of Pigs invasion, 1, 238
Bell, Susan, 60, 272n91
Bender, Lauretta, 56
Berman, Edgar F., 1, 2
Better Homes and Gardens (magazine), 84, 99
Bicycles, 15
"Bikini," 128
Biology, women's: role of, in shaping menopause, 2–5, 9–13, 81, 134, 187, 236–239; and positions of responsibility, 1–2, 32–34, 38, 39, 134–135, 139, 163–164, 236, 238; and women's fate, 102, 158, 172. *See also* Fertility; Menopause; Menstruation; Motherhood

315